ATLAS OF
VETERINARY
HEMATOLOGY

ATLAS OF VETERINARY HEMATOLOGY

BLOOD AND BONE MARROW OF DOMESTIC ANIMALS

JOHN W. HARVEY, D.V.M., Ph.D., D.A.C.V.P.

Professor and Chair
Department of Physiological Sciences
College of Veterinary Medicine
University of Florida
Gainesville, Florida

W.B. SAUNDERS COMPANY
A Harcourt Health Sciences Company
Philadelphia   London   New York   St. Louis   Sydney   Toronto

W.B. SAUNDERS COMPANY
A Harcourt Health Sciences Company

The Curtis Center
Independence Square West
Philadelphia, Pennsylvania 19106

Library of Congress Cataloging-in-Publication Data

Harvey, John W.
    Atlas of veterinary hematology: blood and bone marrow of domestic animals / John W. Harvey.

        p. cm.

    Includes bibliographical references (p.).

    ISBN 0–7216–6334–6
        1. Veterinary hematology—Atlases.   2. Blood cells—Atlases.   3. Bone marrow—Atlases.
    I. Title.

    SF769.5.H37 2001
    636.089'615—dc21   00–063569

ATLAS OF VETERINARY HEMATOLOGY   ISBN 0–7216–6334–6

Printed in the United States of America

Last digit is the print number: 9   8   7   6   5   4   3   2   1

To Liz

Preface

This color atlas is designed as a reference book for the morphologic aspects of veterinary hematology of common domestic animals, excluding birds. Species covered include dogs, cats, horses, cattle, sheep, goats, pigs, and llamas. The atlas is divided into two sections, blood and bone marrow. It includes basic material for the novice, as well as material of primary interest to those with advanced training. Techniques for the collection and preparation of blood and bone marrow smears and bone marrow core biopsies are discussed, in addition to the morphology of the tissues collected. Often, more than one example of a cell type or abnormal condition is shown, because cells and conditions can vary in morphology. Veterinary technologists will likely find the blood section and the techniques part of the bone marrow section to be most helpful. Veterinary students and practicing veterinarians should benefit from the complete book, even if they are not directly involved in bone marrow evaluation, because it provides a basis for understanding diseases affecting the marrow. The bone marrow aspirate smear cytology and core biopsy histology section will be most useful to clinical pathologists, anatomic pathologists, and residents in training for these disciplines. This is not a complete hematology textbook, but rather a reference book in which the text explains the significance of the morphologic abnormalities shown in the color photographs. Readers interested in learning more about a given topic will hopefully appreciate the extensive bibliography provided.

John Harvey

Acknowledgments

I want to acknowledge those most responsible for my education as a clinical pathologist. Few people have the opportunity to receive training from the giants of their profession, but I was blessed in being trained by Jerry Kaneko, the father of veterinary clinical biochemistry, and Oscar Schalm, the father of veterinary hematology. Many other colleagues have contributed to my development as a hematologist, with Victor Perman and Alan Rebar being particularly noteworthy, as we have challenged one another with unknown hematology slides in front of various audiences. I thank Denny Meyer for his encouragement in taking on the task of preparing this atlas and Rose Raskin, Leo McSherry, and Shashi Ramaiah for their conscientious reviews and helpful suggestions. I appreciate Melanie Pate's careful editorial review and am grateful to Ray Kersey at W.B. Saunders Co. for his remarkable patience and persistent support in this endeavor.

John Harvey

Editor's Note

The purpose of this text/atlas is to provide veterinarians, veterinary students, veterinary technicians and veterinary technology students with a complete treatise on the cytology of blood and bone marrow.

The subjects will be covered in a user friendly way utilizing color photographs and appropriate text that clarifies diagnostic implications. Therapy will be discussed only when diagnosis can be confirmed by response to treatment. Ninety percent of the information will focus on commonly recognized diseases.

Contents

BLOOD

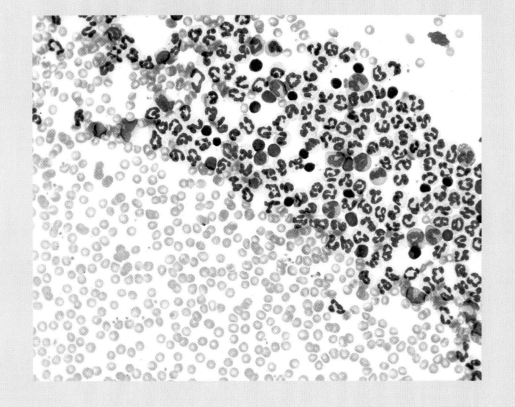

CHAPTER 1

Examination
of Blood Samples

▨ SAMPLE COLLECTION AND HANDLING

An overnight fast avoids postprandial lipemia in monogastric animals, which can interfere with plasma protein, fibrinogen, and hemoglobin determinations. Ethylenediaminetetraacetic acid (EDTA) is the preferred anticoagulant for complete blood count (CBC) determination in most species, but blood from some birds and reptiles hemolyzes when collected into EDTA.[1] In those species, heparin is often used as the anticoagulant. The disadvantage of heparin is that leukocytes do not stain as well (presumably because heparin binds to leukocytes),[2] and platelets generally clump more than they do in blood collected with EDTA. However, as will be discussed later, platelet aggregates and leukocyte aggregates may occur even in properly collected EDTA-anticoagulated blood samples.[3–8] In those cases, collection of blood using another anticoagulant (e.g., citrate) may prevent the formation of cell aggregates. Cell aggregation tends to be more pronounced as blood is cooled and stored; consequently, processing samples as rapidly as possible after collection may minimize the formation of leukocyte and/or platelet aggregates.

Collection of blood directly into a vacuum tube is preferred to collection of blood by syringe and transfer to a vacuum tube. This method reduces platelet clumping and clot formation in samples for CBC determinations. Even small clots render a sample unusable. Platelet counts are markedly reduced, and significant reduction can sometimes occur in hematocrit (HCT) and leukocyte counts as well. Also, when the tube is allowed to fill based on the vacuum within the tube, the proper sample to anticoagulant ratio will be present. Inadequate sample size results in decreased HCT due to excessive EDTA solution. Care should be taken to avoid iatrogenic hemolysis, which interferes with plasma protein, fibrinogen, and various erythrocyte measurements. Samples should be submitted to the laboratory as rapidly as is feasible, and blood films should be made as soon as possible and rapidly dried to minimize morphologic changes.

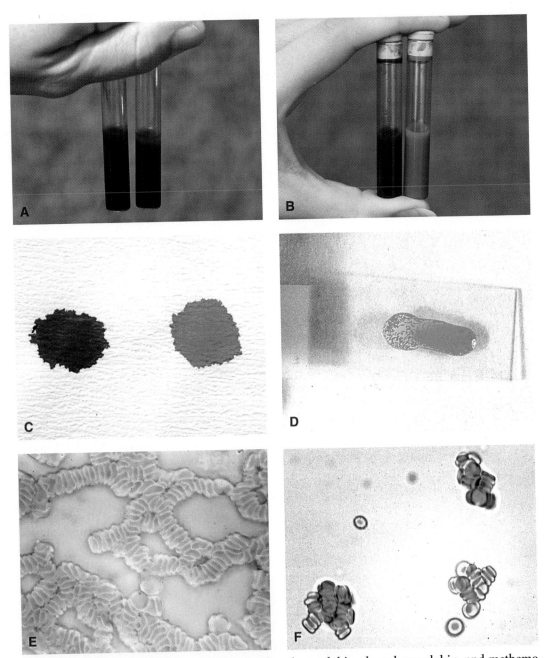

FIGURE 1. Gross appearance of mixtures of oxyhemoglobin, deoxyhemoglobin, and methemo-globin and differentiation of erythrocyte agglutination from rouleau formation. **A.** Venous blood sample from a cat with 28% methemoglobin (left sample) compared to a normal cat with less than 1% methemoglobin (right sample). Both samples also contain a mixture of oxyhemoglobin and deoxyhemo-globin. **B.** Oxygenated blood sample from a cat with 28% methemoglobin (left sample)

(Continued)

■ GROSS EXAMINATION

Samples are checked for clots and mixed well (gently inverted 20 times) immediately before removing aliquots for hematology procedures. Horse erythrocytes settle especially rapidly because of rouleau formation (adhesion of erythrocytes together like a stack of coins). Blood should be examined grossly for color and evidence of erythrocyte agglutination. The presence of marked lipemia may result in a blood sample with a milky red color resembling "tomato soup" when oxygenated.

Methemoglobinemia

Hemoglobin is a protein consisting of four polypeptide globin chains, each of which contains a heme prosthetic group within a hydrophobic pocket. Heme is composed of a tetrapyrrole with a central iron molecule that must be maintained in the ferrous (+2) state to reversibly bind oxygen. Methemoglobin differs from hemoglobin only in that the iron molecule of the heme group has been oxidized to the ferric (+3) state and it is no longer able to bind oxygen.[9] The presence of large amounts of deoxyhemoglobin accounts for the dark, bluish color of normal venous blood samples. Methemoglobinemia may not be recognized in venous blood samples, because the brownish color of methemoglobin is not readily apparent when mixed with deoxyhemoglobin (Fig. 1A). When deoxyhemoglobin binds oxygen to form oxyhemoglobin, it becomes bright red; consequently, the brownish coloration of methemoglobin becomes more apparent in the oxygenated samples (Fig. 1B). A simple spot test provides a rapid way to oxygenate a venous blood sample and determine if clinically significant levels of methemoglobin are present. One drop of blood from the patient is placed on a piece of absorbent white paper and a drop of normal control blood is placed next to it. If the methemoglobin content is 10% or greater, the patient's blood will have a noticeably brown color, compared to the bright red color of control blood (Fig. 1C).[9] Accurate determination of methemoglobin content requires that blood be submitted to a laboratory that has this test available.[10]

Methemoglobinemia results from either increased production of methemoglobin by oxidants or decreased reduction of methemoglobin associated with a deficiency in the erythrocyte methemoglobin reductase enzyme. Experimental studies indicate that many drugs can produce methemoglobinemia in animals.

---

compared to a normal cat with less than 1% methemoglobin (right sample). The sample on the left contains a mixture of oxyhemoglobin and methemoglobin, and the one on the right contains almost exclusively oxyhemoglobin.   **C.**   A drop of blood from a methemoglobin reductase–deficient cat with 50% methemoglobin (left) is placed on absorbent white paper next to a drop of normal cat blood with less than 1% methemoglobin.   **D.**   Grossly visible agglutination in blood from a dog with immune-mediated hemolytic anemia.   **E.**   Microscopic rouleaux in an unstained wet mount preparation of normal cat blood.   **F.**   Microscopic agglutination in an unstained wet mount preparation of saline-washed erythrocytes from a foal with neonatal isoerythrolysis.

Significant methemoglobinemia has been associated with clinical cases of benzo-
caine, acetaminophen, and phenazopyridine toxicities in cats and dogs; nitrite
toxicity in cattle; copper toxicity in sheep and goats; and red maple toxicity in
horses.[9]

Agglutination

The appearance of red granules in a well-mixed blood sample (Fig. 1D) suggests
the presence of erythrocyte agglutination, the aggregation or clumping of erythrocytes together in clusters. Agglutination is caused by the occurrence of immunoglobulins bound to erythrocyte surfaces. It must be differentiated from rouleaux, the adhesion of erythrocytes together like a stack of coins, which can be
seen in blood from healthy horses and cats (Fig. 1E). Agglutination can be
differentiated from rouleaux by washing erythrocytes in physiologic saline or by
adding equal drops of physiologic saline and blood together to see if the
aggregation of erythrocytes is dispersed (rouleaux) or remains (agglutination).
The microscopic appearance of agglutination in a sample of washed erythrocytes is shown (Fig. 1F).

▦ MICROHEMATOCRIT TUBE EVALUATION

When blood is submitted for a CBC, most commercial laboratories determine
the HCT electronically. This efficiency negates the need to centrifuge a microhematocrit tube filled with blood. Unfortunately, useful information concerning
the appearance of plasma is missed unless a serum or a plasma sample is also
prepared for clinical chemistry tests.

Packed Cells

In addition to determining the HCT, the buffy coat is evaluated. The buffy coat
contains platelets and leukocytes. It may appear reddish due to the presence of
marked reticulocytosis. In some species, certain leukocytes may also be present
in the top portion of the packed erythrocyte column (e.g., neutrophils in
cattle). A large buffy coat suggests leukocytosis (Fig. 2A) or thrombocytosis and
a small one suggests low numbers of these cells may be present.

Plasma Appearance

Plasma is normally clear in all species. It is nearly colorless in small animals,
pigs, and sheep but light yellow in horses, because they naturally have higher
bilirubin concentrations.[11] Plasma varies from colorless to light yellow (carot-
enoid pigments) in cattle, depending on their diet. Increased yellow coloration
usually indicates increased bilirubin concentration. This increase often occurs
secondarily to anorexia (fasting hyperbilirubinemia) in horses due to reduced

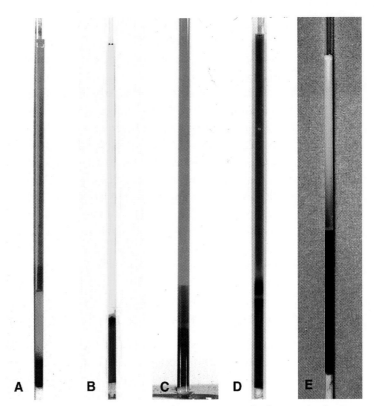

FIGURE 2. Gross appearance of microhematocrit tubes demonstrating leukocytosis, icterus, hemolysis, and lipemia.   A. Microhematocrit tube from a markedly anemic cat with a large buffy coat resulting from an acute myeloid leukemia with a total leukocyte count of 236,000 leukocytes/μL. Hemolysis is present in plasma because the blood sample was sent through the mail and was several days old.   **B.** Microhematocrit tube from an anemic cat, with icteric plasma secondary to hepatic lipidosis. **C.** Microhematocrit tube with evidence of hemolysis in plasma from a cat with acetaminophen-induced Heinz-body hemolytic anemia. Less-dense erythrocyte "ghosts" can be seen above the packed intact erythrocytes.   **D.** Microhematocrit tube with evidence of hemolysis in plasma from a horse with intravascular hemolysis induced by the inadvertent intravenous and intraperitoneal administration of hypotonic fluid. Less-dense erythrocyte ghosts can be seen above the buffy coat.   **E.** Microhematocrit tube with marked lipemia in plasma from a dog with hypothyroidism that was also being treated with prednisone for an allergic dermatitis. It was unclear from the medical record if this was a fasting blood sample.

removal of unconjugated bilirubin by the liver.[12] In other species, yellow plasma with a normal HCT suggests hyperbilirubinemia secondary to liver disease. Hyperbilirubinemia associated with a marked decrease in the HCT suggests an increased destruction of erythrocytes; however, the concomitant occurrence of liver disease and a nonhemolytic anemia could produce a similar finding (Fig. 2B).

Red discoloration of plasma indicates the presence of hemolysis. This discoloration may represent either true hemoglobinemia, resulting from intravascular hemolysis (Figs. 2C, 2D), or the hemolysis may have occurred after sample collection due to such causes as rough handling, fragile cells, lipemia, or prolonged storage. The hematocrit value may help differentiate these two possibilities, with red plasma and a normal hematocrit suggesting *in vitro* hemolysis. The concomitant occurrence of hemoglobinuria indicates the presence of intravascular hemolysis.

Lipemia is recognized as a white opaque appearance caused by chylomicrons and very-low-density lipoproteins (VLDL). The presence of chylomicrons may also result in a white layer at the top of the plasma column (Fig. 2E). The presence of lipemia is frequently the result of a recent meal (postprandial lipemia), but diseases including diabetes mellitus, pancreatitis, and hypothyroidism may result in lipemia in dogs. Hereditary causes include lipoprotein lipase deficiency in cats and dogs and idiopathic hyperlipidemia in miniature schnauzer dogs.[13,14] Ponies (especially obese ones), miniature horses, and donkeys are susceptible to developing lipemia associated with pregnancy, lactation, and/or anorexia.[15,16] These conditions result in the mobilization of unesterified fatty acids from adipose tissue and the subsequent overproduction of VLDL by the liver.

Plasma Protein Determination

After the HCT is measured and the appearance of the plasma and buffy coat are noted, the microhematocrit capillary tube is broken just above the buffy coat, and the plasma is placed in a refractometer for plasma protein determination. Plasma protein values in newborn animals (approximately 4.5 to 5.5 g/dL) are lower than adult values and increase to the adult range by 3 to 4 months of age.[11] The presence of lipemia or hemolysis will falsely increase the measured plasma protein value. Maximum information can be gained by interpretation of the HCT and plasma protein concentrations simultaneously.[1]

Fibrinogen Determination

Fibrinogen can be measured in a hematocrit tube because it readily precipitates from plasma when heated to 56° to 58°C for 3 minutes. The difference between the total protein of the plasma and the total protein of the defibrinogenated (heated) plasma gives an estimate of the fibrinogen concentration in the plasma.[17] This method is useful in identifying high-fibrinogen concentrations, but not accurate in identifying low-fibrinogen concentrations.[18,19]

■ BLOOD FILM PREPARATION

Blood films should be prepared within a couple of hours of blood sample collection to avoid artifactual changes that will distort the morphology of blood cells. Blood films are prepared in various ways including the slide (wedge) method, coverslip method, and automated slide spinner methods. It is essential that a monolayer of intact cells be present on the slide so that accurate examination and differential leukocyte counts can be made.

Slide Blood Film Method

A clean glass slide is placed on a flat surface and a small drop of well-mixed blood is placed on one end of the slide (Fig. 3A). This slide is held in place with one hand and a second glass slide (spreader slide) is placed on the first slide and held between the thumb and forefinger with the other hand at about a 30-degree angle in front of the drop of blood. The spreader slide is then backed into the drop of blood, and as soon as the blood flows along the back side of the spreader slide (Fig. 3B), the spreader slide is rapidly pushed forward (Fig. 3C). The thickness of the smear is influenced by the viscosity of the sample. The angle between the two slides may be increased when the blood is less viscous (low HCT) and decreased when the blood is more viscous (high HCT) than normal to produce a smear of appropriate thickness.

If the drop of blood is the proper size, all blood will remain on the slide, and a smear will be prepared that is thick at the back of the slide, where the drop of blood was placed, and thin at the front (feathered) edge of the slide. If the drop of blood is too large, some of the blood will be pushed off the end of the slide, causing potential problems. Often these blood films will be too thick for accurate evaluation. Secondly, clumps of cells tend to be pushed off the slide, making them unavailable for examination.

Once prepared, the slide is immediately dried by waving it in the air or by holding it in front of a hair dryer set on a warm-air setting. Holding the slide close to a dryer set on a hot-air setting can result in fragmentation of cells. Slides are identified by writing on the thick end of the smear or the frosted end of the slide with a graphite pencil or a pen containing ink that is not removed by alcohol fixation.

Coverslip Blood Film Method

Two 22-mm square, No. 1½ coverslips are required to make coverslip blood films (Fig. 3D). A camel's-hair brush is used to remove particles from the surfaces that will contact blood. One coverslip is held between the thumb and index finger of one hand, and a small drop of blood is placed in the middle of the coverslip using a microhematocrit tube. The drop of blood should be as perfectly round as possible to produce even spreading between coverslips. The second coverslip is dropped on top of the first in a crosswise position. After the blood spreads evenly between the two coverslips and a feathered edge forms at the periphery, the coverslips are rapidly separated by grasping an exposed corner of the top coverslip with the other hand and pulling apart in a smooth, horizontal manner. Coverslips are immediately dried as described above and then identified by marking on the thick end of the smears with a graphite pencil or a pen containing ink that is not removed by alcohol fixation.

If the drop of blood used is too large, a feathered edge will not form and the blood film will be too thick. Multiple coverslip blood films may be stained in small, slotted coplin jars or in ceramic staining baskets that are placed in beakers of fixative and stain.

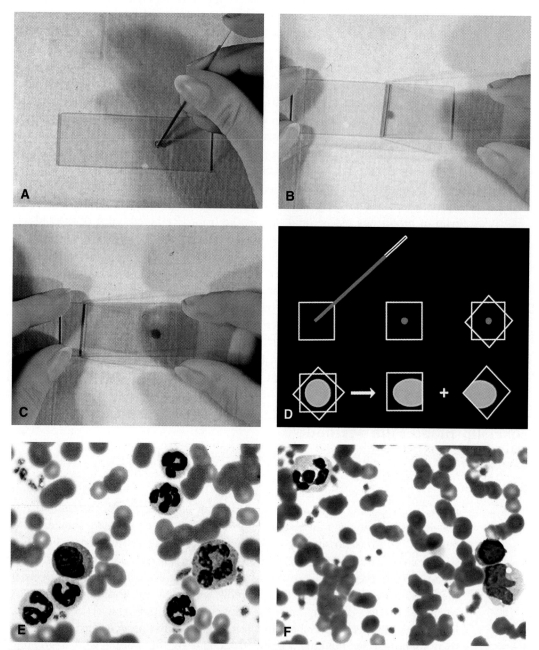

FIGURE 3. **Techniques for glass-slide and coverslip blood film preparations and the appear-ance of stained blood films.** **A.** Slide blood film preparation—step 1. A small drop of well-mixed blood is placed on one end of clean glass slide. **B.** Slide blood film preparation—step 2. A second glass slide (spreader slide) is placed on the first slide at about a 30-degree angle in front of the drop of blood and then backed into the drop of blood. **C.** Slide blood film preparation—step 3. As soon as

(Continued)

◾ BLOOD FILM STAINING PROCEDURES

Romanowsky-Type Stains

Blood films are routinely stained with a Romanowsky-type stain (e.g., Wright or Wright-Giemsa) either manually or using an automatic slide stainer. Romanowsky-type stains are composed of a mixture of eosin and oxidized methylene blue (azure) dyes. The azure dyes stain acids, resulting in blue to purple colors, and eosin stains bases, resulting in red coloration (Fig. 3E). These staining characteristics depend on the pH of the stains and rinse water as well as the nature of the cells present (Fig. 3F). Pale staining cells can result from inadequate staining time, degraded stains, or excessive washing.

Blood films may have an overall blue tint if stored unfixed for weeks before staining or if the unfixed blood films are exposed to formalin vapors, as occurs when blood films are shipped to the laboratory in a package that also contains formalin-fixed tissue. Blood films prepared from blood collected with heparin as the anticoagulant have an overall magenta tint due to the mucopolysaccharides present.

Various problems can occur during the drying, fixation, and staining of blood films that result in poor-quality films. Drying or fixation problems can result in variably shaped refractile inclusions in erythrocytes that may be confused with erythrocyte parasites (Fig. 4A). The presence of stain precipitation can make identification of leukocytes and blood parasites difficult (Fig. 4B). Precipitated stain may be present because the stain(s) needed to be filtered, the staining procedure was too long, or washing was not sufficient. Carboxymethylcellulose has been infused into the peritoneal cavity of horses and cattle in an attempt to prevent abdominal adhesions after surgery. This material can appear as a precipitate between cells in blood that resembles stain precipitation (Fig. 4C).[20]

Various rapid stains are available. The quality of the stained blood films is generally somewhat lower than that obtained by longer staining procedures. The Diff-Quik stain is a commonly used Wright-type rapid blood stain. The quality of this staining procedure is improved considerably by allowing the blood film to remain in the fixative for several minutes. One limitation of this stain is that it does not stain basophil or mast cell granules well. However, it is superior to Wright or Wright-Giemsa stains in staining distemper inclusions in canine blood cells.[21]

---

the blood flows along the back side of the spreader slide, the spreader slide is rapidly pushed forward. **D.** Steps used in preparing coverslip blood films are described in the text. **E.** Normal cat blood stained with Wright-Giemsa and rinsed in distilled water. Four neutrophils, a basophil (far right), and a lymphocyte (round nucleus) are present. Erythrocytes exhibit rouleaux, a normal finding in cats. **F.** Normal cat blood stained with Wright-Giemsa and rinsed in tap water. A neutrophil (left), monocyte (bottom right), and lymphocyte (top right) are present. The blue color of the erythrocytes results from using water with inappropriate pH.

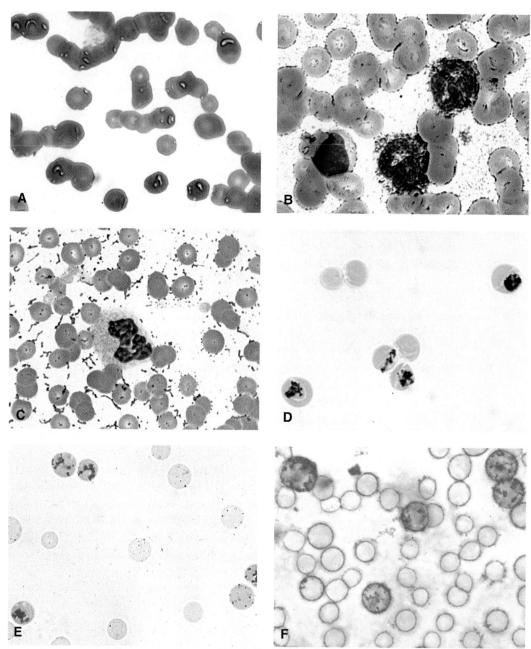

FIGURE 4.   Staining artifacts, the appearance of carboxymethylcellulose, and reticulocyte morphology in blood films.   **A.**   Refractile inclusions in erythrocytes from a horse are artifacts resulting from drying or fixation problems. Erythrocytes exhibit rouleaux, a normal finding in horses. Wright-Giemsa stain.   **B.**   Stain precipitation in blood from a dog. The two neutrophils present might be mistaken for basophils because of the adherent precipitated stain. Wright-Giemsa stain.   **C.**   The blue to purple

(Continued)

Reticulocyte Stains

Reticulocyte stains are commercially available. Those wishing to prepare their own stain can do so by dissolving 0.5 g of new methylene blue and 1.6 g of potassium oxalate in 100 mL of distilled water. Following filtrations, equal volumes of blood and stain are mixed together in a test tube and incubated at room temperature for 10 to 20 minutes. After incubation, blood films are made and reticulocyte counts are performed by examining 1,000 erythrocytes and determining the percentage that are reticulocytes.[17] The use of a Miller's disc in one of the microscope oculars saves time in performing the reticulocyte count.

The blue-staining aggregates or "reticulum" seen in reticulocytes (Fig. 4D) does not occur as such in living cells but results from the precipitation of ribosomal ribonucleic acid (RNA; the same RNA that causes the bluish color seen in polychromatophilic erythrocytes) in immature erythrocytes during the staining process.[11] As a reticulocyte matures, the number of ribosomes decreases until only small punctate (dotlike) inclusions are observed in erythrocytes (punctate reticulocytes) stained with the reticulocyte stain (Fig. 4E). To reduce the chance that a staining artifact would result in misclassifying a mature erythrocyte as a punctate reticulocyte using a reticulocyte stain, the cell in question should have two or more discrete blue granules that are visible without requiring fine-focus adjustment of the cell being evaluated to be classified as a punctate reticulocyte.

In normal cats, as well as in cats with regenerative anemia, the number of punctate reticulocytes is much greater than that seen in other species.[22] This apparently occurs because the maturation (loss of ribosomes) of reticulocytes in cats is slower than that in other species. Consequently, reticulocytes in cats are classified as aggregate (if coarse clumping is observed) or punctate (if small individual inclusions are present). Percentages of both types should be reported. Based on composite results from several authors, normal cats generally have from 0% to 0.5% aggregate and 1% to 10% punctate reticulocytes when determined by manual means. Higher punctate numbers of 2% to 17% have been reported using flow cytometry.[23]

The percentages of aggregate reticulocytes in cats correlate directly with the percentages of polychromatophilic erythrocytes observed in blood films

---

precipitate present between erythrocytes in this horse blood results from treatment with carboxymethylcellulose. Photograph of a stained blood film from a 1994 ASVCP slide review case submitted by M.J. Burkhard, M.A. Thrall, and G. Weiser. Wright-Giemsa Stain.   **D.**   Four reticulocytes (with blue-staining material) and three mature erythrocytes in blood from a dog with a regenerative anemia. New methylene blue reticulocyte stain.   **E.**   Three whole aggregate reticulocytes (containing blue-staining aggregates of RNA) and one half of an aggregate reticulocyte (far right) in blood from a cat with a markedly regenerative anemia. A majority of the remaining cells are punctate reticulocytes containing discrete dotlike inclusions. New methylene blue reticulocyte stain   **F.**   Five reticulocytes (with blue-staining material) in blood from a dog with a regenerative anemia in a new methylene blue stained wet preparation. Note the difference in morphology compared to reticulocytes stained with a standard reticulocyte stain (Fig. 4D). New methylene blue stained wet preparation.

stained with Wright-Giemsa stain.[22] Aggregate reticulocytes mature to punctate types in a day or less. Several more days are required for maturation (total disappearance of ribosomes) of punctate reticulocytes in cats.[24,25]

In contrast to those of the cat, most reticulocytes in other species are of the aggregate type. Consequently, no attempts are made to differentiate stages of reticulocytes in species other than the cat. The percentage of reticulocytes in most species correlates directly with the percentage of polychromatophilic erythrocytes observed on routinely stained blood films.

Heinz bodies are composed of denatured, precipitated hemoglobin. They are spherical, stain pale blue with reticulocyte stains, and are usually found at the periphery of the erythrocyte.

New Methylene Blue "Wet Mounts"

A new methylene blue "wet mount" preparation can be used for rapid information concerning the number of reticulocytes, platelets, and Heinz bodies present. The stain consists of 0.5% new methylene blue dissolved in 0.85% NaCl. One mL of formalin is added per 100 mL of stain as a preservative. This stain is filtered after preparation and stored in dropper bottles. Alternately, the stain may be stored in a plastic syringe with a 0.2 μm syringe filter attached so that the stain is filtered as it is used. Dry unfixed blood films are stained by placing a drop of stain between the coverslip and a glass slide. This preparation is not permanent and does not stain mature erythrocytes or eosinophil granules. Punctate reticulocytes are not demonstrated, but aggregate reticulocytes appear as erythrocyte ghosts containing blue to purple granular material (Fig. 4F). Platelets stain blue to purple, and Heinz bodies appear as refractile inclusions within erythrocyte ghosts. Although this staining method is not optimal for differential leukocyte counts, the number and type of leukocytes present can be appreciated.

Iron Stains

An iron stain such as the Prussian blue stain is used to verify the presence of iron-containing (siderotic) inclusions in blood and bone marrow cells and to evaluate bone marrow iron stores. Smears may be sent to a commercial laboratory for this stain, or a stain kit can be purchased and applied in-house (Harleco Ferric Iron Histochemical Reaction Set, #6498693, EM Diagnostic Systems, Gibbstown, NJ). When this stain is applied, iron-positive material stains blue, in contrast to the dark pink color of the cells and background.

The presence of focal areas of basophilic stippling within erythrocytes stained with Romanowsky-type blood stains suggests that the stippling may contain iron. Iron-containing erythrocytes are referred to as siderocytes and iron-containing nucleated erythrocytes are called sideroblasts. Neutrophils and monocytes may contain dark bluish-black or greenish iron-positive particles within their cytoplasm when stained with Romanowsky-type stains. Leukocytes containing iron-positive inclusions have been called sideroleukocytes.

Prussian blue stain applied to bone marrow aspirate smears is a useful way to evaluate the amount of storage iron that is present in the marrow. Minimal or no iron is expected in iron deficiency anemia (although cats normally have no stainable iron in the marrow), whereas normal or excess iron may be observed in animals with hemolytic anemia and in animals with anemia resulting from decreased erythrocyte production.

Cytochemical Stains

A variety of cytochemical stains, such as peroxidase, chloroacetate esterase, alkaline phosphatase, and nonspecific esterase, are utilized to classify cells in animals with acute myeloid leukemias.[11,26,27] Reactions vary not only by cell type and stage of maturation but also by species.[28] These stains are done in a limited number of laboratories and special training and/or experience is required to interpret the results. The appearance of positive reactions also varies depending on the reagents used. Because of the complexities of the staining procedures and interpretation of results, minimal information on cytochemical stains will be presented in this atlas.

■ EXAMINATION OF STAINED BLOOD FILMS

An overview and organized method of blood film examination are presented here. Descriptions and photographs of normal and abnormal blood cell morphology, inclusions, and infectious agents will be given in subsequent sections.

Blood films are generally examined following staining with Romanowsky-type stains such as Wright or Wright-Giemsa stains. These stains allow for examination of erythrocyte, leukocyte, and platelet morphology. Blood films should first be scanned using a low-power objective to estimate the total leukocyte count and to look for the presence of erythrocyte agglutination (Fig. 5A), leukocyte aggregates (Fig. 5B), platelet aggregates (Fig. 5C), microfilaria (Fig. 5D), and abnormal cells that might be missed during the differential leukocyte count. It is particularly important that the feathered end of blood films made on glass slides be examined because leukocytes (Fig. 5E) and platelet aggregates (Fig. 5F) may be concentrated in this area. Aggregates of cells tend to be in the center of coverslip blood films rather than at the feathered edge.

When examining a glass-slide blood film, the blood film will be too thick to evaluate blood cell morphology at the back of the slide (Fig. 6A) and too thin at the feathered edge where cells are flattened (Fig. 6C). The optimal area for evaluation is generally in the front half of the smear behind the feathered edge (Fig. 6B). This area should appear as a well-stained monolayer (a field in which erythrocytes are close together with approximately one half touching each other) of cells.

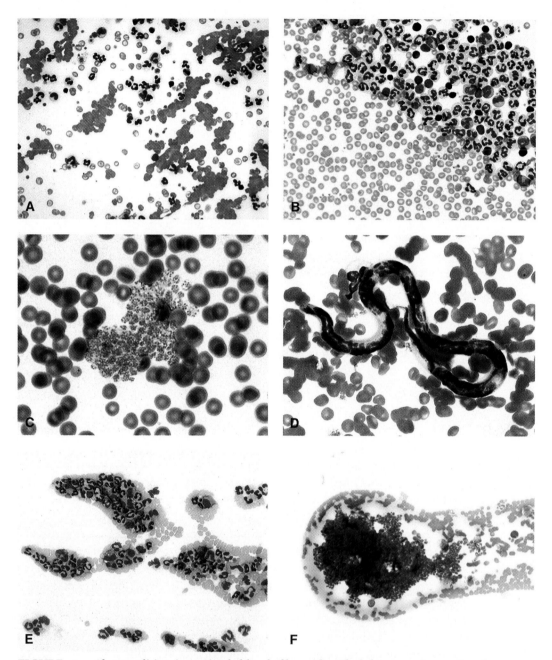

FIGURE 5. Abnormalities in stained blood films identified by scanning using low-power magnification. **A.** Autoagglutination of erythrocytes in blood from a dog with immune-mediated hemolytic anemia and marked leukocytosis. Wright-Giemsa stain. **B.** Leukocyte aggregate in blood from a dog. Leukocyte aggregates were present when EDTA was used as the anticoagulant but not when citrate was used as the anticoagulant. Wright-Giemsa stain. **C.** Platelet aggregate in blood from a cow.

(Continued)

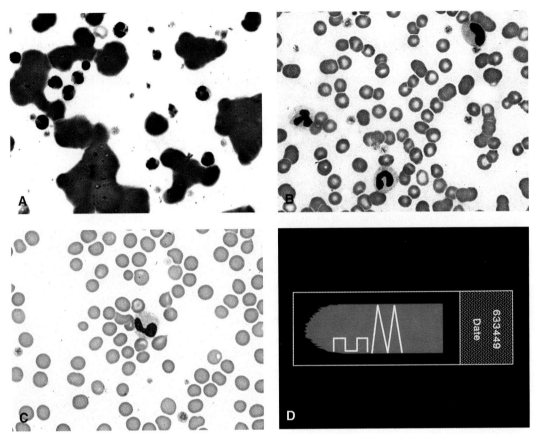

FIGURE 6. **Selection of the appropriate area for blood slide examination and patterns to use to perform a leukocyte differential count.** **A.** Thick area in the back end of a blood film from a dog. The blood film was prepared using glass slides. Wright-Giemsa stain. **B.** Optimal area for morphologic evaluation in the front half of a dog blood film (same blood film as shown in Fig. 6A) prepared using glass slides. Wright-Giemsa stain. **C.** Thin area near the feathered edge of a dog blood film (same blood film as shown in Figures 6A and 6B) prepared using glass slides. Erythrocytes are flattened to the extent that central pallor is not readily apparent. Wright-Giemsa stain. **D.** Patterns of slide blood film examination that may be used to improve the accuracy of differential leukocyte counts.

Wright-Giemsa stain. **D.** *Dirofilaria immitis* microfilaria in blood from a cat with heartworm disease. Wright-Giemsa stain. **E.** Leukocytes concentrated in the feathered edge of a blood film, from a dog. The blood film was prepared using glass slides. Wright-Giemsa stain. **F.** Platelet aggregate in the feathered edge of a blood film from a cat. The blood film was prepared using glass slides. Wright-Giemsa stain.

Leukocyte Evaluation

As a quality-control measure, the number of leukocytes present should be estimated to assure that the number present on the slide is consistent with the total leukocyte count measured. If 10X oculars and a 10X objective are used (100X magnification), the total leukocyte count in blood (cells/μL) may be estimated by determining the average number of leukocytes present per field and multiplying by 100 to 150. If a 20X objective is used, the total leukocyte count may be estimated by multiplying the average number of leukocytes per field by 400 to 600. The correction factor used may vary, depending on the microscope used. Consequently, the appropriate correction factors for the microscope being used should be determined by performing estimates on a number of blood films in which the total leukocyte counts have been accurately determined.

A differential leukocyte count is done by identifying 200 consecutive leukocytes using a 40X or 50X objective. Because neutrophils tend to be pulled to the edges in a wedge-type (glass slide) blood smear and lymphocytes tend to remain in the body of the smear,[17] differential counts are done by examining cells in a pattern that evaluates both the edges and the center of the smear (Fig. 6D). After the count is complete, the percentage of each leukocyte type present is calculated and multiplied by the total leukocyte count to get the absolute number of each cell type present per microliter of blood.

It is the absolute number of each leukocyte type that is important. Relative values (percentages) can be misleading when the total leukocyte count is abnormal. Let us consider two dogs, one with 7% lymphocytes and a total leukocyte count of 40,000/μL, and the other with 70% lymphocytes and a total leukocyte count of 4,000/μL. The first case would be said to have a "relative" lymphopenia and the second case would be said to have a "relative" lymphocytosis, but they both have the same normal absolute lymphocyte count (2,800/μL).

The presence of abnormal leukocyte morphology, such as toxic cytoplasm in neutrophils or increased reactive lymphocytes (e.g., more than 5% of lymphocytes are reactive), should be recorded on the hematology report form. The frequency of degenerative neutrophils is reported as few (5% to 10%), moderate (11% to 30%) or many (>30%) and the severity of degenerative change is recorded as 1+ to 4+ (Table 1).[29]

Erythrocyte Morphology

Erythrocyte morphology should be examined and recorded as either normal or abnormal. Erythrocytes on blood films from normal horses, cats, and pigs often exhibit rouleau formation, and erythrocytes from normal horses and cats may contain a low percentage of small, spherical nuclear remnants called Howell-Jolly bodies. Rouleaux and the presence of Howell-Jolly bodies should be recorded on the hematology form when they appear in blood films from species in which these are not normal findings.

TABLE 1	Semiquantitative Evaluation of Degenerative Changes in Neutrophils.[a]

NEUTROPHILS WITH DEGENERATIVE CHANGE	
Few	5–10 (%)
Moderate	11–30 (%)
Many	>30 (%)
SEVERITY OF DEGENERATIVE CHANGE	
Doehle bodies	1+
Basophilia of cytoplasm	1+
Foamy cytoplasm	2+
Dark blue-gray foamy cytoplasm	3+
Toxic granules	3+
Indistinct nuclear membrane	4+
Karyolysis	4+

[a] Modified from Weiss 1984.[29]

TABLE 2	Semiquantitative Evaluation of Erythrocyte Morphology Based on Average Number of Abnormal Cells per 1000X Microscopic Monolayer Field.[a]			
	1+	2+	3+	4+
Anisocytosis				
Dog	7–15	16–20	21–29	>30
Cat	5–8	9–15	16–20	>20
Cattle	10–20	21–30	31–40	>40
Horse	1–3	4–6	7–10	>10
Polychromasia				
Dog	2–7	8–14	15–29	>30
Cat	1–2	3–8	9–15	>15
Cattle	2–5	6–10	11–20	>20
Horse	rarely observed	—	—	—
Hypochromasia[a]	1–10	11–50	51–200	>200
Poikilocytosis[a]	3–10	11–50	51–200	>200
Codocytes (Dogs)	3–5	6–15	16–30	>30
Spherocytes[b]	5–10	11–50	51–150	>150
Echinocytes[b]	5–10	11–100	101–250	>250
Other shapes[c]	1–2	3–8	9–20	>20

[a] A monolayer field is defined as a field in which erythrocytes are close together with approximately one half touching each other. In severely anemic animals, such monolayers may not be present. When erythrocytes are generally not touching (e.g., tend to be separated by the distance of one cell diameter), then the number of erythrocytes with morphologic abnormalities are counted for two fields. From Weiss 1984.[29]

[b] The same parameters are used for all species. [c] Parameters are used for acanthocytes, schistocytes, keratocytes, elliptocytes, dacrocytes, drepanocytes, and stomatocytes in all species.

Additional observations regarding erythrocyte morphology, such as the degree of polychromasia (presence of polychromatophilic erythrocytes), anisocytosis (variation in size), and poikilocytosis (abnormal shape) should be made. Polychromatophilic erythrocytes are reticulocytes that stain bluish red due to the combined presence of hemoglobin (red staining) and ribosomes (blue staining). Abnormal erythrocyte shapes should be classified as specifically as possible, because specific shape abnormalities can help determine the nature of a disorder that may be present. Examples of abnormal erythrocyte morphology include echinocytes, acanthocytes, schistocytes, keratocytes, dacryocytes, elliptocytes, eccentrocytes, and spherocytes. The number of abnormal cells should be reported in a semiquantitative fashion, such as that shown in Table 2.[29]

Platelets

Platelet numbers should be estimated as low, normal, or increased. Blood smears from most domestic animals normally average between 10 and 30 platelets per field when examined using 10X oculars and the 100X objective (1,000X magnification). As few as 6 platelets per 1,000X field may be present in normal horse blood films.[29] Platelet numbers may be estimated by multiplying the average number per field by 15,000 to 20,000 to get the approximate number of platelets/μL of blood.[29,30] While special attention will be given to the estimation of platelet numbers in animals with hemostatic diatheses, it is important to routinely estimate the platelet numbers on blood films, because many animals with thrombocytopenia exhibit no evidence or past history of bleeding tendencies. If a thrombocytopenia is suspected, it should be confirmed with a platelet count. Dogs and cats have larger platelets than do horses and ruminants. Platelets contain magenta-staining granules, but these granules generally stain poorly in horses. The presence of abnormal platelet morphology (large platelets or hypogranular platelets) should be recorded on the hematology form.

Infectious Agents and Inclusions

Blood films are examined for the presence of infectious agents and intracellular inclusions using the 100X objective. Infectious agents and inclusions that may be seen in blood films include Howell-Jolly bodies, Heinz bodies (unstained), basophilic stippling, canine distemper inclusions, siderotic inclusions, Doehle bodies, *Babesia* spp., *Cytauxzoon felis*, *Haemobartonella* spp., *Ehrlichia* spp., *Hepatozoon* spp., *Trypanosoma* spp., *Theileria* spp., and *Borrelia* spp. The appearance of these agents and inclusions is discussed in subsequent sections.

CHAPTER 2

ERYTHROCYTES

■ ERYTHROCYTE MORPHOLOGY

Erythrocytes from all mammals are anucleated, and most are in the shape of biconcave discs called discocytes.[11] The biconcave shape results in the central pallor of erythrocytes observed in stained blood films (Fig. 7A). Of common domestic animals, biconcavity and central pallor are most pronounced in dogs, which also have the largest erythrocytes (Fig. 7B). Other species do not consistently exhibit central pallor in erythrocytes on stained blood films. The apparent benefit of the biconcave shape is that it gives erythrocytes high surface-area to volume ratios and allows for deformations that must take place as they circulate. Erythrocytes from goats generally have a flat surface with little surface depression; a variety of irregularly shaped erythrocytes (poikilocytes) may be present in clinically normal goats (Fig. 7C). Erythrocytes from animals in the Camelidae family (camels, llamas, vicunas, and alpacas) are thin, elliptical cells termed elliptocytes or ovalocytes (Fig. 7D), and they are not biconcave in shape. Erythrocytes from birds, reptiles, and amphibians are also elliptical in shape, but they contain nuclei and are larger than mammalian erythrocytes.

Rouleaux

Erythrocytes on blood films from healthy horses, cats, and pigs often exhibit rouleau (adhesion of erythrocytes together like a stack of coins) formation (Fig. 7A). Increased concentrations of fibrinogen and globulin proteins potentiate rouleau formation in association with inflammatory conditions. Rouleau formation can also occur in association with some lymphoproliferative disorders in which one or more immunoglobulins are secreted in high amounts (Fig. 7E). Prominent rouleau formation in species other than horses, cats, or pigs should be noted as an abnormal finding.[11]

Agglutination

Aggregation, or clumping, of erythrocytes together in clusters (not in chains as in rouleaux) is termed agglutination (Fig. 7F). Agglutination is caused by the

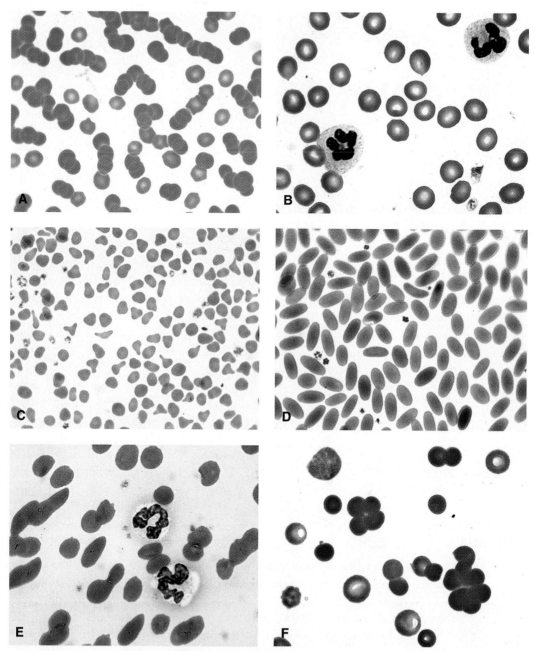

FIGURE 7.   Erythrocyte morphology in domestic animal species.   A.   Blood film from a horse. Most erythrocytes are adhered together like stacks of coins (rouleaux), a normal finding in this species. Individual nonadherent erythrocytes exhibit central pallor as a result of their biconcave shape. Wright-Giemsa stain.   **B.**   Blood from a dog with acute blood-loss anemia and normal erythrocyte morphology. Erythrocytes exhibit prominent central pallor. Two mature neutrophils and two platelets (bottom right corner) are also present. Wright-Giemsa stain.   **C.**   Poikilocytes in blood from a normal goat. Wright-
(Continued)

occurrence of immunoglobulins bound to erythrocyte surfaces. Because of their pentavalent nature, IgM immunoglobulins have the greatest propensity to produce agglutination.[1] High-dose unfractionated heparin treatment in horses also causes erythrocyte agglutination by an undefined mechanism.[31,32]

Polychromasia

The presence of bluish-red erythrocytes in stained blood films is called polychromasia (Fig. 8A). Polychromatophilic erythrocytes are reticulocytes that stain bluish red due to the combined presence of hemoglobin (red staining) and individual ribosomes and polyribosomes (blue staining). Low numbers of polychromatophilic erythrocytes are usually seen in blood from normal dogs and pigs because up to 1.5% reticulocytes may be present in dogs and up to 1% reticulocytes may be present in pigs even when the HCT is normal.[11] Slight polychromasia may be present in normal cats, but many normal cats exhibit no polychromasia in stained blood films. Polychromasia is absent in stained blood films from normal cattle, sheep, goats, and horses because reticulocytes are not normally present in blood in these species.[11]

The most useful approach in the classification of anemia is to determine whether or not evidence of a bone marrow response to the anemia is present in blood. For all species except the horse, this involves determining whether absolute reticulocyte numbers are increased in blood. Horses rarely release reticulocytes from the bone marrow even when an increased production of erythrocytes occurs. When an absolute reticulocytosis is present, the animal is said to have a regenerative anemia. The presence of a regenerative response suggests that the anemia results from either increased erythrocyte destruction or hemorrhage. A nonregenerative anemia generally indicates that the anemia is the result of decreased erythrocyte production (Fig. 8B); however, about 3 to 4 days are required for increased reticulocyte production and release by the bone marrow in response to an acute anemia. Consequently, the anemia appears nonregenerative shortly after hemolysis or hemorrhage has occurred (Fig. 7B).[1]

Increased polychromasia is usually present in regenerative anemias because many reticulocytes stain bluish-red with routine blood stains (Fig. 8A). When the degree of anemia is severe, basophilic macroreticulocytes or so-called stress reticulocytes may be released into the blood (Fig. 8C). It is proposed that one less mitotic division occurs during production, and immature reticulocytes, twice the normal size, are released. There is a direct correlation between the percentage of polychromatophilic erythrocytes and the percentage of reticulo-

Giemsa stain.   **D.** Elliptocytes in blood from a normal llama. Wright-Giemsa stain.   **E.** Rouleau formation in blood from a dog with multiple myeloma and a monoclonal hyperglobulinemia. The cytoplasm of the two neutrophils present is pale compared to the background that stains blue because of the increased protein present. Wright-Giemsa stain.   **F.** Erythrocyte agglutination and spherocyte formation in blood from a dog with von Willebrand's disease after transfusion. A large basophilic erythrocyte (macroreticulocyte or stress reticulocyte) is present in the upper left corner and an echinocyte is present in the lower left corner. Wright-Giemsa stain.

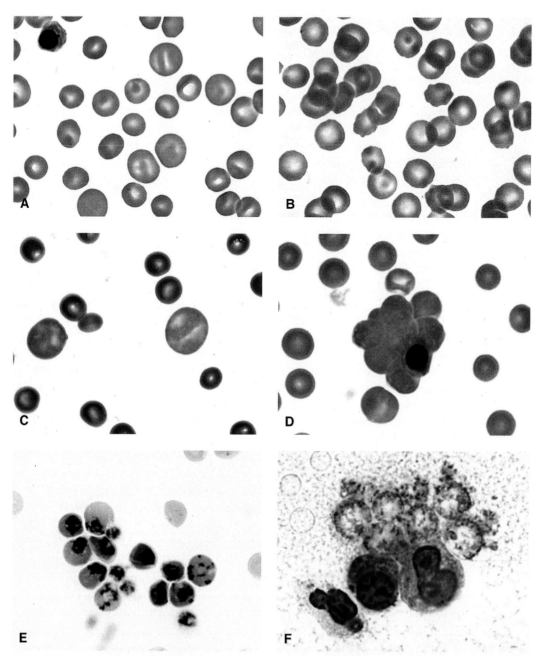

FIGURE 8. Erythrocyte morphology in anemic dogs and cats.   A. Increased polychromasia and anisocytosis in blood from a dog with a hemolytic anemia caused by *Haemobartonella canis*, although no organisms are present in this field. Four large polychromatophilic erythrocytes (reticulocytes) are present in the central area. A nucleated erythrocyte (metarubricyte) is present in the upper left. Wright-Giemsa stain.   **B.** Blood from a dog with a nonregenerative aplastic anemia secondary to trimethoprim-

(Continued)

cytes in dogs (and presumably in pigs) and between the percentage of polychromatophilic erythrocytes and the percentage of aggregate reticulocytes in cats
(Figs. 8D–8F).[22,33] Cats with mild anemia may not release aggregate reticulocytes from the marrow but will release punctate reticulocytes (Fig. 9A).[1] Because
punctate reticulocytes do not contain sufficient numbers of ribosomes within
them to impart a bluish color to the cytoplasm, mild regenerative anemia in
cats may lack polychromasia in stained blood films (Fig. 9B).

Anisocytosis

Variation in erythrocyte diameters in stained blood films is called anisocytosis
(Fig. 9B). It is greater in normal cattle than in other normal domestic animals
(Fig. 9C).[11] Anisocytosis is increased when different populations of cells are
present. It may occur when substantial numbers of smaller than normal cells
are produced, as occurs with iron deficiency, or when substantial numbers of
larger than normal cells are produced as occurs when increased numbers of
reticulocytes are produced. Consequently, increased anisocytosis is usually
present in regenerative anemia (Figs. 8A, 8C, 9B), but it may be present in
some nonregenerative anemia resulting from dyserythropoiesis.[1,34] Anisocytosis,
without polychromasia, may be seen in horses with intensely regenerative anemia (Fig. 9D).

Hypochromasia

The presence of erythrocytes with decreased hemoglobin concentration and
increased central pallor is called hypochromasia (Figs. 10A–10E). Not only is
the center of the cell paler than normal, but the diameter of the area of central
pallor is increased relative to the red-staining periphery of the cell. True hypochromic erythrocytes must be differentiated from torocytes, which have colorless punched-out centers but wider dense red-staining peripheries (Fig.
11A).[11] Torocytes are generally artifacts. Increased hypochromasia is observed in
iron-deficiency anemia.

Erythrocytes from dogs and ruminants with iron-deficiency anemia often
appear hypochromic on stained blood smears (Figs. 10A–10E). Hypochromasia
in iron deficiency results from both decreased hemoglobin concentration within
cells and from the fact that the cells are thin (leptocytes). Because these micro-

---

sulfadiazine therapy. Erythrocyte morphology is normal except for several erythrocytes with scalloped
borders (echinocytes). Wright-Giemsa stain.   **C.** Two exceptionally large basophilic erythrocytes
(macroreticulocytes or stress reticulocytes) are present in blood from a dog with immune-mediated hemolytic anemia. Wright-Giemsa stain.   **D.** Agglutination of polychromatophilic erythrocytes and a metarubricyte in blood from a cat with a Coombs'-positive hemolytic anemia. A reticulocyte stain revealed that
these agglutinated cells are aggregate reticulocytes (Fig. 8E). Wright-Giemsa stain.   **E.** Agglutination of
aggregate reticulocytes in blood from the same cat with a Coombs'-positive hemolytic anemia as shown in
Figure 8D. New methylene blue reticulocyte stain.   **F.** Agglutination of aggregate reticulocytes in blood
from a cat with a Coombs'-positive hemolytic anemia. New methylene blue wet mount preparation.

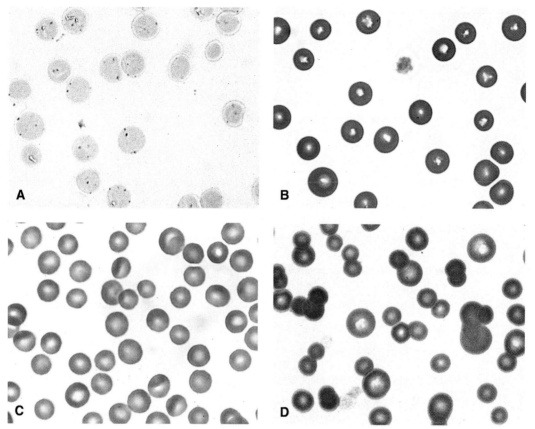

FIGURE 9.   Anisocytosis (variation in erythrocyte size) in blood.   A. Increased punctate reticulocytes (83% uncorrected) in blood from a FeLV-positive cat with a macrocytic normochromic anemia (hematocrit = 23%, MCV = 70 fl, MCHC = 33 g/dL). The uncorrected aggregate reticulocyte count was 0.2%. New methylene blue reticulocyte stain.   **B.** Increased anisocytosis in a blood film made from the same cat blood sample as shown in Figure 9A. Polychromasia is not apparent even though most of the blood cells present are punctate reticulocytes, because there is insufficient RNA present to impart a blue color to the cytoplasm of these cells. Wright-Giemsa stain.   **C.** Anisocytosis in blood from a nonanemic cow. Wright-Giemsa stain.   **D.** Increased anisocytosis in blood from a horse with a regenerative anemia resulting from internal hemorrhage. Horses almost never release reticulocytes in response to anemia; therefore, no polychromasia is present. Wright-Giemsa stain.

cytic leptocytes have increased diameter to volume ratios, they may not appear as small cells when viewed in stained blood films (Fig. 10B).[35] Microcytic erythrocytes from iron-deficient llamas exhibit irregular or eccentric areas of hypochromasia within the cells (Fig. 10E).[36]

Poikilocytosis

Erythrocytes can assume a wide variety of shapes. Poikilocytosis is a general term used to describe the presence of abnormally shaped erythrocytes. Although specific terminology is used for certain abnormal shapes, it is less important to quantify each type of shape change than it is to determine the cause of the shape change.[29] Poikilocytosis may be present in clinically normal goats and young cattle (Figs. 7C, 10F).[37,38] In some instances, these shapes appear to be related to the hemoglobin types present, but an abnormality in protein 4.2 in the membrane has been suggested as a causative factor in calves.[39]

Poikilocytosis forms in various disorders associated with erythrocyte fragmentation.[40] For unknown reasons, severe iron-deficiency anemia in dogs and ruminants may exhibit pronounced poikilocytosis (Figs. 10C, 10D).[35] Poikilocytes can form when oxidant injury results in Heinz body formation and/or membrane injury. One or more blunt erythrocyte surface projections may form as the membrane adheres to Heinz bodies bound to its internal surface.[40] A variety of abnormal erythrocyte shapes have been reported in dogs and cats with doxorubicin toxicity[41,42] and in dogs with dyserythropoiesis.[43]

Echinocytes (Crenated Erythrocytes)

Echinocytes are spiculated erythrocytes in which the spicules are relatively evenly spaced and of similar size.[44] Spicules may be sharp or blunt. When observed in stained blood films, echinocytosis is usually an artifact that results from excess EDTA, improper smear preparation, or prolonged sample storage before blood film preparation. The appearance of the echinocytes can vary depending on the thickness of the blood film (Figs. 11B, 11C). They are common in normal pig blood smears (Fig. 11D), forming *in vitro*.[11] The morphology of echinocytes varies from slightly spiculated echinodiscocytes to highly spiculated spheroechinocytes, which have been called burr cells (Fig. 11E).[17] The most advanced echinocytes are those that have lost most of their spicules and have nearly become spherocytes (Fig. 11F). Echinocytes form when the surface area of the outer lipid monolayer increases relative to the inner monolayer. Echinocytic transformation occurs *in vitro* in the presence of fatty acids, lysophospholipids, and amphipathic drugs that distribute preferentially in the outer half of the lipid bilayer. Echinocytes also form when erythrocytes are dehydrated, pH is increased, erythrocyte adenosine triphosphate (ATP) is depleted (e.g., hypophosphatemia), and intracellular calcium is increased.[9] Transient echinocytosis occurs in dogs following rattlesnake and coral snake envenomation (Figs. 11E, 11F),[45–47] presumably secondary to the action of phospholipases present in venom. Depending on the time course and dose of venom received, either echinocytosis or spherocytosis may be observed after these snake-bites. Echinocytes may occur in uremic animals, immediately after transfusion of stored blood, or in some pyruvate kinase–deficient dogs (Fig. 11G).[40,48] They have been seen with increased frequency in dogs with glomerulonephritis and neoplasia

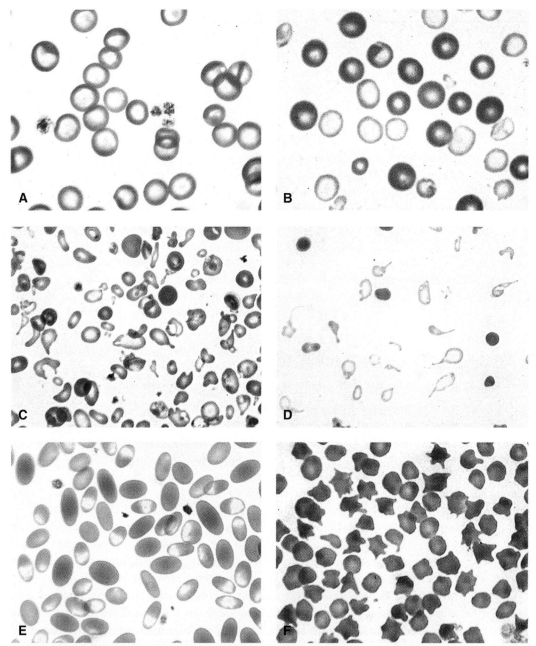

FIGURE 10. Hypochromasia and/or poikilocytosis in blood. **A.** Hypochromic erythrocytes in blood from a dog with iron deficiency secondary to chronic blood loss, resulting from a persistent flea infestation. Not only is the center of each cell paler than normal, but the diameter of the area of central pallor is increased relative to the red-staining periphery of the cell. A polychromatophilic erythrocyte (reticulocyte) is present in the upper left corner. Wright-Giemsa stain. **B.** Blood from a dog with a microcytic hypochromic (MCV = 32 fl, MCHC = 23 g/dL) iron-deficiency anemia was mixed with an equal volume of blood from a normal dog (MCV = 70 fl, MCHC = 34 g/dL) prior to blood film preparation. Because the hypochromic cells are leptocytes, they have diameters similar to normal cells even though they are microcytic cells. Wright-Giemsa stain. **C.** Marked poikilocytosis and hypochromasia in blood from a 6-week-old lamb with microcytic hypochromic iron-deficiency anemia. Wright-Giemsa stain.

(Continued)

(lymphoma, hemangiosarcoma, mast cell tumor, and carcinoma).[44,49] Echinocytosis occurs in horses in which total body depletion of cations has occurred (endurance exercise, furosemide treatment, and systemic disease).[50,51]

Acanthocytes

Erythrocytes with irregularly spaced, variably sized spicules are called acanthocytes or spur cells (Figs. 11H, 11I).[52] Acanthocytes form when erythrocyte membranes contain excess cholesterol compared to phospholipids. Alterations in erythrocyte membrane lipids can result from increased blood cholesterol content or due to the presence of abnormal plasma lipoprotein composition.[53] Acanthocytes have been recognized in animals with liver disease, possibly due to alterations in plasma lipid composition, which can alter erythrocyte lipid composition.[40,54,55] They have also been reported in dogs with disorders that result in erythrocyte fragmentation, such as hemangiosarcoma (Fig. 11I), disseminated intravascular coagulation, and glomerulonephritis.[54]

Marked acanthocytosis is reported to occur in young goats[37] and some young cattle (Fig. 10F).[38,56] Acanthocytosis of young goats occurs as a result of the presence of hemoglobin C at this early stage of development.[57]

Keratocytes

Erythrocytes containing what appear to be one or more intact or ruptured "vesicles" are called keratocytes (Figs. 11J–11M). These nonstaining areas appear to be circular areas of apposed and sealed membrane rather than true vesicles. The removal or rupture of this area results in the formation of one or two projections. Keratocytes have been recognized in various disorders including iron-deficiency anemia,[35] liver disorders,[55] doxorubicin toxicity in cats,[42] and myelodysplastic syndrome[58] and in various disorders in dogs having concomitant echinocytosis or acanthocytosis.[44,54] Keratocyte formation is potentiated by the storage of cat blood collected with EDTA.

Stomatocytes

Cup-shaped erythrocytes that have oval or elongated areas of central pallor when viewed in stained blood films are called stomatocytes (Fig. 11N). They most often occur as artifacts in thick blood film preparations. Stomatocytes form when erythrocyte water content is increased as occurs in hereditary stomatocytosis in dogs (Fig. 11O).[59–61] Stomatocytes also form when amphipathic drugs that distribute preferentially in the inner half of the lipid bilayer are present.[62]

D. Marked poikilocytosis (primarily dacryocytes) and hypochromasia in blood from a goat with microcytic hypochromic iron-deficiency anemia secondary to chronic blood loss, resulting from *Haemonchus* gastrointestinal parasites. Wright-Giemsa stain.   **E.** Microcytic erythrocytes in blood from an iron-deficient llama, exhibiting irregular or eccentric areas of hypochromasia within the cells. Wright-Giemsa stain.   **F.** Poikilocytosis (acanthocytes and echinocytes) in blood from a nonanemic young calf. Wright-Giemsa stain.

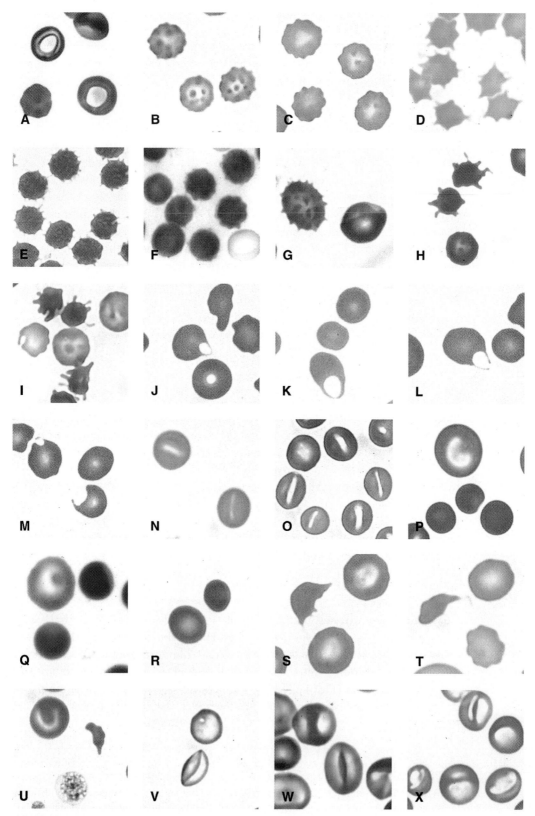

FIGURE 11. *See legend on opposite page.*

Spherocytes

Spherical erythrocytes that result from cell swelling and/or loss of cell membrane are referred to as spherocytes. Spherocytes lack central pallor and have smaller diameters than normal on stained blood films (Fig. 11P). Spherical erythrocytes with slight indentations on one side may be called stomatospherocytes (Fig. 11Q). Spherocytes occur most frequently in association with immune-mediated hemolytic anemia in dogs.[40,63] Other potential causes of sphero-

---

FIGURE 11. Erythrocyte shape abnormalities. **A.** Two torocytes with colorless punched-out centers and wide dense red-staining peripheries in blood from a dog. Wright-Giemsa stain. **B.** Echinocytes with regularly spaced spicules of similar length, in blood from a dog with malignant histiocytosis. Wright-Giemsa stain. **C.** Echinocytes, in a thinner area of the same blood film as shown in Figure 11B, appear as erythrocytes with scalloped borders; consequently, the old term "crenation" from Latin meaning "notched" is used. Wright-Giemsa stain. **D.** Echinocytes in blood from a normal pig. Wright-Giemsa stain. **E.** Highly spiculated echinocytes (burr cells) in blood from a dog following an Eastern diamondback rattlesnake bite. Wright-Giemsa stain. **F.** Spheroechinocytes and a lysed erythrocyte "ghost" (bottom right) in blood from a dog following a coral snake bite. Wright-Giemsa stain. **G.** An echinocyte (left) in blood from a pyruvate kinase–deficient Cairn terrier dog. Wright-Giemsa stain. **H.** Two acanthocytes (above) with irregularly spaced, variably sized spicules in blood from a dog with neoplastic lymphoid infiltrates in the liver. Wright-Giemsa stain. **I.** Three acanthocytes with irregularly spaced, variably sized spicules in blood from a dog with hemangiosarcoma. Wright-Giemsa stain. **J.** A keratocyte with what appears to be a "vesicle" in the cytoplasm of an erythrocyte in blood from a cat with hepatic lipidosis. Wright-Giemsa stain. **K.** A keratocyte with what appears to be a "vesicle" in the cytoplasm of an erythrocyte in blood from a cat with hepatic lipidosis. Wright-Giemsa stain. **L.** A keratocyte, exhibiting what appears to be a ruptured "vesicle" in blood from a cat with hepatic lipidosis. Wright-Giemsa stain. **M.** Two keratocytes, exhibiting what appear to be ruptured "vesicles" in blood from a cat with hepatic lipidosis. Wright-Giemsa stain. **N.** Stomatocytes with elongated areas of central pallor in blood from a cat with hemolytic anemia. The stomatocytes were not uniformly present in the blood film and were considered to be artifacts. Wright-Giemsa stain. **O.** Stomatocytes with elongated areas of central pallor in blood from an asymptomatic Pomeranian dog with persistent stomatocytosis associated with macrocytic hypochromic erythrocytes. Like dogs with hereditary stomatocytosis, erythrocytes were osmotically fragile and had low-reduced glutathione concentration. Wright-Giemsa stain. **P.** Three spherocytes (bottom) and a large polychromatophilic erythrocyte or reticulocyte (top) in blood from a dog with immune-mediated hemolytic anemia. Wright-Giemsa stain. **Q.** A large polychromatophilic erythrocyte or reticulocyte (top left) and two stomatospherocytes in blood from a dog with immune-mediated hemolytic anemia. The two stomatospherocytes are not prefect spheres. Each has a slight indentation on one side. Wright-Giemsa stain. **R.** A spherocyte (top) and a discocyte (bottom) in blood from a foal with immune-mediated neonatal isoerythrolysis. Wright-Giemsa stain. **S.** A fragmented erythrocyte (schistocyte) and two discocytes in blood from a dog with disseminated intravascular hemolysis. Wright-Giemsa stain. **T.** A schistocyte (left), discocyte (top), and echinocyte (bottom) in blood from a dog with disseminated intravascular hemolysis. Wright-Giemsa stain. **U.** A schistocyte (top right), large platelet (bottom right), and polychromatophilic erythrocyte (top left) in blood from a splenectomized pyruvate kinase–deficient Cairn terrier dog. Wright-Giemsa stain. **V.** Two thin flat hypochromic-appearing erythrocytes (leptocytes), with increased membrane-to-volume ratios, are present in blood from a dog with severe iron-deficiency anemia. The bottom leptocyte is folded. Wright-Giemsa stain. **W.** Two triconcave knizocytes (center) are present in a dog with a portosystemic shunt. Wright-Giemsa stain. **X.** Leptocytes, including two knizocytes (top and bottom center), are present in blood of a dog with iron-deficiency anemia. Wright-Giemsa stain.

cyte formation include coral snake and rattlesnake envenomation,[46,47] bee stings,[64] zinc toxicity,[65] erythrocyte parasites, transfusion of stored blood, and a familial dyserythropoiesis.[43] Since erythrocytes from other common domestic animals exhibit less central pallor than those of dogs, it is difficult to be certain when spherocytes are present in these noncanine species (Fig. 11R). Spherocytes have been reported in cattle with anaplasmosis[66] and in Japanese Black cattle with inherited erythrocyte band 3 deficiency.[67]

Schistocytes

Erythrocyte fragmentation may occur when erythrocytes are forced to flow through altered vascular channels or exposed to turbulent blood flow. Erythrocyte fragments with pointed extremities are called schistocytes or schizocytes (Figs. 11S–11U), and they are smaller than normal discocytes. Schistocytes may be seen in dogs with microangiopathic hemolytic anemia associated with disseminated intravascular coagulation (DIC).[40] Mechanical fragmentation occurs as the cells pass through the fibrin meshwork of a microthrombus. Schistocytes are not typically seen in cats or horses with DIC, possibly because the erythrocytes of these species are smaller and less likely to be split by fibrin strands in the circulation. Schistocytes have also been seen in severe iron-deficiency anemia,[35] myelofibrosis,[68–70] liver disease,[55] heart failure, glomerulonephritis, hemophagocytic histiocytic disorders, hemangiosarcoma in dogs, and congenital and acquired dyserythropoiesis in dogs.[40,43,54,58,70,71] Marked poikilocytosis with schizocytes and acanthocytes has been recognized in pyruvate kinase–deficient dogs after splenectomy (Fig. 11U).[72,73] It is assumed that the spleen had previously removed these fragmented erythrocytes.

Leptocytes

These cells are thin, often hypochromic-appearing erythrocytes with increased membrane-to-volume ratios. Some leptocytes appear folded (Fig. 11V), some appear as triconcave knizocytes that give the impression that the erythrocyte has a central bar of hemoglobin (Figs. 11W, 11X), and others appear as codocytes (Figs. 12A–12C). Codocytes (target cells) are bell-shaped cells that exhibit a central density or "bull's-eye" in stained blood films. Small numbers of codocytes are often seen in normal dog blood and both codocytes and knizocytes are increased in regenerative anemia in dogs. Codocytes are especially increased in dogs with a congenital dyserythropoiesis.[43] Leptocytes may be seen in iron-deficiency anemia (Figs. 11V, 12B)[35] and rarely in hepatic insufficiency (Fig. 12C) that results in a balanced accumulation of membrane phospholipids and cholesterol.[74] Polychromatophilic erythrocytes can sometimes appear as leptocytes.

Eccentrocytes (Hemighosts)

An erythrocyte in which the hemoglobin is localized to part of the cell, leaving a hemoglobin-poor area visible in the remaining part of the cell, is termed an eccentrocyte (Figs. 12D, 12E). They are formed by the adhesion of opposing areas of the cytoplasmic face of the erythrocyte membrane. Eccentrocytes that have become spherical with only a small tag of cytoplasm remaining may be called pyknocytes. Eccentrocytes have been seen in animals ingesting or receiving oxidants including onions, acetaminophen, and vitamin K in dogs;[75] red maple leaves in horses;[76] and intravenous hydrogen peroxide as a "home remedy," in a cow.[77] Eccentrocytes have also been seen in a horse with glucose-6-phosphate dehydrogenase (G6PD) deficiency[78] and in a horse with glutathione reductase deficiency secondary to erythrocyte flavin adenine dinucleotide (FAD) deficiency.[79]

Elliptocytes (Ovalocytes)

Erythrocytes from nonmammals and animals in the Camelidae family normally are elliptical or oval in shape (Fig. 7D). They are generally flat rather than biconcave. Abnormal elliptocytes have been recognized in cats with bone marrow abnormalities (myeloproliferative disorders and acute lymphoblastic leukemia),[70] hepatic lipidosis,[55] portosystemic shunts,[80] and doxorubicin toxicity[42] and in dogs with myelofibrosis,[69,81] myelodysplastic syndrome,[58] and glomerulonephritis, in which the elliptocytes may be spiculated (Figs. 12F, 12G).[49] Hereditary elliptocytosis has been reported in a dog with a membrane protein 4.1 deficiency.[82]

Dacryocytes

These erythrocytes are teardrop-shaped with single elongated or pointed extremities (Figs. 12H, 12I). Dacryocytosis is a common feature of myelofibrosis in people, but dacryocytes are not as commonly recognized in dogs with myelofibrosis.[69,70,83] Dacryocytes have also been seen in blood of dogs and cats with myeloproliferative disorders,[11] dogs with glomerulonephritis, and a dog with hypersplenism.[84] Dacryocytes are common erythrocyte shape abnormalities in iron-deficient ruminants, including llamas (Figs. 11J, 11K).[36]

Drepanocytes (Sickle Cells)

Fusiform or spindle-shaped erythrocytes are often observed in blood from normal deer (Fig. 12L) and in blood from people with sickle cell anemia.[85] These drepanocytes develop secondary to hemoglobin polymerization, and drepanocyte shape in deer depends on the hemoglobin types present. It is an *in vitro* phenomenon that occurs when oxygen tension is high and pH is between 7.6 and 7.8.

Polymerization of hemoglobin in tubular filaments occurs in some normal adult Angora goats[57,86] and some breeds of British sheep.[87] The resultant fusiform or spindle-shaped erythrocytes resemble drepanocytes in deer; they have been called acuminocytes by some authors (Fig. 12M).[11] The proportion of fusiform cells in Angora goats varies depending on the individual goat and on

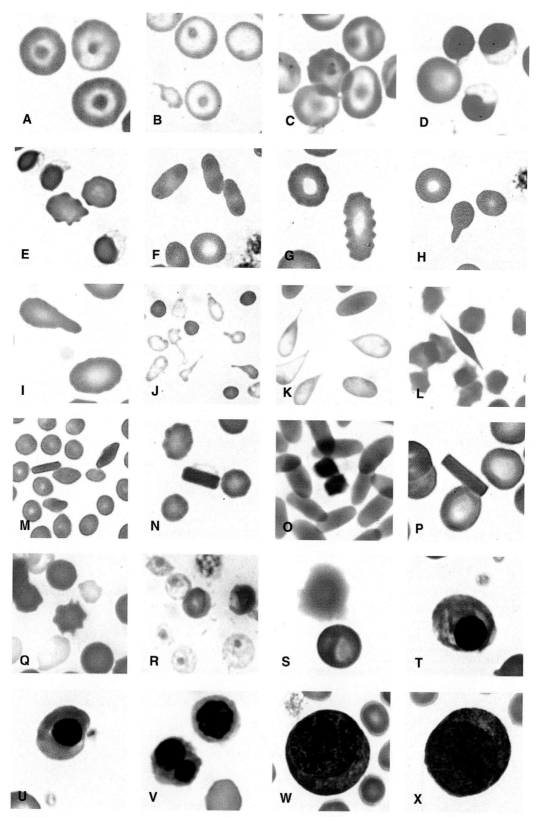

FIGURE 12. *See legend on opposite page.*

in vitro alterations in temperature, pH, and oxygenation. The number of these cells decreases during anemia, probably because of the synthesis of hemoglobin C.[86]

Crystalized Hemoglobin

The presence of large hemoglobin crystals within erythrocytes is commonly recognized in blood films from cats (Fig. 12N)[88–90] and llamas (Fig. 12O)[91,92] and rarely recognized in blood films from dogs (Fig. 12P), primarily pups less than 3 months of age.[93] No hemoglobin abnormalities have been recognized by hemoglobin electrophoresis and no pathologic significance has been attributed to finding hemoglobin crystals in blood films from domestic animals.

FIGURE 12. Erythrocyte shape abnormalities and the appearance of nucleated erythroid precursor cells. **A.** Three codocytes in blood from a Cairn terrier dog with a regenerative anemia and hepatic hemochromatosis secondary to pyruvate kinase–deficiency. These erythrocytes exhibit a central density or "bull's-eye" and are often referred to as target cells. Wright-Giemsa stain. **B.** Two codocytes (top and bottom center) and a schistocyte (bottom left) in blood from a dog with severe iron-deficiency anemia. Wright-Giemsa stain. **C.** Codocytes in blood from a dog with liver disease. Wright-Giemsa stain. **D.** Three eccentrocytes and a discocyte (left) in blood from a dog with oxidant injury induced by the administration of acetaminophen. The cell at top center appears spherical with a small tag of cytoplasm and may be referred to as a pyknocyte. Wright-Giemsa stain. **E.** Three eccentrocytes in blood from a horse with inherited erythrocyte glucose-6-phosphate dehydrogenase deficiency. Wright-Giemsa stain. **F.** Three elliptocytes and a discocyte in blood from a diabetic cat with mild anemia. Radiographs revealed diffuse interstitial lung disease of unknown etiology. Wright-Giemsa stain. **G.** An echinoelliptocyte in blood from a dog with glomerulonephritis. Wright-Giemsa stain. **H.** A dacryocyte (bottom) and two discocytes in blood from a cat. Wright-Giemsa stain. **I.** A dacryocyte (left) and elliptocyte (right) in blood from a dog with glomerulonephritis. Wright-Giemsa stain. **J.** Hypochromic dacryocytes in blood from a goat with severe iron-deficiency anemia. **K.** Hypochromic dacryocytes in blood from a llama with severe iron-deficiency anemia. The presence of the normal llama elliptocyte (above right) is the result of a blood transfusion. Wright-Giemsa stain. **L.** Elongated drepanocyte (sickle cell) in blood from a white-tailed deer. Wright-Giemsa stain. **M.** Erythrocytes containing hemoglobin inclusions in blood from a mixed-breed goat. Some erythrocytes appeared as rectangles but most appeared more fusiform and may represent polymerization of hemoglobin in tubular filaments as occurs in drepanocytes. Wright-Giemsa stain. **N.** Crystalized hemoglobin in an erythrocyte from a cat. Wright-Giemsa stain. **O.** Crystalized hemoglobin in two erythrocytes from a llama. Wright-Giemsa stain. **P.** Crystalized hemoglobin in an erythrocyte from a dog. Wright-Giemsa stain. **Q.** Red-staining intact erythrocytes (echinocyte in the center) and pale-staining erythrocyte ghosts in blood from a horse in which intravascular hemolysis was produced by the intravenous and intraperitoneal administration of hypotonic fluid believed isotonic at the time of administration. Wright-Giemsa stain. **R.** Erythrocyte ghosts, each containing a single red-staining Heinz body, in erythrocytes from a cat with intravascular hemolysis caused by acetaminophen administration. Wright-Giemsa stain. **S.** A lysed erythrocyte (red smudge at top) and discocyte in blood from a dog with lipemia. The lysis occurred during smear preparation. Wright-Giemsa stain. **T.** Orthochromatic metarubricyte in blood from a dog with a regenerative hemolytic anemia. Wright-Giemsa stain. **U.** Polychromatophilic metarubricyte in blood from a dog with a regenerative hemolytic anemia. Wright-Giemsa stain. **V.** Two polychromatophilic rubricytes, one of which has a lobulated nucleus, in blood from a cat with erythroleukemia and a nonregenerative anemia. Wright-Giemsa stain. **W.** Exceptionally large basophilic rubricyte in blood from a cat with myelodysplastic syndrome and a nonregenerative anemia. Wright-Giemsa stain. **X.** Rubriblast in blood from a cat with erythroleukemia and a nonregenerative anemia. Wright-Giemsa stain.

Lysed Erythrocytes

The presence of erythrocyte "ghosts" in peripheral blood films indicates that the cells lysed prior to blood film preparation (Fig. 12Q). Erythrocyte membranes are rapidly cleared from the circulation following intravascular hemolysis; consequently, the presence of erythrocyte ghosts indicates either recent intravascular hemolysis or *in vitro* hemolysis in the blood tube after collection. If the hemolysis is caused by an oxidant, Heinz bodies may be visible within erythrocyte ghosts (Fig. 12R). When erythrocytes lyse during blood film preparation, they appear as red smudges (Fig. 12S). These smudged erythrocytes are commonly seen in lipemic samples.

Nucleated Erythrocytes

Metarubricytes (Figs. 12T, 12U) and rubricytes are seldom present in the blood of normal adult mammals, although low numbers may occur in some normal dogs and cats.[94] These nucleated erythrocytes are often seen in blood (normoblastemia) in association with regenerative anemia; however, their presence does not necessarily indicate a regenerative response is present.[95] Nucleated erythrocytes are rarely seen in horses with regenerative anemia.

Nucleated erythrocytes may be seen in animals with lead poisoning in which there is minimal or no anemia (Fig. 13M)[96,97] and in nonanemic conditions in which bone marrow is damaged, such as septicemia, endotoxic shock, and drug administrations.[94,98] Low numbers of nucleated erythrocytes are seen in a wide variety of conditions in dogs including cardiovascular disease, trauma, hyperadrenocorticism, and various inflammatory conditions.[95]

When frequent nucleated erythrocyte precursors are present in the blood of an animal with nonregenerative anemia (Figs. 12V–12X), conditions including myelodysplasia, hematopoietic neoplasia,[11,95] infiltrative marrow disease,[94,99] impaired splenic function,[94] and inherited dyserythropoietic disorders[43,100] should be considered. The presence of rubriblasts in blood from an animal with nonregenerative anemia strongly suggests that a myeloproliferative disorder is present (Fig. 12X). Erythrocyte nuclei may be lobulated or fragmented in animals with myeloproliferative disorders (Fig. 12V)[101–103] or following vincristine therapy, if nucleated erythrocytes are present in blood (Figs. 13A, 13B). Nucleated erythroid precursors earlier than metarubricytes are capable of division; consequently, mitotic nucleated erythrocytes may be seen in blood (Fig. 13C).

■ INCLUSIONS OF ERYTHROCYTES

Howell-Jolly Bodies

These small, spherical nuclear remnants form in the bone marrow and are removed by the "pitting" action of the spleen. Howell-Jolly Bodies may be present in low numbers in erythrocytes of normal horses and cats (Fig. 13D).

They are often present in association with regenerative anemia or following splenectomy in other species. They may also be increased in animals receiving glucocorticoid therapy (Fig. 13E).[11] Nuclear fragmentation and multiple Howell-Jolly bodies may be present in animals treated with vincristine, if regenerative anemia is present (Figs. 13A, 13B).

Heinz Bodies

These inclusions are large aggregates of oxidized, precipitated hemoglobin that are attached to the internal surfaces of erythrocyte membranes. In contrast to Howell-Jolly bodies, which stain dark blue, Heinz bodies stain red to pale pink with Romanowsky-type stains (Figs. 13F, 13G). They bind to the inner surface of erythrocyte membranes and may be recognized as small surface projections when the membrane binds around much of an inclusion (Fig. 13F). When intravascular hemolysis occurs, they may be visible as red inclusions within erythrocyte ghosts (Figs. 12R, 13F). Heinz bodies appear light blue with reticulocyte stains (Fig. 13H). They can also be visualized as dark refractile inclusions in new methylene blue "wet mount" preparations (Fig. 13I). In contrast to other domestic animal species, normal cats may have up to 5% Heinz bodies within their erythrocytes.[104] Not only is cat hemoglobin more susceptible to denaturation by endogenous oxidants,[9] but the cat spleen is less efficient in the removal (pitting) of Heinz bodies from erythrocytes than are spleens of other species.[105] Increased numbers of Heinz bodies may occur with minimal anemia in cats with spontaneous diseases, such as diabetes mellitus (especially when ketoacidosis is present), hyperthyroidism, and lymphoma.[104,106] Small Heinz bodies may be seen in other species following splenectomy.[11]

Dietary causes of Heinz body hemolytic anemia include consumption of onions in small and large animals, consumption of kale and other *Brassica* species by ruminants, consumption of lush winter rye by cattle, and consumption of red maple leaves by horses.[9,75,107] Heinz bodies have been recognized in erythrocytes from selenium-deficient Florida cattle grazing on St. Augustine grass pastures and in postparturient New Zealand cattle grazing primarily on perennial ryegrass. Copper toxicity results in Heinz body formation in sheep and goats. Heinz body formation has been reported in dogs ingesting zinc-containing objects (e.g., U.S. pennies minted after 1982).[9] Naphthalene ingestion may have caused Heinz body formation in a dog.[108] Heinz body hemolytic anemia has occurred following the administration of a variety of drugs including acetaminophen and methylene blue in cats and dogs, methionine and phenazopyridine in cats, menadione (vitamin K_3) in dogs, and phenothiazine in horses.[9,75]

Basophilic Stippling

Reticulocytes usually stain as polychromatophilic erythrocytes with Romanowsky-type blood stains due to the presence of dispersed ribosomes and polyribosomes, but sometimes the ribosomes and polyribosomes aggregate to-

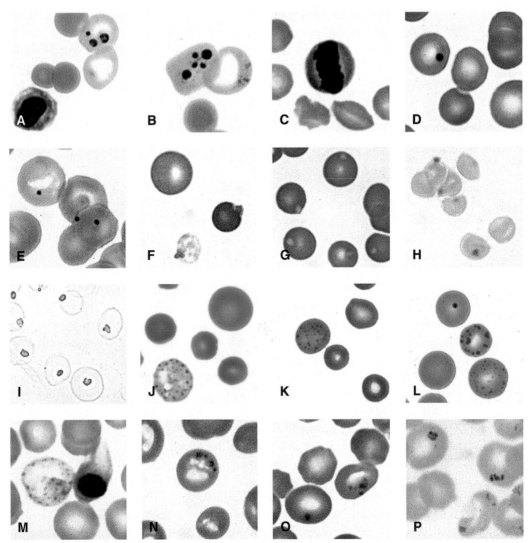

FIGURE 13. Erythrocyte inclusions and the appearance of a mitotic erythroid precursor cell.
A. Polychromatophilic metarubricyte with elongated nucleus and erythrocyte containing nuclear fragments in blood from a dog with immune-mediated hemolytic anemia and thrombocytopenia 5 days after treatment with vincristine. Wright-Giemsa stain.   **B.** Erythrocyte containing nuclear fragments in blood from a dog with immune-mediated hemolytic anemia and thrombocytopenia 5 days after treatment with vincristine. Wright-Giemsa stain.   **C.** Mitotic rubricyte in blood from a dog with hemangiosarcoma and a regenerative anemia. Wright-Giemsa stain.   **D.** Erythrocyte (left) containing a Howell-Jolly body (spherical nuclear remnant) in blood from a cat. Wright-Giemsa stain.   **E.** Three Howell-Jolly bodies in blood from a dog being treated with glucocorticoid steroids. Wright-Giemsa stain.   **F.** A large polychromatophilic erythrocyte (top), erythrocyte "ghost" containing a Heinz body (bottom), and an intact erythrocyte containing a Heinz body projecting from its surface (right) in blood from a dog with a hemolytic anemia resulting from the ingestion of several pennies containing zinc. Wright-Giemsa stain.   **G.** Heinz bodies in blood from a cat appearing as pale "spots" within erythrocytes. Wright-Giemsa stain.   **H.** Heinz bodies in blood from a cat. New methylene blue reticulocyte stain.   **I.** Heinz bodies in blood from a cat. New methylene blue wet mount preparation.   **J.** Diffuse basophilic stippling (bottom left) in
(Continued)

gether, forming blue-staining punctate inclusions referred to as basophilic stippling (Figs. 13J–13M).[52] These aggregates are similar to those produced using reticulocyte stains, but they form during the process of cell drying prior to staining with Romanowsky-type blood stains. Diffuse basophilic stippling commonly occurs in regenerative anemia in ruminants (Figs. 13J, 13K) and occasionally occurs in regenerative anemia in other species (Fig. 13L).[11] Basophilic stippling may be prominent in any species with lead poisoning (Fig. 13M).[96,97]

Siderotic Inclusions

Siderotic inclusions contain iron. In contrast to basophilic stippling, which is distributed throughout the erythrocyte, siderotic inclusions generally appear as focal basophilic inclusions located near the periphery of the erythrocyte. These inclusions have been called Pappenheimer bodies when visible in routinely stained blood films (Figs. 13N, 13O).[52] Electron microscopy of these bodies in human erythrocytes reveals that the iron is often contained within autophagic vacuoles (lysosomes) that also contain degenerating mitochondria.[52]

A Prussian blue staining procedure is used to verify the presence of iron-positive material (Fig. 13P). Erythrocytes containing these inclusions are called siderocytes. Siderocytes are rare or absent in the blood of normal animals but may occur with lead toxicity,[96] hemolytic anemia, dyserythropoiesis, myeloproliferative diseases, chloramphenicol therapy, and experimental pyridoxine deficiency in pigs.[9,58] Siderotic inclusions have been recognized in a dog with zinc toxicity,[109] but it is unclear whether this was a result of the zinc toxicity per se, or was associated with the accompanying hemolytic anemia. Finally, large numbers of Pappenheimer bodies have rarely been seen in nonanemic dogs (Figs. 13O, 13P) in which the causes were unclear. A common factor in two of these dogs was treatment with hydroxyzine; however, hematologic abnormalities have not previously been reported with this drug.[109,110]

---

a macrocytic polychromatophilic erythrocyte, a macrocytic erythrocyte (top right), and three normal-sized erythrocytes in blood from a cow with anaplasmosis (no organisms present) and a subsequent regenerative anemia. Wright-Giemsa stain.   **K.**   Diffuse basophilic stippling in a large erythrocyte (left) in blood from a sheep with a regenerative anemia. Wright-Giemsa stain.   **L.**   Erythrocytes containing a Howell-Jolly body (top), diffuse coarse basophilic stippling (middle) and diffuse fine basophilic stippling (bottom) in blood from a cat with hemobartonellosis (no organisms present) and a regenerative anemia. Wright-Giemsa stain.   **M.**   A polychromatophilic erythrocyte with basophilic stippling (left) and a polychromatophilic metarubricyte (right) in blood from a dog with lead toxicity. Wright-Giemsa stain.   **N.**   Focal basophilic stippling in an erythrocyte (siderocyte) in blood from a dog treated with chloramphenicol. The inclusions were shown to contain iron using the Prussian blue staining procedure. Wright-Giemsa Stain.   **O.**   Focal basophilic stippling in two erythrocytes (siderocytes) in blood from a male Sheltie dog that had many siderocytes in his blood when examined several times over 4 years. Erythrocytes were microcytic, but the dog was not anemic. Abnormalities in copper, zinc, and pyridoxine metabolism were ruled out, as was lead toxicity. Blood samples and case information provided by M. Plier. Wright-Giemsa stain.   **P.**   Iron-positive inclusions in erythrocytes (siderocytes) in blood from the same dog as shown in Figure 13O. Prussian blue stain.

■ INFECTIOUS AGENTS OF ERYTHROCYTES

A number of infectious agents are recognized to occur in or on erythrocytes. These include intracellular protozoal parasites (*Babesia* species, *Theileria* species, and *Cytauxzoon felis*), intracellular rickettsial organisms (*Anaplasma* species), and epicellular mycoplasma organisms (*Haemobartonella* species and *Eperythrozoon* species). The protozoal organisms each have a nucleus within their cytoplasm. The rickettsia and mycoplasma organisms are bacteria and, therefore, lack nuclei. These infectious agents generally cause mild to severe hemolytic anemia, depending on the pathogenicity of the organism and the susceptibility of the host. Distemper virus inclusions may also be seen in dog erythrocytes.

Babesia Species

Many species of *Babesia* infect animals worldwide.[111-113] When stained with Romanowsky-type blood stains, a babesial organism generally has colorless to light-blue cytoplasm with a red to purple nucleus (Figs. 14A–14E). Babesial parasites vary considerably in size from large, easily visualized *Babesia canis* parasites (Fig. 14A) to small, difficult to see *Babesia gibsoni* (Fig. 14B) and *Babesia felis* (Fig. 14C) parasites. Large babesial organisms generally appear pear-shaped and commonly occur in pairs. Small babesial organisms are more often round in shape.

Theileria Species

Theilerial organisms appear similar to babesial organisms when observed on stained blood films (Fig. 14F). The genus *Theileria* differs from the genus *Babesia* in that the *Theileria* species have a tissue phase as well as an erythrocyte stage of development. Schizonts develop in lymphoid cells and when mature, release merozoites, which enter erythrocytes. *Babesia* organisms proliferate only in erythrocytes. Theilerial species cause important diseases in ruminants in Africa, Asia, and the Middle East; however, the theilerial organisms present in ruminants in the United States are usually nonpathogenic.[114,115] Organisms are most commonly observed in deer blood in the United States (Fig.14G).

Cytauxzoon Felis

Cytauxzoon felis (Figs. 14H, 14I), as its name implies, infects feline erythrocytes.[116] It is similar in morphology to *Babesia felis* (Fig. 14C). Like *Theileria*, the genus *Cytauxzoon* has both a tissue phase and an erythrocyte phase. In contrast to *Theileria*, the schizonts of *Cytauxzoon* develop in macrophages rather than in lymphocytes.

Anaplasma Species

Anaplasma organisms appear as round to oval basophilic inclusions in ruminant erythrocytes (Figs. 14J–14L), which must be differentiated from Howell-Jolly bodies.[117] Although morulae are not appreciated by light microscopy, the inclusions consist of one to several subunits within a membrane-lined vesicle. The size of an inclusion seen by light microscopy is directly related to the number of subunits present. Unlike Howell-Jolly bodies, *Anaplasma* organisms are generally not perfect spheres, and most are smaller than Howell-Jolly bodies.

Distemper Inclusions

Viral inclusions may be seen in the blood cells of some dogs during the viremic stage of canine distemper virus infection.[118,119] These inclusions can be difficult to visualize when routine Wright or Giemsa stains are used. In erythrocytes, they appear as variably sized round, oval, or irregular, blue-gray inclusions that most often occur in polychromatophilic cells (Fig. 14M). For an unknown reason, distemper inclusions typically stain red and are easier to see in erythrocytes stained with the Diff-Quik stain (Fig. 14N), which is a rapid, modified Wright stain.[21]

Distemper inclusions are composed of aggregates of viral nucleocapsids. The presence of viral inclusions in anucleated cells is explained by the fact that they form within nucleated erythroid precursors in the bone marrow and persist following expulsion of the nucleus.[119]

Haemobartonella Species

These epicellular organisms attach to the external surface of erythrocytes.[120] *Haemobartonella felis* organisms appear as small blue-staining cocci, rings, or rods on feline erythrocytes (Figs. 14O, 14P). Organisms are quite pleomorphic and vary in size, but most are between 0.5 and 1.5 microns in diameter or length. Organisms occur in cyclic parasitemias; consequently, they are not always identifiable in blood even during acute infections. *Haemobartonella canis* organisms commonly form chains of organisms that appear as filamentous structures on the surface of canine erythrocytes (Fig. 14Q). Reticulocyte stains cannot be used to search for *Haemobartonella* organisms, because the basophilic ribosomal material in reticulocytes can appear similar to the parasites. *Haemobartonella* organisms were classified as rickettsia for many years, but molecular biology studies have shown that they are mycoplasmal organisms.[121,122]

Eperythrozoon Species

Eperythrozoon species appear as small delicate basophilic rings upon or between erythrocytes. *Eperythrozoon* infections occur in pigs, sheep, cattle, and llamas (Figs. 14R–14U).[123–126] These organisms can cause significant anemia in pigs and sheep (primarily young animals), but not usually in cattle or llamas.

Differentiation of the genera *Haemobartonella* and *Eperythrozoon* is purportedly based on the fact that *Haemobartonella* organisms rarely occur as ring forms while *Eperythrozoon* organisms frequently do. Differentiation is also based on the fact that *Eperythrozoon* organisms occur with about equal frequency on

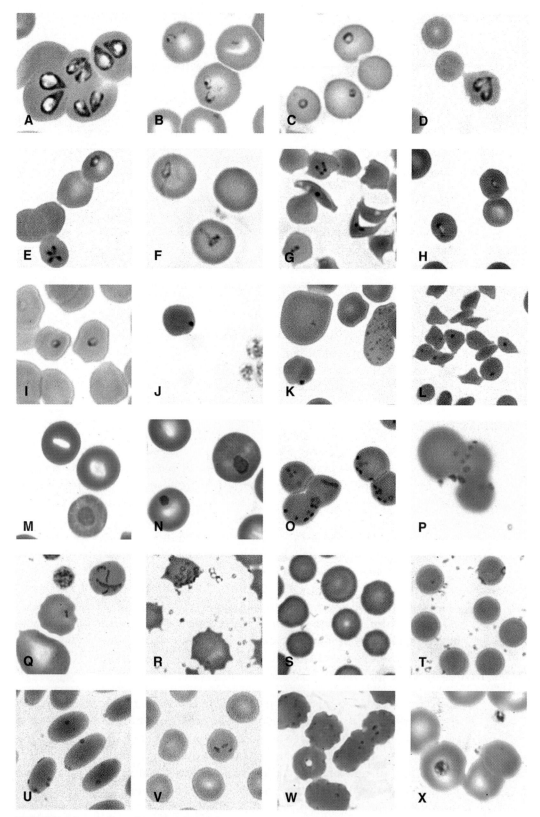

FIGURE 14. *See legend on opposite page.*

FIGURE 14.   Infectious agents of erythrocytes.   A. Two pear-shaped *Babesia canis* organisms in each of four erythrocytes in blood from a puppy with hemolytic anemia. Infected erythrocytes often were seen adhered to one another. Wright-Giemsa stain.   **B.**   Two small *Babesia gibsoni* organisms in one erythrocyte (top) and a single organism in another erythrocyte (bottom right) in blood from a dog. Photograph of a stained blood film from a 1999 ASVCP slide review case submitted by A.R. Irizarry-Rovira, J. Stephens, D.B. DeNicola, J. Christian, and P. Conrad. Wright Stain.   **C.**   Single *Babesia felis* organisms in three erythrocytes in blood from a domestic cat from South Africa. Wright stain.   **D.**   Two *Babesia bigemina* organisms in an erythrocyte from a cow. Wright-Giemsa stain.   **E.**   A single *Babesia equi* organism in one erythrocyte (top) and a Maltese cross of four organisms in another erythrocyte (bottom) in blood from a horse. Wright-Giemsa stain.   **F.** Single *Theileria buffeli*–like organisms in two erythrocytes in blood from a pregnant Simmental cow. Photograph of a stained blood film from a 1997 ASVCP slide review case submitted by S.L. Stockham, D.A. Schmidt, M.A. Scott, J.W. Tyler, G.C. Johnson, P.A. Conrad, and P. Cuddihee. Wright-Giemsa Stain.   **G.**   *Theileria cervi* organisms in erythrocytes in blood from a white-tailed deer. Several drepanocytes (sickle erythrocytes) are present. Wright-Giemsa stain.   **H.**   Two erythrocytes, each containing a *Cytauxzoon felis* organism, are present in blood from a cat. Wright-Giemsa stain.   **I.**   Two erythrocytes, each containing a *Cytauxzoon felis* organism, are present in blood from a cat. Wright-Giemsa stain.   **J.**   *Anaplasma marginale* organism located within an erythrocyte in blood from a Holstein cow. Three platelets are also visible (right). Wright-Giemsa stain.   **K.**   An erythrocyte containing an *Anaplasma marginale* organism (bottom left), a macrocytic erythrocyte (top left), and an abnormally shaped erythrocyte with basophilic stippling (right) in blood from a Holstein cow. Wright-Giemsa stain.   **L.**   *Anaplasma ovis* organisms in blood from a 6-month-old goat with esophageal perforation and intestinal *Trichostrongylus* infestation. Wright-Giemsa stain.   **M.**   Round blue-gray distemper inclusion in a polychromatophilic erythrocyte (bottom) in blood from a dog. Wright-Giemsa stain.   **N.**   Two round reddish distemper inclusions in erythrocytes in blood from the same dog as shown in Figure 14M. The inclusion at top right is in a large polychromatophilic erythrocyte. Diff-Quik stain.   **O.** *Haemobartonella felis* organisms located on the outside of erythrocytes in blood from a cat. A chain of organisms is out of focus in the center erythrocyte. Wright-Giemsa stain.   **P.**   *Haemobartonella felis* organisms located on the surface of erythrocytes in blood from a cat. Some organisms appear as rings, including the unattached one at the bottom right. Wright-Giemsa stain.   **Q.**   *Haemobartonella canis* organisms located on the outside of erythrocytes in blood from a dog. One erythrocyte (center) has a rod-shaped structure on its surface that is probably composed of two closely associated organisms, while another erythrocyte (top right) has many organisms forming filamentous chains in deep grooves on its surface. A platelet and large polychromatophilic erythrocyte are also present. Wright-Giemsa stain.   **R.**   *Eperythrozoon suis* organisms on the surface of erythrocytes and between erythrocytes in blood from a splenectomized pig. Erythrocytes appear as echinocytes, a normal finding in pig blood. A large polychromatophilic erythrocyte is located at the bottom. Photograph of a stained blood film from a 1980 ASVCP slide review case submitted by G. Searcy. Wright stain.   **S.**   *Eperythrozoon wenyoni* organisms between erythrocytes in blood from a Charolais bull. Photograph of a stained blood film from a 1993 ASVCP slide review case submitted by E.G. Welles, J.W. Tyler, and D.F. Wolfe. Wright stain.   **T.**   *Eperythrozoon ovis* organisms between erythrocytes in blood from a sheep. Wright-Giemsa stain.   **U.**   *Eperythrozoon* organisms on the surface of erythrocytes and between erythrocytes in blood from a llama. Wright-Giemsa stain.   **V.** *Bartonella henselae* organisms in an erythrocyte (center right) from a confirmed bacteremic cat. In addition to blood culture, organisms were identified in fixed erythrocytes using a fluorescent-labeled antibody. Photograph was provided by Dr. Rose E. Raskin. Wright-Giemsa stain.   **W.**   Drying artifact and precipitated stain present in this blood film from a cat may be confused with blood parasites. Wright-Giemsa stain.   **X.**   A platelet overlaying an erythrocyte (bottom left) may be confused with a blood parasite in this blood film from a dog. Wright-Giemsa stain.

the erythrocytes and occur free in plasma, while *Haemobartonella* organisms are firmly attached to erythrocytes. These criteria seem inadequate for the establishment of two genera, especially since the frequency of ring forms and the number of free organisms can be influenced to some degree simply by the manner in which a blood film is prepared. Like *Haemobartonella*, organisms in this genus are mycoplasmas.[121,127]

Bartonella Species

Members of the *Bartonella* species are small, gram-negative bacteria. Although the names sound similar, *Bartonella* and *Haemobartonella* organisms are not closely related organisms. *Bartonella (Rochalimaea) henselae* appears to be the primary cause of cat scratch disease in people. This organism causes mild illness and anemia in cats during the initial infection, but subsequently, cats become carriers without evidence of disease.[128] This small rod-shaped bacterium occurs within erythrocytes[129] but is rarely appreciated in blood films of bacteremic cats (Fig. 14V), even though the organism can be cultured from the blood of many healthy cats.[128]

Artifacts Resembling Infectious Agents

Erythrocyte parasites (especially *Haemobartonella* and *Eperythrozoon* species) must be differentiated from precipitated stain, refractile drying or fixation artifacts (Figs. 4A, 14W), poorly staining Howell-Jolly bodies, and basophilic stippling (Figs. 13J–13O). Platelets overlying erythrocytes (Fig. 14X) may also be confused with erythrocyte parasites, especially *Babesia* species.

CHAPTER 3

Leukocytes

■ NEUTROPHIL MORPHOLOGY

Mammalian leukocytes, or white blood cells, have been classified as either polymorphonuclear (PMN) or mononuclear leukocytes. The polymorphonuclear leukocytes have condensed, segmented nuclei. They are commonly referred to as granulocytes because they contain large numbers of cytoplasmic granules. The granules in these cells are lysosomes containing hydrolytic enzymes, antibacterial agents, and other compounds. Primary granules are synthesized in the cytoplasm of late myeloblasts or early promyelocytes. They appear reddish purple when stained with routine blood stains such as Wright-Giemsa. Secondary (specific) granules appear at the myelocyte stage of development in the bone marrow. Three types of granulocytes (neutrophils, eosinophils, and basophils) are identified by the staining characteristics of their secondary granules.

Normal Neutrophil Morphology

Normal neutrophil morphology is similar in common domestic mammalian species. The chromatin of the nucleus is condensed (dark-staining clumped areas separated by lighter-staining areas) and segmented (lobulated) and stains blue to purple (Fig. 15A). Nuclear lobes may be joined by fine filaments, but generally there is simply a narrowing of the nucleus between lobes without true filament formation. When an area of the nucleus has a diameter less than two-thirds the diameter of any other area of the nucleus, the neutrophil is classified as mature, even if only two lobes are present (Fig. 15B). The nuclear outline is more scalloped (jagged) in horses than in other species (Fig. 15C). The background cytoplasm generally appears colorless but may appear pale pink or faintly basophilic (Fig. 15D). Neutrophil granules either do not stain, or appear as light pink rods with routine blood stains. A Barr body (sex chromatin lobe or drumstick) is present in a low percentage of neutrophils from females (Figs. 15E , 15F).[11] This round, basophilic body is attached to the nucleus by a thin chromatin strand. It represents the pyknotic inactivated remains of one of the two X chromosomes.

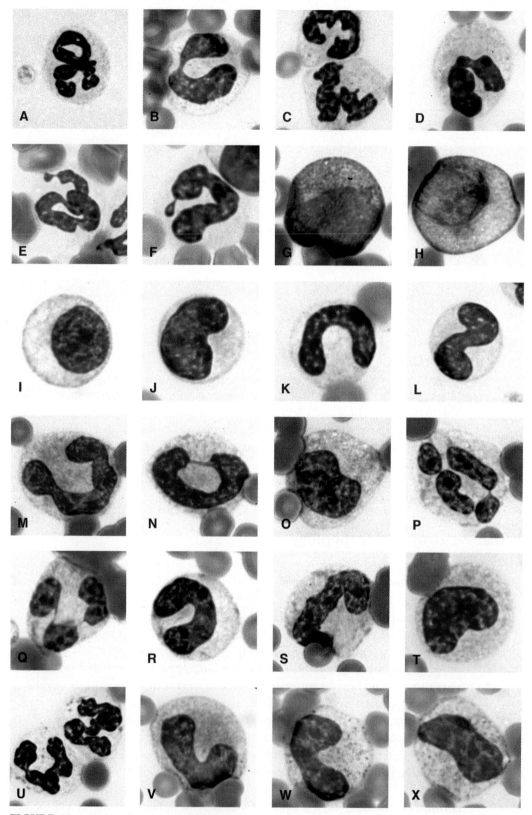

FIGURE 15. *See legend on opposite page.*

Morphology of Left Shifts

Mature segmented neutrophils and, sometimes, low numbers of band neutrophils are released from bone marrow into blood in normal animals. When increased numbers of nonsegmented neutrophilic cells are present in blood, their presence is referred to as a left shift.

Band neutrophils are commonly seen in blood, with metamyelocytes and myelocytes present less often and promyelocytes and myeloblasts rarely encountered. Morphologic changes that occur as cells of the granulocytic series undergo maturation from myeloblasts to mature granulocytes in bone marrow include slight diminution in size, decrease in nucleus:cytoplasm (N:C) ratio, progressive nuclear condensation, changes in nuclear shape, and the appearance of cytoplasmic granules. The background (i.e., nongranular) cytoplasm color changes from gray-blue in myeloblasts to nearly colorless in mature neutrophils, in the absence of toxicity. However, cytoplasmic toxicity is often present in animals with pronounced left shifts in blood.

FIGURE 15. Neutrophils and their precursor cells.   A. Neutrophil in blood from a dog. Wright-Giemsa stain.   **B.** Bilobed neutrophil in blood from a cow. Wright-Giemsa stain.   **C.** Two neutrophils in blood from a horse. Wright-Giemsa stain.   **D.** Neutrophil with slightly pink cytoplasm in blood from a cow. Wright-Giemsa stain.   **E.** Neutrophil in blood from a female dog exhibiting a sex chromatin lobe or Barr body. Wright-Giemsa stain.   **F.** Neutrophil in blood from a female cat exhibiting a sex chromatin lobe or Barr body. Wright-Giemsa stain.   **G.** Promyelocyte with purple cytoplasmic granules in blood from a dog with acute myelomonocytic leukemia (AML-M4). Wright-Giemsa stain.   **H.** Promyelocyte with faintly staining purple cytoplasmic granules in blood from a cat with a marked left shift (leukemoid reaction) secondary to a bacterial infection that resulted in the formation of multiple draining abscesses. Wright-Giemsa stain.   **I.** Neutrophilic myelocyte in blood from a dog with chronic myeloid leukemia. Wright-Giemsa stain.   **J.** Neutrophilic metamyelocyte in blood from a dog with chronic myeloid leukemia. Wright-Giemsa stain.   **K.** Band neutrophil in blood from a dog with immune-mediated hemolytic anemia. Wright-Giemsa stain.   **L.** S-shaped band neutrophil in blood from a dog with immune-mediated hemolytic anemia. Wright-Giemsa stain.   **M.** Neutrophil with foamy basophilia (toxicity) of the cytoplasm in blood from a cat with septic peritonitis. Wright-Giemsa stain.   **N.** Neutrophil with doughnut-shaped nucleus and foamy basophilia (toxicity) of the cytoplasm in blood from a cat with septic peritonitis. Wright-Giemsa stain.   **O.** Toxic metamyelocyte with foamy basophilia of the cytoplasm in blood from a cat with septic peritonitis. Wright-Giemsa stain.   **P.** Toxic neutrophil with foamy basophilia and Doehle bodies (angular blue inclusions) in the cytoplasm in blood from a cat with septic peritonitis. Wright-Giemsa stain.   **Q.** Toxic neutrophil with foamy basophilia and Doehle bodies in the cytoplasm in blood from a cat with a marked left shift (leukemoid reaction) secondary to a bacterial infection that resulted in the formation of multiple draining abscesses. Wright-Giemsa stain.   **R.** Band neutrophil with lightly basophilic cytoplasm containing Doehle bodies in blood from a horse. Wright-Giemsa stain.   **S.** Toxic band neutrophil with foamy basophilia and Doehle bodies in the cytoplasm in blood from a cat with septic peritonitis. Wright-Giemsa stain.   **T.** Toxic neutrophilic metamyelocyte with foamy basophilia and faintly staining Doehle bodies in the cytoplasm in blood from a cat with a marked left shift (leukemoid reaction) secondary to a bacterial infection that resulted in the formation of multiple draining abscesses. Wright-Giemsa stain.   **U.** Doehle bodies in the cytoplasm of two neutrophils in blood from a cat, without other cytoplasmic evidence of toxicity. Wright-Giemsa stain.   **V.** Band neutrophil with toxic granulation in blood from a horse with acute salmonellosis. Wright-Giemsa stain.   **W.** Band neutrophil with toxic granulation in blood from a Holstein cow with a bacterial infection. Wright-Giemsa stain.   **X.** Neutrophilic metamyelocyte with toxic granulation in blood from a Holstein cow with a bacterial infection. Wright-Giemsa stain.

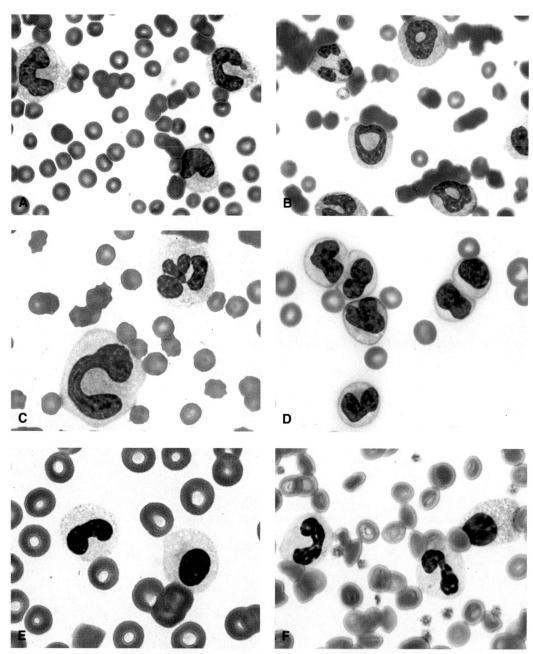

FIGURE 16.   Neutrophils and their precursor cells.   A. Two toxic band neutrophils and a toxic neutrophilic metamyelocyte (bottom) with foamy basophilic cytoplasm in blood from a cat. The band on the right appears to have a fragmented nuclear membrane forming a nuclear vesicle. Wright-Giemsa stain. **B.** Toxic left shift in the blood of a cat with a leukemoid reaction secondary to a bacterial infection that resulted in the formation of multiple draining abscesses. Two neutrophilic cells have doughnut-shaped nuclei. Wright-Giemsa stain.   **C.** Giant neutrophil (bottom) in the blood of a cat with a leukemoid

(Continued)

Myeloblasts. The morphology of myeloblasts is described in the section on blast cells in blood (Fig. 24). Their presence indicates the likelihood of a myeloproliferative disorder.

Promyelocytes. Promyelocytes or progranulocytes have round to oval nuclei with lacy to coarse chromatin. Although nucleoli or nucleolar rings may be seen in some promyelocytes, most exhibit no evidence of nucleolar structures. Their most identifiable characteristic is the presence of many magenta-staining primary granules within light-blue cytoplasm (Figs. 15G, 15H).

Myelocytes. Myelocytes have round nuclei (Fig. 15I), but they are generally smaller with more nuclear condensation and lighter-blue cytoplasm than promyelocytes. Primary, magenta-staining granules characteristic of promyelocytes are no longer visible in myelocytes. Secondary granules that characterize neutrophils are present, but difficult to visualize because of their neutral-staining characteristics.

Metamyelocytes. Nuclei with slight indentations are still classified as myelocytes, but once the nuclear indentation extends more than 25% into the nucleus, the cell is called a metamyelocyte (Fig. 15J). Nuclear condensation becomes readily apparent at this stage of maturation.

Band Cells. Cells with thinner, rod-shaped nuclei with parallel sides are called bands (Fig. 15K). No area of the nucleus has a diameter less than two thirds the diameter of any other area of the nucleus. Band cell nuclei twist to conform to the space within the cytoplasm, and U-shaped or S-shaped nuclei (Fig. 15L) are common. Chromatin condensation is prominent, and the cytoplasm appearance is essentially the same as that seen in mature neutrophils. Once nuclear segments form, the cell is called a mature neutrophil, even if only two lobes are present (Fig. 15B).

Disorders with Left Shifts

Left shifts are usually associated with inflammatory conditions. These inflammatory conditions are often infectious but may be noninfectious, such as in immune-mediated disorders and infiltrative marrow disease.[1,99] Left shifts are also present in animals with chronic myeloid leukemia and Pelger-Huet anomaly.

Inflammation. The presence of a significant left shift in animals with an inflammatory disorder indicates that the stimulus for release of neutrophils from bone marrow is greater than can be accommodated by release from

---

reaction secondary to a bacterial infection that resulted in the formation of multiple draining abscesses. Wright-Giemsa stain.   **D.** Left shift in the blood of a dog with chronic myeloid leukemia. Band neutrophils, neutrophilic metamyelocytes, and a neutrophilic myelocyte are present. Wright-Giemsa stain. **E.** Band neutrophil (left) and neutrophilic myelocyte (right) in the blood of a dog with Pelger-Huet anomaly. Wright-Giemsa stain.   **F.** Band neutrophil (left), bilobed neutrophil (center), and eosinophilic myelocyte (right) in the blood of a cat with Pelger-Huet anomaly. Wright-Giemsa stain.

mature neutrophil stores alone. The magnitude of a left shift in response to inflammation can vary from slightly increased numbers of bands to severe left shifts with metamyelocytes, myelocytes, and, rarely, even promyelocytes present in blood. The total neutrophil count may be low, normal, or high, depending on the number of these cells released from the bone marrow versus the number utilized in the inflammatory process. Toxic cytoplasm is often present in animals with left shifts in response to inflammatory disorders (Fig. 16A). Other abnormalities that may be present include donut-shaped nuclei and giant neutrophils (Figs. 16B, 16C).

A marked leukocytosis (total leukocyte count of 50,000 to 100,000/μL) with a marked left shift back to at least myelocytes associated with an inflammatory condition is called a leukemoid reaction, because it resembles the blood pattern seen in chronic myeloid leukemia. Left shifts associated with leukemoid reactions are usually orderly, with mature segmented neutrophils being the most numerous neutrophilic cells present, bands being the next most numerous, metamyelocytes being less numerous, and myelocytes being present in low numbers. When a leukemoid response is present, a localized purulent inflammatory condition such as pyometra is suspected.

Chronic Myeloid Leukemia. Chronic myeloid leukemia (CML) presents with a high total leukocyte count (usually greater than 50,000/μL) with marked neutrophilic left shift in blood (Fig. 16D).[130–132] In domestic animals, CML is primarily seen in dogs. Increased numbers of monocytes, eosinophils, and/or basophils may also be present. Myeloblasts are either absent or present in low numbers in blood. CML is suspected when no inflammatory disorder can be found to explain the extreme left shift. The left shift present in CML is usually less orderly than those seen in leukemoid reactions. The presence of dysplastic abnormalities in other blood cell types also supports a diagnosis of CML. On the other hand, the presence of moderate to marked cytoplasmic toxicity, increased inflammatory plasma proteins, and physical evidence of inflammation suggest a leukemoid reaction is present, rather than CML.

Pelger-Huet Anomaly. The term hyposegmentation refers to a left shift with condensed nuclear chromatin without nuclear constrictions (Figs. 16E, 16F). It occurs as an inherited trait in the Pelger-Huet anomaly in dogs and cats.[133,134] Eosinophils and basophils may also be affected. No clinical signs are associated with animals that are heterozygous for this disorder. A pseudo-Pelger-Huet anomaly may occur transiently with chronic infections and rarely following the administration of certain drugs or in animals with myeloproliferative disorders.[103]

Toxic Cytoplasm

When the cytoplasm of a neutrophilic cell has increased basophilia, has foamy vacuolation, and/or contains Doehle bodies, it is said to be toxic. These morphologic abnormalities develop in neutrophilic cells within the bone marrow prior to their release into the circulation.[135,136]

Foamy Basophilia.   Foamy basophilia often occurs with severe bacterial infections but can occur with other causes of toxemia (Figs. 15M–15T). When viewed by electron microscopy, foamy vacuolation appears as irregular, electron-lucent areas that are not membrane bound. Cytoplasmic basophilia results from the persistence of large amounts of rough endoplasmic reticulum and polyribosomes.[135]

Doehle Bodies.   Doehle bodies are bluish, angular cytoplasmic inclusions of neutrophils and their precursors (Figs. 15P–15U). They are composed of retained aggregates of rough endoplasmic reticulum.[52] By themselves, these inclusions represent mild evidence of toxicity and are sometimes seen in neutrophils of cats that do not exhibit signs of illness (Fig. 15U). Doehle bodies must be differentiated from iron-positive granules, distemper inclusions in dogs, and granules present in neutrophils from cats with inherited Chediak-Higashi syndrome.

Toxic Granulation.   Toxic granulation refers to the presence of magenta-staining cytoplasmic granules (Figs. 15V–15X, 17A).[52] These granules consist of primary granules that have retained the staining intensity normally observed in promyelocytes in the bone marrow. The presence of toxic granulation and cytoplasmic basophilia suggests severe toxemia. Toxic granulation may be seen in horses, cattle, and sheep but is rarely seen in dogs and cats. Toxic granulation should not be confused with the pink staining of secondary granules which is not a sign of toxicity. Toxic granulation must be differentiated from the granules present in some Birman cats, granules in animals with certain lysosomal storage disorders, and miscellaneous granules and inclusions to be discussed subsequently.

Granules and Inclusions

Normal Foals.   Purple granules are often seen in neutrophils from foals without other evidence of cytoplasmic toxicity (Fig. 17B),[109] the clinical significance of which is unclear. It is assumed that, like toxic granulation, these granules are primary granules that have retained the staining intensity normally observed in promyelocytes in the bone marrow.

Lipemia in a Horse.   Purple granules were present in neutrophils from a Paso Fino mare with hyperlipidemia and hepatic lipidosis (Fig. 17C).[137] Like in the normal foals described above, no other cytoplasmic evidence of toxicity was present. Consequently, caution must be exercised in using the term "toxic granulation" in horses.

Lysosomal Storage Diseases.   The lysosomal system is the principal site of intracellular degradation. Lysosomes are membrane-bound organelles that contain more than 40 acid hydrolases capable of degrading most biologically important macromolecules. An inherited deficiency in one of these enzymes can result in the accumulation of undegraded substances (e.g., glycosaminoglycans, complex oligosaccharides, cerebrosides, etc.) within lysosomes—hence the name

(text continued on page 54)

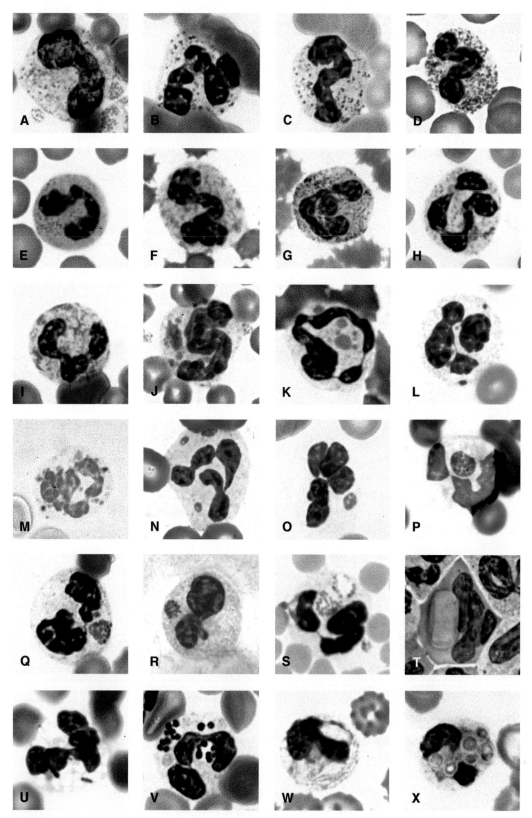

FIGURE 17. *See legend on opposite page.*

FIGURE 17.   Granules, inclusions, and infectious agents of neutrophils.   A. Band neutrophil with basophilic cytoplasm and toxic granulation in blood from a Holstein cow with a bacterial infection. Wright-Giemsa stain.   **B.** Neutrophil with basophilic cytoplasmic granules in the blood of a normal foal. Wright-Giemsa stain.   **C.** Neutrophil with cytoplasmic granules in the blood of a hyperlipemic 7-year-old Paso Fino mare with hepatic lipidosis. Photograph of a stained blood film from a 1983 ASVCP slide review case submitted by J.R. Duncan and E.A. Mahaffey. Wright stain.   **D.** Neutrophil with cytoplasmic granules in the blood of a 7-month-old miniature schnauzer dog with mucopolysaccharidosis type VI. Photograph of a stained blood film from a 1995 ASVCP slide review case submitted by P.R. Avery, D.E. Brown, M.A. Thrall, and D.A. Wenger. Wright-Giemsa stain.   **E.** Neutrophil with cytoplasmic granules in the blood of a 1-year-old domestic shorthair cat with inherited mucopolysaccharidosis type VI. Photograph of a stained blood film from a 1995 ASVCP slide review case submitted by D.A. Andrews, D.B. DeNicola, S. Jakovljevic, J. Turek, and U. Giger. Wright stain.   **F.** Neutrophil with cytoplasmic granules in the blood of an 8-month-old domestic shorthair cat with inherited mucopolysaccharidosis type VII. Photograph of a stained blood film from a 1996 ASVCP slide review case submitted by M.A. Thrall, L. Vap, S. Gardner, and D. Wenger. Wright stain.   **G.** Neutrophil with cytoplasmic granules in the blood of a 3-month-old German shepherd dog with inherited mucopolysaccharidosis type VII. Photograph of a stained blood film from a 1997 ASVCP slide review case submitted by D.I. Bounous, D.C. Silverstein, K.S. Latimer, and K.P. Carmichael. Wright stain.   **H.** Neutrophil with cytoplasmic granules in the blood of a korat cat with inherited GM$_2$-gangliosidosis. Wright-Giemsa stain.   **I.** Neutrophil with reddish cytoplasmic granulation in blood from a Siamese cat without clinical signs attributable to a lysosomal storage disease. Wright-Giemsa stain.   **J.** Neutrophil with large cytoplasmic granules in blood from a 15-month-old Hereford female with Chediak-Higashi syndrome. Photograph of a stained blood film from a 1987 ASVCP slide review case submitted by M. Menard and K.J. Wardrop. Wright stain.   **K.** Neutrophil with large cytoplasmic granules in blood from a Persian cat with Chediak-Higashi syndrome. Photograph taken from a stained slide provided by J. Kramer. Wright stain.   **L.** Neutrophil with siderotic cytoplasmic inclusions in blood from a horse with equine infectious anemia. Wright-Giemsa stain.   **M.** Neutrophil with siderotic cytoplasmic inclusions in blood from a horse with equine infectious anemia (same blood sample as shown in Figure 17L). Blue-staining inclusions indicate the presence of iron. Prussian blue stain.   **N.** Three reddish distemper inclusions in the cytoplasm of a neutrophil in blood from a dog with canine distemper. Diff-Quik stain.   **O.** *Ehrlichia ewingii* morula in the cytoplasm of a neutrophil in blood from a dog, determined by a 16S rRNA sequence following polymerase chain reaction amplification. Wright-Giemsa stain.   **P.** *Ehrlichia* morula in the cytoplasm of a neutrophil in blood from a dog of unknown species. Serology was positive for *E. canis* and negative for *E. equi*. Specific assays for *E. ewingii*, which might have cross-reacting antibodies with *E. canis*, were not done. Wright-Giemsa stain.   **Q.** *Ehrlichia equi* morula in the cytoplasm of a neutrophil in blood from a horse. Wright-Giemsa stain.   **R.** *Ehrlichia equi* morula in the cytoplasm of a neutrophil in blood from a horse stained using the new methylene blue wet mount procedure.   **S.** Two *Ehrlichia phagocytophila* morulae in the cytoplasm of a neutrophil in blood from a goat. Wright-Giemsa stain.   **T.** *Hepatozoon americanum* gamont in the cytoplasm of a neutrophil in blood from a dog. Photograph taken from a slide provided by K.A. Gossett. Wright stain.   **U.** Bacterial rods phagocytized by a neutrophil in a buffy coat smear prepared from blood from a cat with a leukopenia and septicemia. Wright-Giemsa stain.   **V.** Bacterial cocci phagocytized by a neutrophil in blood from a dog with urolithiasis, pyelonephritis, and septicemia. *Staphylococcus intermedius* was cultured from blood and urine. Wright-Giemsa stain.   **W.** *Mycobacterium* organisms in the cytoplasm of a neutrophil in blood from a dog. These organisms do not stain, and they appear as linear clear areas. Photograph of a stained blood film from a 1988 ASVCP slide review case submitted by H. Tvedten. Wright stain.   **X.** *Histoplasma capsulatum* organisms in the cytoplasm of a neutrophil from an adult dog. Photograph of a stained blood film from a 1987 ASVCP slide review case submitted by J.H. Meinkoth, R.L. Cowell, K.D. Clinkenbeard, and R.D. Tyler. Wright stain.

lysosomal storage disease.[138] Blue to magenta–staining granulation occurs in the cytoplasm of neutrophils from animals with certain lysosomal storage disorders including mucopolysaccharidosis type VI (Figs. 17D, 17E),[139–141] mucopolysaccharidosis type VII (Figs. 17F, 17G),[142–144] and GM$_2$-gangliosidosis (Fig. 17H).[145,146]

Birman Cats.   Small reddish granules have been reported as an inherited anomaly in Birman cats without evidence of illness.[147] These granules were of normal size when examined by transmission electron microscopy. They did not stain with alcian blue or toluidine blue, indicating that the animals did not have an inherited mucopolysaccharidosis.

Reddish Granulation in Cats.   We have observed persistent reddish granulation in neutrophils of four cats (Fig. 17I) that appeared similar to that reported in Birman cats. Affected animals included a 10-year-old male Siamese, a 6-year-old male Siamese, a 13-year-old female Siamese, and a 2-year-old male Himalayan. Granules were negative when stained with toluidine blue. No clinical signs could be associated with the presence of the granules, which were present even when animals were healthy.

Chediak-Higashi Syndrome.   The Chediak-Higashi syndrome is an inherited disorder characterized by partial oculocutaneous albinism, increased susceptibility to infections, hemorrhagic tendencies, and the presence of enlarged membrane-bound granules in many cell types including blood leukocytes. Neutrophils from affected cattle[148–150] and Persian cats[134] contain large pink to purple granules (Figs. 17J, 17K). The giant granules may arise from unregulated fusion of primary lysosomes during cell development.

Siderotic Inclusions.   Iron-positive inclusions (hemosiderin) may be seen in neutrophils and monocytes from animals with hemolytic anemia. Prior to the development of definitive serologic tests, the presence of these inclusions in equine leukocytes (sideroleukocytes) was used to support a diagnosis of equine infectious anemia (Figs. 17L, 17M).[151,152] These inclusions can be differentiated from Doehle bodies using the Prussian blue staining procedure, because Doehle bodies do not stain positively for iron.

Infectious Agents

Distemper Inclusions.   These viral inclusions are formed in bone marrow precursor cells and may be present in blood cells during the acute viremic stage of the disease.[118,119,153] These viral inclusions can be difficult to visualize in the cytoplasm of neutrophils in Wright- or Giemsa-stained blood films but can easily be seen as homogeneous round, oval, or irregularly shaped 1- to 4-μm red inclusions when stained with Diff-Quik (Fig. 17N).[21]

Ehrlichia Species.   Morulae of *Ehrlichia* species appear as tightly packed basophilic clusters of organisms within the cytoplasm (Figs. 17O–17S). Granulocytic *Ehrlichia* species recognized to infect animals include *E. ewingii*, and closely related members of the *Ehrlichia phagocytophila* genogroup, including *E. equi, E. phagocytophila*, and a human granulocytic ehrlichia (HGE).[154,155] Morulae are regularly found in neutrophils during the acute stage of infection. In addition to blood neutrophils, morulae may also be found in a low percentage of neutrophils within the joint fluid of *E. ewingii*–infected dogs with polyarthritis.[156] E. equi and HGE infections cause similar clinical syndromes in horses,[157–160] and both agents can infect other species including dogs.[161–164] *E. phagocytophila* is the etiologic agent of ehrlichiosis in cattle and sheep in Europe.[165] A granulocytic ehrlichial organism in the *Ehrlichia phagocytophila* genogroup has also been reported in a llama.[166]

Hepatozoon *Species*.   Hepatozoonosis is a severe protozoal disease in dogs in the United States, but *Hepatozoon* infections typically cause mild or inapparent disease in dogs in other areas of the world.[167] Based on clinical findings, histopathologic findings, gamont size and ultrastructure, serology results, and tick infectivity, the species present in the United States has been classified as *Hepatozoon americanum*, with the classification of *Hepatozoon canis* used for organisms present outside the United States.[168] Gamonts of the organism *H. americanum* may rarely be seen in the cytoplasm of circulating neutrophils (Fig. 17T) and monocytes. They appear as large oblong structures. The nucleus of a gamont usually stains poorly with routine blood stains.[169] *Hepatozoon* organisms of undetermined species have been recognized in domestic cats and various wild carnivores throughout the world.[170]

Miscellaneous Bacteria, Fungi, and Protozoa.   Although a bacteremia is common, microorganisms are seldom numerous enough to be found in stained blood films. Because blood stains are easily contaminated with bacteria (especially when they are also used to stain exfoliative cytology), it is important that the bacteria be found phagocytized within cells before a diagnosis of a bacteremia is made (Figs. 17U, 17V). *Mycobacterium* organisms appear as unstained rods within the cytoplasm (Fig. 17W).[171,172] In addition to mononuclear phagocytes, neutrophils may rarely contain phagocytized organisms in animals with systemic histoplasmosis (Fig. 17X)[173,174] and dogs with leishmaniasis.[175,176]

Hypersegmentation

Hypersegmentation (right shift) refers to the presence of five or more distinct nuclear lobes within neutrophils (Figs. 18A, 18B). It occurs as a normal aging process and may reflect prolonged transit time in blood as can occur with resolving chronic inflammation, glucocorticoid administration,[177] or hyperadrenocorticism. It may develop *in vitro* when blood film preparation is delayed for a number of hours. Hypersegmentation may be present in myeloproliferative disorders.[58,178] Idiopathic hypersegmentation has been reported in a horse without evidence of clinical disease.[179] It has also been described in dogs with an inherited defect in cobalamin absorption[180] and in a cat with folate deficiency.[181]

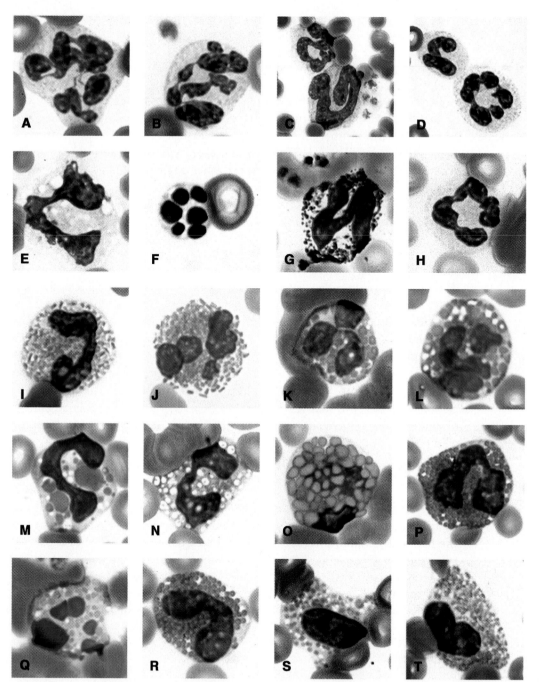

FIGURE 18. Morphologic abnormalities of neutrophils and species differences in eosinophil morphology. **A.** Hypersegmented neutrophil in blood from a dog with systemic mastocytosis treated with vincristine and prednisone. Wright-Giemsa stain. **B.** Hypersegmented neutrophil in blood from a dog with AML-M4. Wright-Giemsa stain. **C.** Giant neutrophil in blood from a cat with septic peritonitis. Wright-Giemsa stain. **D.** Giant hypersegmented neutrophil in blood from a dog with lymphoma. Wright-Giemsa stain. **E.** Toxic neutrophil exhibiting karyolysis (nuclear lysis) in blood from an FIV-positive leukopenic cat. Wright-Giemsa stain. **F.** Pyknosis and karyorrhexis in a neutrophil in blood from a dog with acute lymphoblastic leukemia (ALL). Wright-Giemsa stain. **G.** Stain precipitation associated with a neutrophil in blood from a dog. Wright-Giemsa stain. **H.** Normal-appearing neutrophil in blood from a dog three oil immersion fields away from the neutrophil shown

(Continued)

Miscellaneous Morphologic Abnormalities

Giant Neutrophils. Large neutrophils may occur in animals (especially cats) with inflammatory diseases and/or dysgranulopoiesis.[11] They may exhibit normal nuclear morphology (Fig. 18C) or appear hypersegmented (Fig. 18D). Dysgranulopoiesis is seen in acute myeloid leukemias, myelodysplastic syndromes, feline leukemia virus (FeLV) infections, and feline immunodeficiency virus (FIV) infections. It may also occur transiently in animals responding to granulocytic hypoplasia, such as panleukopenia in cats.

Karyolysis. The dissolution of the nucleus resulting in nuclear swelling and loss of affinity for basic dyes is referred to as karyolysis (Fig. 18E). It is frequently observed in neutrophils present in septic exudates and may be observed in the blood of animals with infectious processes.

Pyknosis and Karyorrhexis. Neutrophils that undergo programmed cell death (apoptosis) exhibit pyknosis and karyorrhexis. Pyknosis involves shrinkage or condensation of a cell with increased nuclear compactness or density; karyorrhexis refers to the subsequent fragmentation (Fig. 18F). Pyknosis and karyorrhexis are often observed in nonseptic exudates and may be seen in blood neutrophils that have had prolonged time in the circulation.

Cytoplasmic Vacuoles. Foamy vacuolation occurs in toxic neutrophils, but clear, discrete vacuoles, in the absence of cytoplasmic basophilia, usually represent an *in vitro* artifact. In addition to discrete vacuolation, uneven distribution of granules, irregular cell membranes, and pyknosis may occur in neutrophils in blood samples that have been collected in EDTA and kept at room temperature for several hours.[182] These artifacts are avoided by preparing blood films quickly after blood collection.

Stain Precipitation. To an inexperienced observer, neutrophils with precipitated stain may be confused with basophils (Figs. 18G, 18H). When this artifact is unevenly distributed, other areas of the blood film that stain normally can be found.

---

in Figure 18G. Wright-Giemsa stain.   **I.** Eosinophil with rod-shaped granules in blood from a cat. Wright-Giemsa stain.   **J.** Eosinophil with rod-shaped granules in blood from a cat. Wright-Giemsa stain.   **K.** Eosinophil with round granules and a few small cytoplasmic vacuoles in blood from a dog. Wright-Giemsa stain.   **L.** Eosinophil with round granules and a several cytoplasmic vacuoles in blood from a dog. Wright-Giemsa stain.   **M.** Eosinophil with two exceptionally large granules in blood from a dog. Wright-Giemsa stain.   **N.** Heavily vacuolated eosinophil in blood from a Greyhound dog. Wright-Giemsa stain.   **O.** Eosinophil in blood from a horse, exhibiting numerous large granules typical of this species. Wright-Giemsa stain.   **P.** Eosinophil in blood from a cow, exhibiting numerous small round granules typical of this species. Wright-Giemsa stain.   **Q.** Eosinophil in 2-day-old blood from a dog exhibiting pyknosis and karyorrhexis. Wright-Giemsa stain.   **R.** Band eosinophil with numerous small granules in blood from a cow. Wright-Giemsa stain.   **S.** Eosinophilic metamyelocyte in blood from a dog with Pelger-Huet anomaly. Wright-Giemsa stain.   **T.** Eosinophilic metamyelocyte in blood from a cat with Pelger-Huet anomaly. Wright-Giemsa stain.

■ EOSINOPHIL MORPHOLOGY

Eosinophils are so named because their granules have an affinity for eosin, the red dye in routine blood stains. The size, shape, and number of eosinophil granules vary considerably. In most animal species, eosinophils have round granules, but those from domestic cats have rod-shaped granules (Figs. 18I, 18J). Eosinophils from dogs often exhibit a few cytoplasmic vacuoles (Figs. 18K, 18L), and the granules can occasionally be exceptionally large (Fig. 18M). Eosinophils from greyhound dogs, and occasionally from individual animals in other breeds, appear highly vacuolated (Fig. 18N) and may be mistaken for vacuolated neutrophils by inexperienced observers. Horse eosinophils have especially large granules (Fig. 18O). Granules in ruminant and pig eosinophils are small (Fig. 18P). The cytoplasm between the granules is usually faintly blue in color. The nucleus of eosinophils is similar to that of neutrophils but tends to be less lobulated (often divided into only two lobes) and may be partially obscured by granules in some species, most notably the horse (Fig. 18O). Pyknosis and karyorrhexis may occur in eosinophils (Fig. 18Q) as discussed previously for neutrophils.

Band eosinophils are common in some animals (Fig. 18R). They are not usually separated from segmented eosinophils during differential counts because they are generally of little clinical significance and may be difficult to identify with certainty when granules obscure the nucleus. Eosinophil maturation stages may be differentiated when extreme eosinophilia is present, in an attempt to help separate hyperplastic from neoplastic disorders. A more pronounced left shift may be expected in an animal with eosinophilic leukemia than in an animal with an inflammatory eosinophilia. Eosinophilic leukemia is considered a variant of CML.[183] It is a rare disorder that occurs primarily in cats, where it is difficult to differentiate from the hypereosinophilic syndrome.[184–186] As in neutrophils, a pronounced left shift is present in eosinophils in the blood of animals with Pelger-Huet anomaly (Figs. 16F, 18S, 18T). Increased numbers of hyposegmented (pseudo-Pelger-Huet) band eosinophils have been reported in a family of Samoyed dogs with accompanying ocular and skeletal abnormalities.[187]

Ehrlichia organisms have rarely been seen in eosinophils from dogs and horses,[156,157] and *Histoplasma* organisms have been identified in blood eosinophils from a dog.[188]

■ BASOPHIL MORPHOLOGY

The cytoplasm of basophils is generally pale blue in color, and basophil nuclei are often less segmented than are neutrophil nuclei. Basophil granules are acidic and consequently have an affinity for the basic (blue) dyes in routine blood stains. The number, size, and staining characteristics of the granules vary considerably by species. Granules in dog basophils generally appear purple and are not numerous enough to fill the cytoplasm (Figs. 19A–19C). Degranulated

(text continued on page 60)

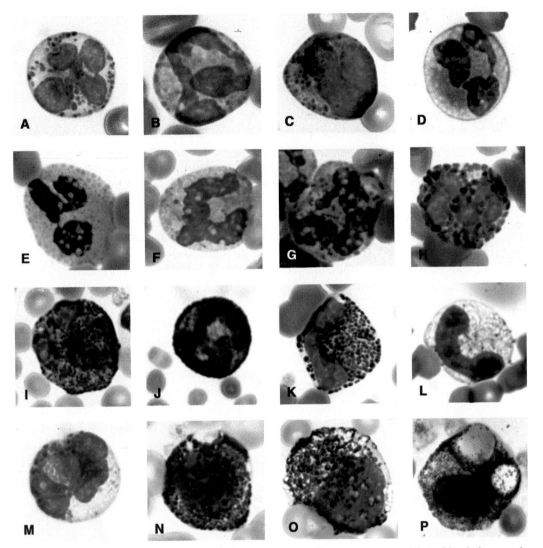

FIGURE 19. Morphology of basophils and mast cells. **A.** Basophil in blood from a dog. Wright-Giemsa stain. **B.** Basophil in blood from a dog. The nucleus is ribbonlike in shape and few granules are present. Wright-Giemsa stain. **C.** Band basophil in the blood of a dog with a basophilia. Wright-Giemsa stain. **D.** Degranulated basophil in blood from a dog with a basophilia. Wright-Giemsa stain. **E.** Basophil in blood from a cat with light-lavender granules filling the cytoplasm and giving the nucleus a moth-eaten appearance. Wright-Giemsa stain. **F.** Band basophil in blood from a cat with light-lavender granules filling the cytoplasm and giving the nucleus a moth-eaten appearance. A single purple-staining granule is also present. Wright-Giemsa stain. **G.** Basophil in blood from a cat with a mixture of light-lavender and purple granules filling the cytoplasm. Wright-Giemsa stain. **H.** Basophil with reddish purple granules filling the cytoplasm in blood from the same Siamese cat as described in Figure 17I. Wright-Giemsa stain. **I.** Basophil in blood from a cow. The granules are so numerous that they prevent evaluation of nuclear shape. Wright-Giemsa stain. **J.** Basophil in the blood of a goat. Few granules are visible, but the cytoplasm stains purple. Wright-Giemsa stain. **K.** Band basophil in the blood of a horse. Wright-Giemsa stain. **L.** Band basophil in blood from a horse. Most granules are not stained. Diff-Quik stain. **M.** Basophil with an *Ehrlichia* morula of unknown species in blood from a dog. The dog had a basophilia and organisms were found in several basophils. Wright-Giemsa stain. **N.** Mast cell in blood from a dog with a noncutaneous mast cell tumor. Wright-Giemsa stain. **O.** Large mast cell with cytoplasmic vacuoles in addition to granules in blood from a dog with a noncutaneous mast cell neoplasm. Wright-Giemsa stain. **P.** Large mast cell exhibiting erythrophagocytosis in blood from a cat with a noncutaneous mast cell neoplasm. Wright-Giemsa stain.

basophils may have purple-staining cytoplasm in the absence of granules (Fig. 19D).

The basophils of domestic cats are distinctive. Most of their granules are round or oval and stain light lavender (or mauve) in color (Figs. 19E, 19F). Some basophils have large purple granules in addition to the light lavender ones (Fig. 19G), as are seen in basophil precursors in the bone marrow. The granules typically fill the cytoplasm, giving the cat basophil nucleus a moth-eaten appearance. All of the granules stained dark purple in a cat with mucopolysaccharidosis type VI[141] and in two cats with reddish granulation of neutrophils of unknown etiology (Fig. 19H).

Granules are often so numerous in ruminant and pig basophils that the nuclear shape is obscured (Fig. 19I). In some instances, discrete granules are not seen, but the cytoplasm stains purple (Fig. 19J). Variable numbers of purple granules are present in horse basophils (Fig. 19K). Basophils can be difficult to recognize in Diff-Quik-stained blood films because granules do not stain as well with this stain (Fig. 19L). *Ehrlichia* morulae have been recognized in basophils from a dog (Fig. 19M).

Band basophils are not usually separated from segmented basophils during differential counts because they are generally of little clinical significance, and, except in dogs, they may be difficult to identify with certainty when granules obscure the nucleus. Basophilic cell stages may be differentiated when extreme basophilia is present, in an attempt to help separate hyperplastic from neoplastic disorders. A more pronounced left shift is expected in an animal with chronic basophilic leukemia (a variant of CML) than in an animal with an inflammatory basophilia.[189,190]

■ MAST CELLS

Mast cells are not normally found in blood. They develop in tissues from precursor cells produced in the bone marrow. Mast cells and basophils have similar biochemical characteristics and probably share a common progenitor cell in bone marrow, but they are clearly different cell types. Basophils have segmented nuclei and mast cells have round nuclei (Figs. 19N, 19O). Mast cells usually have more cytoplasmic granules than do basophils. In cats, both primary and secondary granules in basophils are morphologically different from mast cell granules. Mastocytemia occurs in association with noncutaneous and metastatic cutaneous mast cell tumors.[191,192] Rarely, mast cells have been seen to phagocytize erythrocytes (Fig. 19P).[193,194] Mast cells may also be present in the blood of animals with inflammatory diseases, necrosis, tissue injury, and severe regenerative anemia.[195–198]

■ MONOCYTE MORPHOLOGY

Mononuclear leukocytes in blood are classified as either lymphocytes or monocytes. These cells are not devoid of granules but rather have lower numbers of cytoplasmic granules than do granulocytes. Monocytes are usually larger than lymphocytes and have nuclei that are more variable in shape and N:C ratios of 1.0 or less.

The monocyte nucleus may be round, kidney-shaped, band-shaped, or convoluted (ameboid) with chromatin that is diffuse or mildly clumped (Figs. 20A–20I, 21A–21D). The cytoplasm is typically blue-gray and often contains variably sized vacuoles. Less often, dustlike pinkish or reddish purple granules may be visible in the cytoplasm (Figs. 20G, 20H).

Monocytes in dogs often have band-shaped nuclei (Fig. 20I); consequently, they may be confused with band neutrophils. The cytoplasmic staining of the mature neutrophils should be examined. If no toxicity is present, the cells with band-shaped nuclei and blue-gray cytoplasm are identified as monocytes. Other potentially helpful criteria include the following: the ends of the bandlike nucleus of the monocyte are often enlarged and knoblike and the nuclear chromatin of the monocyte is not clumped in the dark-light pattern to the degree commonly seen in band neutrophils. If marked toxicity is present in the cytoplasm of neutrophilic cells, differentiation becomes much more difficult.

Differentiation of monocytes with round nuclei from large lymphocytes can be difficult, especially in ruminants. The N:C ratio is typically greater than 1.0 for large lymphocytes.

Monocytes develop into macrophages after they leave the blood and enter tissue. In some disorders, mononuclear phagocytes in blood become activated and enlarged and resemble macrophages (Figs. 20J–20L). Erythrophagocytosis may be present in primary or secondary immune-mediated anemia (Figs. 20M, 20N). Monocytes may also contain hemosiderin, which stains gray-to-black with routine blood stains (Fig. 20O). Iron-positive inclusions may be seen in association with hemolytic anemia and/or marked inflammatory responses. Mononuclear phagocytes containing melanin granules (melanophages) may rarely occur with malignant melanoma (Fig. 20P).

Ehrlichial organisms that infect mononuclear phagocytes include *E. canis*, *E. risticii*, and *E. chaffeensis*. In contrast to granulocytic *Ehrlichia* species, morulae of monocytic *Ehrlichia* species are rarely found in blood leukocytes. When present, these morulae appear as tightly packed basophilic clusters of organisms within the cytoplasm (Figs. 20Q, 20R). *E. canis* causes mild-to-severe disease in dogs. *E. chaffeensis* (human monocytic ehrlichiosis) infects dogs but does not cause evidence of disease. *E. risticii* is primarily pathogenic to horses (Potomac horse fever),[199,200] but it can also infect dogs and cats.[201–203]

Other infectious agents that may rarely be seen in blood mononuclear phagocytes include *Histoplasma capsulatum* (Fig. 20S),[204] *Mycobacterium* species,[172,205] *Leishmania infantum*,[176] and remarkably large schizonts of *Cytauxzoon felis* (Fig. 20T).[116]

(text continued on page 65)

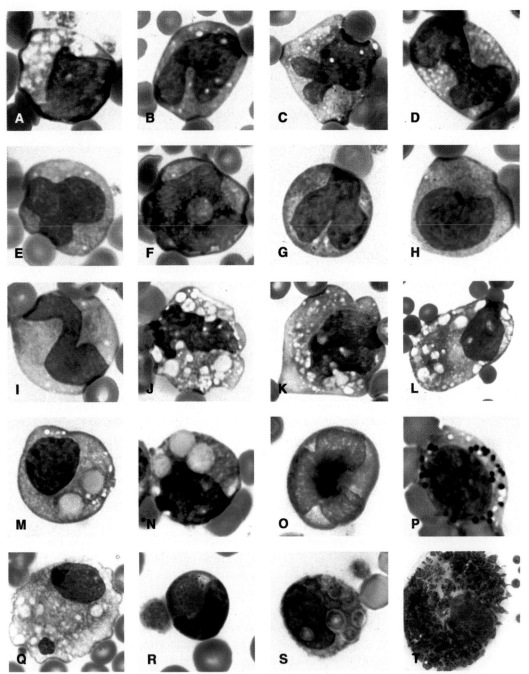

FIGURE 20. Normal and abnormal morphology of monocytes and macrophages. **A.** Monocyte in blood from a cat with a round nucleus and prominent cytoplasmic vacuoles. Wright-Giemsa stain. **B.** Monocyte in blood from a cow with a band-shaped nucleus and basophilic cytoplasm with prominent vacuoles. Wright-Giemsa stain. **C.** Monocyte in blood from a horse with a pleomorphic nucleus and basophilic cytoplasm containing vacuoles. Wright-Giemsa stain. **D.** Monocyte in blood from a horse with basophilic cytoplasm containing vacuoles. Wright-Giemsa stain. **E.** Monocyte in blood from a cow with a pleomorphic nucleus and basophilic cytoplasm. Wright-Giemsa stain. **F.** Monocyte with doughnut-shaped nucleus and basophilic cytoplasm in blood from a cow. Wright-Giemsa stain. **G.** Monocyte in blood from a dog with band-shaped nucleus and basophilic cytoplasm containing magenta-staining granules. Wright-Giemsa stain. **H.** Monocyte in blood from a horse with a

(Continued)

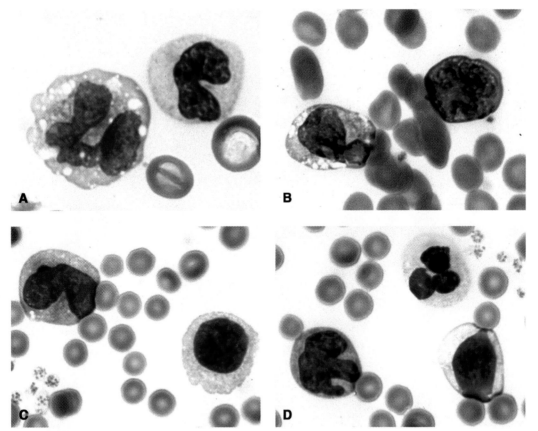

FIGURE 21.   Comparisons of band neutrophil, monocyte, and lymphocyte morphology.   A. Monocyte with prominent cytoplasmic vacuolation (left) and a band neutrophil (right) in blood from a dog with chronic myeloid leukemia. Wright-Giemsa stain.   **B.**   Monocyte (left) and a reactive lymphocyte with intensely basophilic cytoplasm (right) in blood from a dog after vaccination. Wright-Giemsa stain.   **C.**   Monocyte (left) and large lymphocyte (right) in blood from a cow. Wright-Giemsa stain.   **D.** Monocyte (left), lymphocyte (right), and neutrophil (top) in blood from a cow. Wright-Giemsa stain.

---

kidney-shaped nucleus and basophilic cytoplasm containing magenta-staining granules. Wright-Giemsa stain. **I.**   Monocyte in blood from a dog with a band-shaped nucleus and basophilic cytoplasm. Wright-Giemsa stain.   **J.**   Activated monocyte with prominent vacuolation in blood from a dog with babesiosis. Wright-Giemsa stain.   **K.**   Activated monocyte in blood from a cow with bacteremia. Wright-Giemsa stain. **L.**   Macrophage in blood from a cat with hemobartonellosis. Lower magnification than other images in this figure except Figure 20T. Wright-Giemsa stain.   **M.**   Monocyte with erythrophagocytosis in blood from a foal with neonatal isoerythrolysis. Wright-Giemsa stain.   **N.**   Monocyte with erythrophagocytosis in blood from a cat with hemobartonellosis. Wright-Giemsa stain.   **O.**   Monocyte containing hemosiderin (dark material in the center) in blood from a dog. Wright-Giemsa stain.   **P.**   Mononuclear cell containing melanin granules (presumably a melanophage) in blood from an aged gray Arabian gelding with disseminated malignant melanoma. Photograph of a stained blood film from a 1999 ASVCP slide review case submitted by J. Tarrant, T. Stokol, J. Bartol, and J. Wakshlag. Wright stain.   **Q.**   Macrophage with an *Ehrlichia canis* morula in the cytoplasm in a buffy coat smear from a dog. Wright-Giemsa stain.   **R.** *Ehrlichia canis* morula in the cytoplasm of a mononuclear cell that was presumed to be a monocyte. Wright-Giemsa stain.   **S.**   *Histoplasma capsulatum* in the cytoplasm of a monocyte in blood from a cat. Photograph of a stained blood film from a 1980 ASVCP slide review case submitted by D.A. Schmidt. Wright stain.   **T.**   *Cytauxzoon felis* schizont development in a large macrophage in blood from a cat. Note the small size of the erythrocytes compared to the macrophage in this low-magnification image. Wright-Giemsa stain.

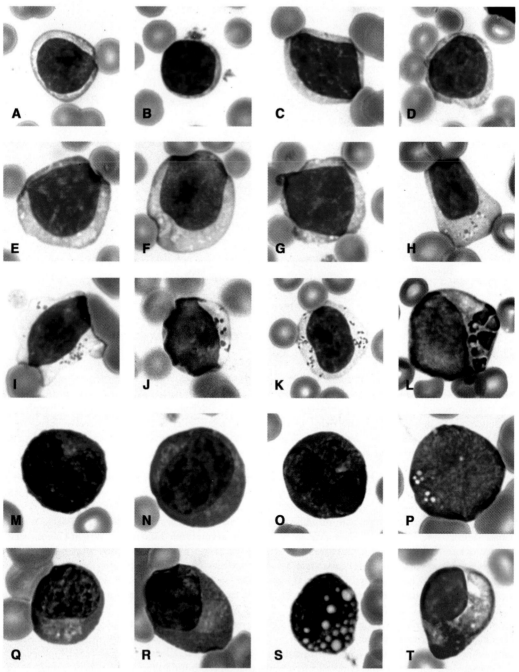

FIGURE 22. Normal and abnormal morphology of lymphocytes.   **A.**   Small lymphocyte in blood from a cat. Wright-Giemsa stain.   **B.**   Small lymphocyte in blood from a cow. Wright-Giemsa stain.   **C.**   Medium-sized lymphocyte in blood from a horse. Wright-Giemsa stain.   **D.**   Medium-sized lymphocyte in blood from a cow. The ringlike clumped chromatin patterns in the nucleus may be confused with nucleoli. Wright-Giemsa stain.   **E.**   Medium to large lymphocyte in blood from a cow. Wright-Giemsa stain.   **F.**   Large lymphocyte in blood from a cow. Wright-Giemsa stain.   **G.**   Me-

(Continued)

LYMPHOCYTE MORPHOLOGY

Most lymphocytes reside within lymphoid organs (lymph nodes, thymus, spleen, and bone marrow). A small number of lymphocytes circulate in blood. Most lymphocytes in blood have come from peripheral lymphoid organs, primarily lymph nodes. Depending on the species and individual variability, about 50% to 75% of blood lymphocytes are T lymphocytes, and about 20% to 35% are B lymphocytes. T lymphocytes and B lymphocytes cannot be differentiated from one another based on morphology in stained blood films. Many blood lymphocytes are memory cells, which are thought to be antigen primed and in a resting state. They naturally express levels of adhesion molecules that allow them to circulate from blood through tissue and then back into blood.

Normal Blood Lymphocyte Morphology

Lymphocytes have high N:C ratios, and they vary considerably in size, with the highest N:C ratios in the smaller cells (Figs. 21C, 21D, 22A–22G). The cytoplasm of resting (e.g., not stimulated) blood lymphocytes is usually pale blue in color, and their nuclei are usually round but may be oval or slightly indented. Nuclear chromatin varies from condensed and densely staining to a pattern of light and dark staining areas to lighter-staining nuclei with a smooth chromatin pattern. Lymphocytes in healthy ruminants may have ringlike clumped chromatin patterns in the nucleus that may be confused with nucleoli (Figs. 22D, 22G). Consequently, caution should be taken in making a diagnosis of lymphoid neoplasia in cattle based on a finding of what appear to be low numbers of lymphoblasts in blood. Most lymphocytes in the blood of domestic animals are small to medium in size, but some large lymphocytes may be present. Lymphocytes in ruminants are often larger with more cytoplasm than is seen in other species, sometimes making these cells difficult to differentiate from monocytes

---

dium to large lymphocyte in blood from a cow. The ringlike clumped chromatin patterns in the nucleus may be confused with nucleoli. Wright-Giemsa stain. **H.** Granular lymphocyte in blood from a dog. Wright-Giemsa stain. **I.** Granular lymphocyte in blood from a horse. Wright-Giemsa stain. **J.** Granular lymphocyte in blood from a cow. Wright-Giemsa stain. **K.** Granular lymphocyte in blood from a cat. Wright-Giemsa stain. **L.** Neoplastic large granular lymphocyte in blood from a cat with large granular lymphoma. Note the large size of the granules compared to the normal granular lymphocyte as shown in Figure 22K. Wright-Giemsa stain. **M.** Reactive lymphocyte with kidney-shaped nucleus and intensely basophilic cytoplasm in blood from a dog with hemobartonellosis. Wright-Giemsa stain. **N.** Reactive lymphocyte with intensely basophilic cytoplasm in blood from a cow infected with bovine leukemia virus. Wright-Giemsa stain. **O.** Reactive lymphocyte with a convoluted nucleus and intensely basophilic cytoplasm in blood from a cat with a bacterial infection. Wright-Giemsa stain. **P.** Reactive lymphocyte with a convoluted nucleus and intensely basophilic cytoplasm in blood from a dog with mild cough. Wright-Giemsa stain. **Q.** Plasmacytoid lymphocyte with intensely basophilic cytoplasm in blood from a dog with babesiosis. Wright-Giemsa stain. **R.** Plasmacytoid lymphocyte with intensely basophilic cytoplasm in blood from a horse with granulocytic ehrlichiosis. Wright-Giemsa stain. **S.** Lymphocyte containing Russell bodies in the cytoplasm in blood from a horse. Wright-Giemsa stain. **T.** Plasma cell with eccentric nucleus in blood from a dog with multiple myeloma. Wright-Giemsa stain.

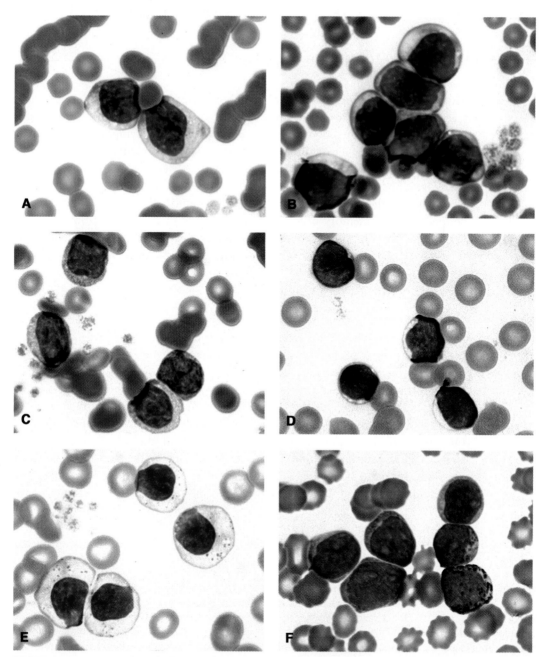

FIGURE 23. Normal and abnormal morphology of lymphocytes. **A.** Normal-appearing medium and large lymphocyte in blood from a cow. Wright-Giemsa stain. **B.** Non-neoplastic lymphocytosis in blood from a cow infected with bovine leukemia virus. Lymphocytes are medium to large in size with increased cytoplasmic basophilia. Wright-Giemsa stain. **C.** Chronic lymphocytic leukemia (CLL) in blood from a cat with normal-appearing lymphocytes. Wright-Giemsa stain. **D.** CLL involving normal-appearing small lymphocytes with scant cytoplasm in blood from a dog. Wright-Giemsa stain. **E.** CLL involving granular lymphocytes with abundant cytoplasm in blood from a dog. Wright-Giemsa stain. **F.** Acute lymphoblastic leukemia (ALL) involving granular lymphocytes in blood from a dog. Lymphoblasts with fine nuclear chromatin and nucleoli are present. Some of these cells contain cytoplasmic granules. Photograph of a stained blood film from a 1989 ASVCP slide review case submitted by M. Wellman and G. Kociba. Wright stain.

(Figs. 21C, 22F, 23A).[206] If it is unclear whether a cell is a lymphocyte or a monocyte, it is classified as a lymphocyte, because this cell type is usually much more numerous in blood than is the monocyte.

Marked lymphocytosis, involving normal-appearing small to medium–sized lymphocytes, is present in the blood of animals with chronic lymphocytic leukemia (CLL) (Figs. 23C, 23D).[191,207,208] Although normal in appearance, these cells have abnormal function. CLL is rare and is reported most often in older dogs.[209–211] A persistent lymphocytosis with some normal-appearing lymphocytes and some reactive lymphocytes (see subsequent discussion) may occur in animals with chronic viremias,[11] of which the persistent lymphocytosis found in cattle with bovine leukemia virus (BLV) infection is most common (Fig. 23B).[212]

Granular Lymphocytes

A low percentage of lymphocytes in blood have red- or purple-staining (generally focal) granules within the cytoplasm (Figs. 22H–22K). These cells are generally medium to large in size with more cytoplasm and lower N:C ratios than small lymphocytes. Granular lymphocytes appear to be either natural killer (NK) cells or cytotoxic T lymphocytes. A lymphocytosis consisting of granular lymphocytes may occur in neoplastic and nonneoplastic inflammatory (e.g., canine ehrlichiosis) disorders.[213,214]

Leukemias involving granular lymphocytes have been reported in dogs.[210,211,215] In most cases, the cells involved appear well-differentiated (Fig. 23E), and the disorder usually behaves as a form of CLL, being indolent and slowly progressive. In other cases, the cells appear less well-differentiated, with fine nuclear chromatin, and the disorder behaves more like acute lymphoblastic leukemia, being fulminant and rapidly fatal (Fig. 23F).[211,214] A large granular lymphocyte leukemia has been reported in a horse.[216]

Neoplasms involving mononuclear cells with large cytoplasmic magenta granules in cats have been termed large granular lymphomas, globule leukocyte tumors, and granulated round cell tumors.[214,217–219] Most of these large granular lymphomas appear to originate as intestinal tumors composed of cytotoxic T lymphocytes. As with other lymphomas, neoplastic cells may sometimes be present in blood (Fig. 22L) and bone marrow.[217,219]

Reactive Lymphocytes

Lymphocytes proliferate in response to antigenic stimulation. They increase in size and exhibit increased cytoplasmic basophilia (Figs. 21B, 22M–22R, 23B). Most of these antigenically stimulated cells remain in peripheral lymphoid tissues, but some may enter the circulation, although usually in low numbers. Various terms including reactive lymphocytes, transformed lymphocytes, and immunocytes have been used to describe them. Some reactive lymphocytes are large with convoluted nuclei (Figs. 21B, 22O, 22P). They resemble monocytes,

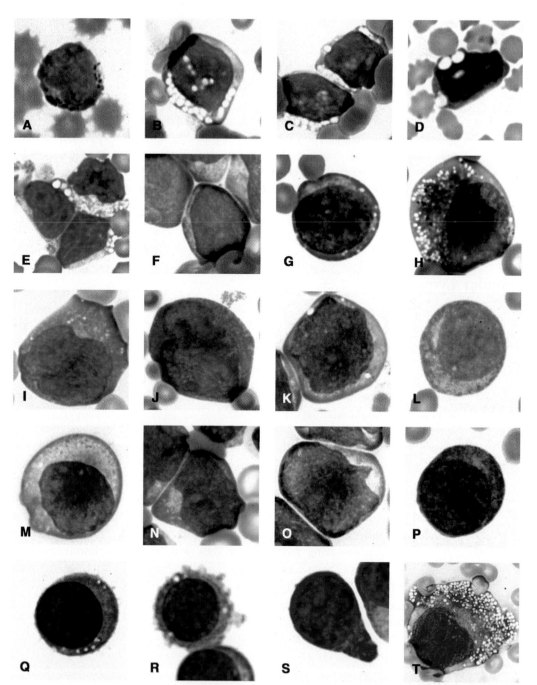

FIGURE 24. Lymphocytes containing granules and vacuoles and blast cells of various types.
A. Lymphocyte containing basophilic granules in the blood of a 3-month-old German shepherd dog with inherited mucopolysaccharidosis type VII. Photograph of a stained blood film from a 1997 ASVCP slide review case submitted by D.I. Bounous, D.C. Silverstein, K.S. Latimer, and K.P. Carmichael. Wright stain.
B. One of many lymphocytes containing cytoplasmic vacuoles in blood from an 8-week-old foal with *Corynebacterium equi* pneumonia. Lymphocytes appeared normal after treatment and recovery. Wright-Giemsa stain. **C.** Lymphocytes with cytoplasmic vacuoles in the blood of a korat cat with inherited GM_2-gangliosidosis. Wright-Giemsa stain. **D.** Lymphocytes with cytoplasmic vacuoles in the blood of a goat with presumptive diagnosis of inherited β-mannosidosis. Photograph of a stained blood film from a

(Continued)

68

except that their cytoplasm is more basophilic (navy blue color) than cytoplasm seen in monocytes (Fig. 21B). These cells can also be difficult to differentiate from some neoplastic lymphocytes. When it is not possible to decide whether a basophilic lymphocyte is reactive or neoplastic, the term "atypical lymphocyte" is sometimes used. Basophilic erythroid precursors may be confused with reactive lymphocytes. Some reactive lymphocytes are plasmacytoid (plasma-cell-like) in appearance (Figs. 22Q, 22R) and may rarely contain pinkish or bluish globules (Russell bodies) within the cytoplasm (Fig. 22S). These inclusions are composed of dilated endoplasmic reticulum—containing immunoglobulins.[11]

Plasma Cells

Plasma cells are present in lymphoid organs (except the thymus), but they are rarely observed in blood even when plasma cell neoplasia (e.g., multiple myeloma) is present (Fig. 22T). Plasma cells have lower N:C ratios and greater cytoplasmic basophilia than resting lymphocytes. The presence of prominent Golgi may create a pale perinuclear area in the cytoplasm. Plasma cells typically have eccentrically located nuclei with coarse chromatin clumping in a mosaic pattern.

1990 ASVCP slide review case submitted by W. Vernau. Wright stain.   **E.** Lymphocytes with cytoplasmic vacuoles in the blood of a domestic shorthair cat with inherited Niemann-Pick disease type C. Photograph of a stained blood film from a 1993 ASVCP slide review case submitted by D.E. Brown and M.A. Thrall. Wright-Giemsa stain.   **F.** Lymphoblast in blood from a dog with ALL. Wright-Giemsa stain.   **G.** Lymphoblast in blood from a cat with ALL. Wright-Giemsa stain.   **H.** Large lymphoblast in blood from a dog with lymphoma. The basophilic cytoplasm is abundant and contains small discrete vacuoles. Wright-Giemsa stain.   **I.** Large lymphoblast in blood from a dog with lymphoma. Wright-Giemsa stain.   **J.** Large lymphoblast in blood from a cow with lymphoma. Wright-Giemsa stain.   **K.** Large lymphoblast in blood from a goat with lymphoma. Wright-Giemsa stain.   **L.** Myeloblast in blood from a cat with erythroleukemia (AML-M6). This neoplastic cell has a round nucleus and gray-blue cytoplasm. A nucleolus is visible in the right side of the nucleus. Wright-Giemsa stain.   **M.** Myeloblast in blood from a dog with myeloblastic leukemia (AML-M2). This cell may be classified as a type II myeloblast because it contains a few small magenta-staining granules in the gray-blue cytoplasm near the top of the cell. Wright-Giemsa stain.   **N.** Monoblast in blood from a dog with acute myelomonocytic leukemia (AML-M4). The nucleus is more irregular than typically seen in myeloblasts.   **O.** Monoblast in blood from a dog with acute monocytic leukemia (AML-M5b). The nucleus is more irregular than typically seen in myeloblasts. Wright-Giemsa stain.   **P.** Rubriblast in blood from a cat with erythroleukemia (AML-M6Er). This neoplastic cell has a remarkably round nucleus with intensely basophilic cytoplasm. Wright-Giemsa stain.   **Q.** Megakaryoblast in blood from a dog with megakaryoblastic leukemia (AML-M7). The neoplastic cell has a remarkably round nucleus with cytoplasm that contains almost imperceptible pink granules and vacuoles. Wright-Giemsa stain.   **R.** Megakaryoblast in blood from a dog with AML-M7. The neoplastic cell has a remarkably round nucleus with pinkish cytoplasm that contains vacuoles and has surface projections. Wright-Giemsa stain.   **S.** Unclassified neoplastic cell in blood from a cat with acute unclassified leukemia (AUL). Pseudopod formation was commonly seen in neoplastic cells in blood from this cat. Wright-Giemsa stain.   **T.** Giant nonhematopoietic neoplastic cell in blood from a dog with widespread metastasis. Although this tumor was highly anaplastic, a pancreatic carcinoma was considered the likely tumor type based on necropsy findings. Wright-Giemsa stain.

Cytoplasmic Granules, Vacuoles, and Inclusions

A low percentage of lymphocytes in blood from normal animals contain cytoplasmic granules (see previous discussion of granular lymphocytes). Basophilic granules may be seen in the lymphocytes from animals with certain lysosomal storage diseases (Fig. 24A), including mucopolysaccharidosis type VI[139,140] and type VII[142,144] in dogs and cats and GM_2-gangliosidosis in pigs.[146]

Cytoplasmic vacuoles may be seen in lymphocytes from a variety of neoplastic and nonneoplastic disorders (Fig. 24B). Discrete vacuoles may occur in the cytoplasm of lymphocytes from animals with inherited lysosomal storage diseases (Figs. 24C–24E), including mucopolysaccharidosis type VII in cats,[143] GM_2-gangliosidosis in cats,[145,220] GM_1-gangliosidosis in cats and dogs,[221,222] α-mannosidosis in cats,[140] β-mannosidosis in goats,[223] Niemann-Pick type C in cats,[224] and α-L-fucosidase in dogs.[225] Basophilic granules and vacuoles may not become apparent in some lysosomal disorders until the affected animal reaches adulthood.

Lymphocytes may also contain distemper inclusions as in other blood cell types.

■ BLAST CELLS OR POORLY DIFFERENTIATED CELLS

Blast cells in blood generally have single round nuclei with finely stippled or smooth chromatin containing one or more distinct or indistinct nucleoli. The N:C ratio is generally high, and the cytoplasm varies from lightly to darkly basophilic. The similarities in appearance of different types of blast cells can make a specific diagnosis difficult or impossible based on routinely stained blood and bone marrow smears. This problem not withstanding, the morphologic appearance of the blast cells can be helpful in reaching a presumptive diagnosis. Blast cells may also be tentatively identified by the company they keep. Consequently, the type(s) of easily identifiable cells that are increased in blood may be helpful in reaching a diagnosis (e.g., increased monocytes in monocytic or myelomonocytic leukemias and increased nucleated erythrocytes in erythroleukemia). Specific diagnosis often requires special histochemical stains and/or immunophenotyping.[26,211]

Lymphoblasts

Lymphoblasts are larger than the normal small lymphocytes present in blood. The nucleus is generally round but may be indented or convoluted. The chromatin is usually finely stippled but may be coarsely granular. One or more nucleoli are present in the nucleus, but they are often difficult to see in routinely stained blood films (Fig. 24F). The cytoplasm is more basophilic than is seen in most blood lymphocytes and sometimes contains vacuoles. Rare lymphoblasts may be observed in disorders with increased antigenic stimulation, but when several of these cells are found during a differential count, lymphoid neoplasia is suspected.

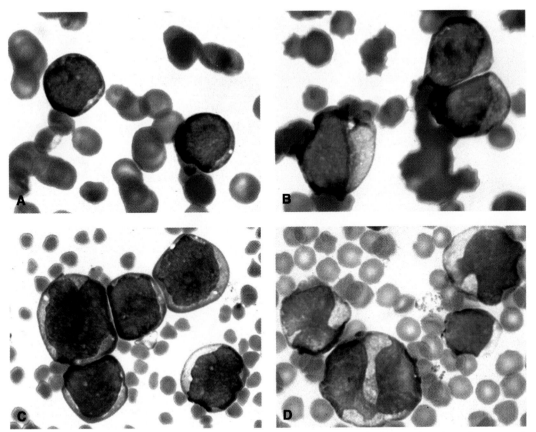

FIGURE 25. **Neoplastic lymphoid cells in acute lymphoblastic leukemia (ALL) and metastatic lymphoma.** **A.** Two lymphoblasts in blood from a dog with ALL. Wright-Giemsa stain. **B.** Three lymphoblasts in blood from a horse with a metastatic lymphoma. Wright-Giemsa stain. **C.** Five lymphoblasts in blood from a goat with metastatic lymphoma. Wright-Giemsa stain. **D.** A small normal-appearing lymphocyte and three large monocytoid neoplastic lymphocytes in blood from a cow with metastatic lymphoma. Wright-Giemsa stain.

Acute lymphoblastic leukemia (ALL) originates from bone marrow and lymphoblasts are generally, although not invariably, present in blood from animals with ALL (Figs. 24F, 24G, 25A).[208,209,226–228] Lymphoblasts are also released into blood in some animals with a lymphoma (Figs. 24H–24K, 25B–25D),[11,229,230] in addition to ALL that originates from the bone marrow. When present in blood this pattern is sometimes called leukemic lymphoma or lymphosarcoma cell leukemia. The morphology of the neoplastic lymphoid cells in blood from animals with lymphoma is quite variable. One or more morphologic features that may be present include exceptionally large size, abundant

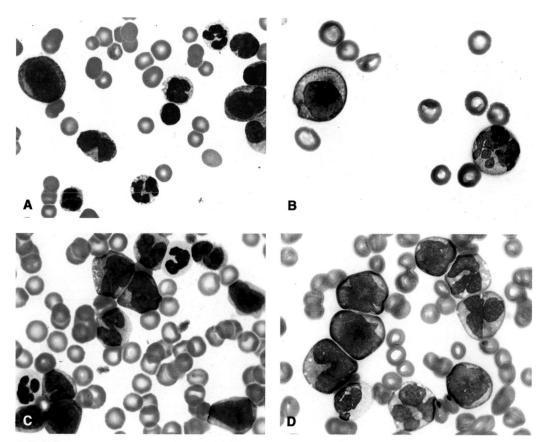

FIGURE 26. Leukemias including chronic myeloid leukemia (CML), myeloblastic leukemia (AML-M2), acute myelomonocytic leukemia (AML-M4), and acute monocytic leukemia (AML-M5). **A.** Blood from a cat with a presumptive diagnosis of chronic myeloid leukemia (CML) exhibiting marked neutrophilia with a prominent left shift. A bone marrow biopsy was not done to confirm the diagnosis. Rare myeloblasts (cell at top left) were seen in the blood film. Wright-Giemsa stain. **B.** Type II myeloblast (left) and a hypersegmented neutrophil (right) in blood from a dog with AML-M2. Wright-Giemsa stain. **C.** Blood from a dog with AML-M4. A mixture of neutrophils, monocytes, and precursors of both cell types are present. Wright-Giemsa stain. **D.** Blood from a dog with AML-M5. All cells present, except a neutrophil at bottom left, are monocyte precursors or mature monocytes. Wright-Giemsa stain.

cytoplasm, heavily vacuolated cytoplasm, and monocytoid-appearing nuclei. Cells present in leukemic lymphoma in cattle often appear monocytoid (Fig. 25D).[231] Nuclei may be especially convoluted (cerebriform) in dogs and cats with mycosis fungoides, a T-lymphocyte type lymphoma of the skin.[232] When these neoplastic cells with convoluted nuclei are present in blood, they have been referred to as Sézary cells, and this presentation of cutaneous T-lymphocyte lymphoma with leukemia has been referred to as the Sézary syndrome.[233–235]

Myeloblasts

Type I myeloblasts appear as large round cells with round to oval nuclei that are generally centrally located in the cell. The N:C ratio is high (>1.5), and the nuclear outline is usually regular and smooth (Figs. 24L, 24M). Nuclear chromatin is finely stippled, containing one or more nucleoli or nucleolar rings. The cytoplasm is generally moderately basophilic but not as dark as rubriblasts. Some myeloblasts may contain a few (<15) small, magenta-staining granules in the cytoplasm and may be classified as type II myeloblasts (Fig. 24M).[236] Myeloblasts may be present in blood in low numbers in CML (Fig. 26A). They are more often present in blood with various forms of acute myeloid leukemia (AML), including myeloblastic leukemia (AML–M1 and AML-M2) (Fig. 26B), myelomonocytic leukemia (AML-M4), and erythroleukemia (AML-M6) (Fig. 27B).[183,236,237] Myeloblasts, promyelocytes, and myelocytes in blood all have round nuclei and resemble lymphoid cells, but cytochemical stains or recognition of surface markers can help differentiate these cell types in leukemic animals.[26,211]

Monoblasts

Monoblasts resemble myeloblasts except that their nuclear shape is irregularly round or convoluted in appearance (Figs. 24N, 24O). A clear area in the cytoplasm, representing the Golgi zone, is often observed, especially near the site of nuclear indentation. The N:C ratio is high but may be somewhat lower than that in myeloblasts.[236] Monoblasts may be present in blood in animals with acute myelomonocytic leukemia (AML-M4) (Fig. 26C) and acute monocytic leukemia (AML-M5) (Fig. 26D).[183,237,238] Although rare, most horses reported with AML have had either AML-M4 or AML-M5.[239,240]

Rubriblasts

Rubriblasts have more basophilic cytoplasm than myeloblasts, monoblasts, and most lymphoblasts (Fig. 24P). Although the other blasts mentioned have nuclei that are generally round in shape, the nucleus of a rubriblast is usually nearly perfectly round. The chromatin is generally finely granular, with one or more nucleoli. Rubriblasts are not usually seen in the blood of animals with regenerative anemia. They may be present in variable numbers in the blood of animals with erythroleukemia (AML-M6 or AML-M6Er) (Figs. 27A, 27B).[183,237]

Megakaryoblasts

Megakaryoblasts occur in the blood of animals with megakaryoblastic leukemia (AML-M7). Nuclei of megakaryoblasts are nearly as round as rubriblast nuclei, but their cytoplasm is typically less basophilic and may contain magenta-staining granules (Figs. 24Q, 24R). Unique features present in some of these cells include multiple discrete vacuoles (Fig. 27C)[241,242] and cytoplasmic projections (Fig. 24R).[183,243,244]

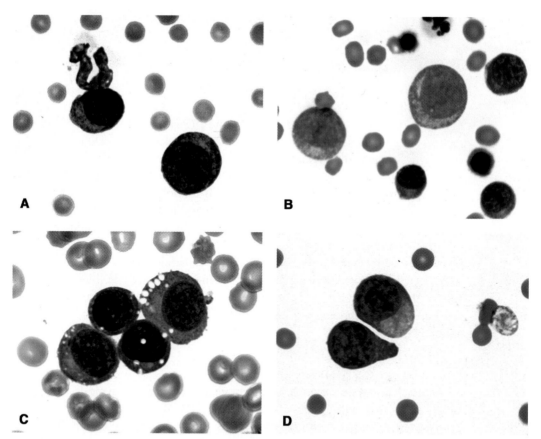

FIGURE 27. Acute myeloid leukemia including erythroleukemia, megakaryoblastic leukemia (AML-M7), and acute unclassified leukemia (AUL). **A.** Blood from a cat with erythroleukemia (AML-M6Er). A neutrophil and two rubriblasts with basophilic cytoplasm are present. Wright-Giemsa stain. **B.** Blood from a cat with erythroleukemia (AML-M6). The two largest cells with pale-blue cytoplasm are myeloblasts. The smaller round cells are all erythroid precursors. Wright-Giemsa stain. **C.** Blood from a dog with AML-M7. Four neoplastic megakaryoblasts with prominent cytoplasmic vacuoles are present. Wright-Giemsa stain. **D.** Blood from a cat with AUL. Two unclassified neoplastic cells are present. Wright-Giemsa stain.

Unclassified Blast Cells

Primitive cells that cannot be classified with certainty are listed as unclassified during differential cell counts. When unclassified cells predominate in bone marrow (and sometimes blood), a diagnosis of acute unclassified leukemia (AUL) is made (Figs. 24S, 27D).[236]

Metastatic Blast Cells

Although metastasis of tumors from nonhematopoietic organs is common, these neoplastic cells are rarely recognized in blood (except for malignant mast cells). When present, these blast cells are typically much larger than hematopoietic blast cells (Fig. 24T).

CHAPTER 4

Platelets

■ NORMAL PLATELET MORPHOLOGY

Blood platelets (thrombocytes) in mammals are small, round-to-oval anucleated cell fragments (thin discs when unstimulated) that form from cylinders of megakaryocyte cytoplasm. Platelet cytoplasm appears light blue with many small reddish purple granules when visualized using routine blood stains (Figs. 28A, 28B). Equine platelets often stain poorly with Wright-Giemsa stain (Fig. 28C) but generally stain well with Diff-Quik (Fig. 28D). Platelets typically stain uniformly purple with the new methylene blue wet preparation (Fig. 29A).

The diameter of platelets varies depending on the species, with cats having larger platelets than other domestic animals (Fig. 28E). Cat platelets appear especially sensitive to activation during blood sample collection and handling, resulting in degranulated platelet aggregates, which may be overlooked by an inexperienced observer (Fig. 28F). Some of the precipitated cryoglobulin recognized in blood from a cat with a monoclonal cryoglobulinemia (Fig. 28G) also resembled aggregates of degranulated platelets.

Newly formed platelets have higher RNA content and have been termed reticulated platelets. They cannot be quantified by morphology but can be counted using flow cytometry following labeling of RNA with a fluorescent dye.[245,246]

Platelet morphology is typically normal in animals with thrombocythemia, a chronic myeloproliferative disorder in which platelet counts typically exceed $1 \times 10^6/\mu L$ (Fig. 29B). However, increased mean platelet volumes (MPV) have been reported in two dogs believed to have thrombocythemia.[247]

■ ABNORMAL PLATELET MORPHOLOGY

Macroplatelets

Platelets that are as large, or larger, in diameter as erythrocytes are called macroplatelets, megaplatelets, or macrothrombocytes (Figs. 28H–28L). They may be seen in low numbers in normal cats. The presence of frequent macro-

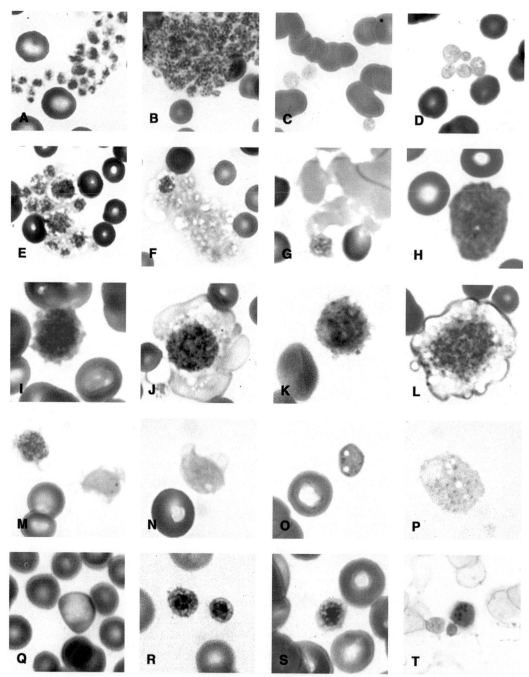

FIGURE 28. Normal and abnormal morphology of platelets.   A. An aggregate of platelets in blood from a dog. Wright-Giemsa stain.   **B.** An aggregate of platelets in blood from a cow. Wright-Giemsa stain.   **C.** Three pale-staining platelets in blood from a horse. An erythrocyte contains a Howell-Jolly body. Wright-Giemsa stain.   **D.** Five platelets in blood from a horse. Diff-Quik stain. **E.** An aggregate of platelets in blood from a cat, demonstrating the presence of large platelets characteristic of this species. Wright-Giemsa stain.   **F.** An aggregate of activated and degranulated platelets in blood

(Continued)

platelets in a thrombocytopenic animal suggests that enhanced thrombopoiesis is present,[1] but macroplatelets may also be present in thrombocytopenic animals with myelodysplastic or myeloproliferative disorders.[131] Macroplatelets may be present in nonthrombocytopenic animals that have recently recovered from thrombocytopenia (Figs. 29C, 29D). A population of macroplatelets may be seen in healthy King Charles spaniel dogs[248] and in otter hound dogs with a hereditary platelet function defect.[249]

Activated Platelets

Partially activated platelets are no longer discs but have thin cytoplasmic processes extending from a spherical cell body. When platelets are more fully activated, their granules are crushed together by a surrounding web of microtubules and microfilaments. This central aggregate of platelet granules may be mistaken for a nucleus (Fig. 28J). Platelet aggregates form following platelet activation *in vitro*. If degranulation occurs, aggregates may be difficult to recognize, appearing as light-blue material on stained blood films (Figs. 28F, 29E). The presence of platelet aggregates should be recorded because the platelet count may be erroneously decreased.

Hypogranular Platelets

Hypogranular platelets may result from platelet activation and secretion, but they have also been seen in animals with myeloproliferative disorders (Figs.

---

from a cat. Only a single platelet in the upper left of the aggregate still contains visible granules. Wright-Giemsa stain.   **G.**   Blue-staining homogenous globules of cryoglobulin in blood from an American domestic shorthair cat with multiple myeloma and an IgG monoclonal cryoglobulinemia. The precipitated globules sometimes mimic the appearance of an aggregate of degranulated platelets. A single platelet is present at the bottom between two erythrocytes. Photograph of a stained blood film from a 1999 ASVCP slide review case submitted by T. Stokol, J. Blue, F. Hickford, Y. von Gessel, and J. Billings. Wright stain.   **H.**   Macroplatelet in blood from a dog with immune-mediated thrombocytopenia. Wright-Giemsa stain.   **I.**   Macroplatelet in blood from a dog with *Ehrlichia platys* infection and thrombocytopenia. Wright-Giemsa stain.   **J.**   Macroplatelet with aggregated granules that may be mistaken for a nucleus in blood from a cat with an abdominal abscess and toxic left shift in the blood. Wright-Giemsa stain.   **K.**   Macroplatelet in blood from a dog with CML. Wright-Giemsa stain.   **L.**   Macroplatelet with centrally located granules in blood from a cat with myelodysplastic syndrome. Wright-Giemsa stain.   **M.**   Platelet with granules (top left) and a hypogranular platelet (right) in blood from a dog with CML. Both platelets exhibit thin cytoplasmic processes. Wright-Giemsa stain.   **N.**   Hypogranular platelet in blood from a dog with CML, exhibiting thin cytoplasmic processes. Wright-Giemsa stain.   **O.**   Hypogranular platelet in blood from a dog with erythroleukemia (AML-M6Er). Wright-Giemsa stain.   **P.**   Hypogranular macroplatelet in blood from a dog with CML. Wright-Giemsa stain.   **Q.**   Cytoplasmic fragment in blood from a cow with leukemic lymphoma. The fragment might be confused with a hypogranular platelet. Wright-Giemsa stain.   **R.**   Two platelets containing *Ehrlichia platys* morulae, which stain dark-blue in contrast to the normal magenta-staining granules, in blood from a dog. Wright-Giemsa stain.   **S.**   Platelet containing an *Ehrlichia platys* morula, which stains dark-blue in contrast to the normal magenta-staining granules, in blood from a dog. Wright-Giemsa stain.   **T.**   Large platelet containing what appears to be two *Ehrlichia platys* morulae, each with multiple subunits, in blood from a dog. New methylene blue wet mount preparation.

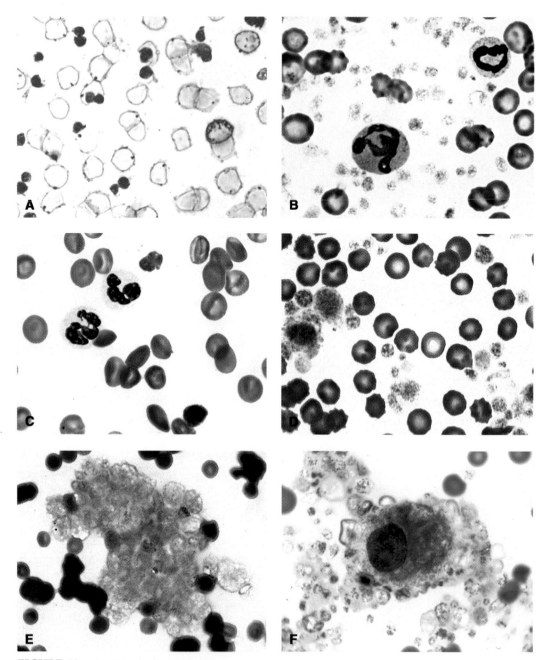

FIGURE 29. *See legend on opposite page.*

28M–28P).[131,250] Hypogranular platelets must be differentiated from cytoplasmic fragments from other cells, as has been reported in ruminants with leukemic lymphomas (Fig. 28Q).[251]

Ehrlichia Platys Infection

Ehrlichia platys is a rickettsial parasite that specifically infects platelets in dogs. Morulae appear as tightly packed basophilic clusters of organisms within the cytoplasm of platelets (Figs. 28R–28T).[252] Similar-appearing inclusions have been seen in platelets from a cat.[253]

FIGURE 29.   Abnormalities of platelets and a dwarf megakaryocyte.   A. Mild thrombocytosis following splenectomy in blood from a dog. Platelets appear as small purple cells and erythrocytes appear as unstained "ghosts." Single small Heinz bodies in many erythrocytes appear as basophilic "dots." A reticulocyte is present at center right. New methylene blue wet mount staining procedure.   **B.** Markedly increased platelet numbers in blood from a dog with thrombocythemia. A basophil (bottom) and neutrophil (top right) are also present. Photograph of a stained blood film from a 1987 ASVCP slide review case submitted by C.P. Mandell, N.C. Jain, J.G. Zinkl. Wright stain.   **C.** Lack of platelets in blood from a dog with immune-mediated thrombocytopenia (platelets = 20 × 10³/μL) and regenerative anemia. Polychromatophilic erythrocytes, a metarubricyte (bottom), and two neutrophils are present. Wright-Giemsa stain.   **D.** Thrombocytosis (platelets = 950 × 10³/μL) with several macroplatelets in blood from the same dog as shown in Figure 29C a week after beginning prednisone therapy. Wright-Giemsa stain.   **E.** A large platelet aggregate in blood from a cat with thrombocytosis. The presence of many platelet aggregates in the blood sample resulted in an erroneously high total leukocyte count measured electronically using impedance technology. Wright-Giemsa stain.   **F.** Dwarf megakaryocyte and many platelets in the buffy coat of a cat with myelodysplastic syndrome. Wright-Giemsa stain.

CHAPTER 5

Miscellaneous Cells and Parasites

■ PYKNOSIS AND KARYORRHEXIS

Cells that undergo programmed cell death (apoptosis) exhibit pyknosis and karyorrhexis (Figs. 30A–30D). Pyknosis involves shrinkage or condensation of a cell with increased nuclear compactness or density. Karyorrhexis refers to the subsequent fragmentation. It may not be possible to determine the cell of origin.

■ MITOTIC CELLS

Mitotic cells may be present in the blood of animals with malignant neoplasia (Fig. 30E), but they may also occur in nonneoplastic disorders, such as lymphocytes undergoing blast transformation (Fig. 30F), nucleated erythroid precursors in regenerative anemia, and activated mononuclear phagocytes.

■ FREE NUCLEI

When cells are lysed during blood film preparation, free nuclei (nuclei without cytoplasm) may be seen (Fig. 30G). When a free nucleus is spread thin on the blood film, it appears as a netlike pinkish structure that has been referred to as a basket "cell" (Fig. 30H). This term is a misnomer, because a basket cell is not truly a cell but only the distorted nucleus of a cell. Lymphocytes are the most likely blood cell type to lyse during blood film preparation.

■ ENDOTHELIAL CELLS

Spindle-shaped endothelial cells with elongated nuclei may sometimes be seen in blood films (Fig. 30I). Endothelial cells line vessels and may become dislodged as the needle enters the vein during blood sample collection.

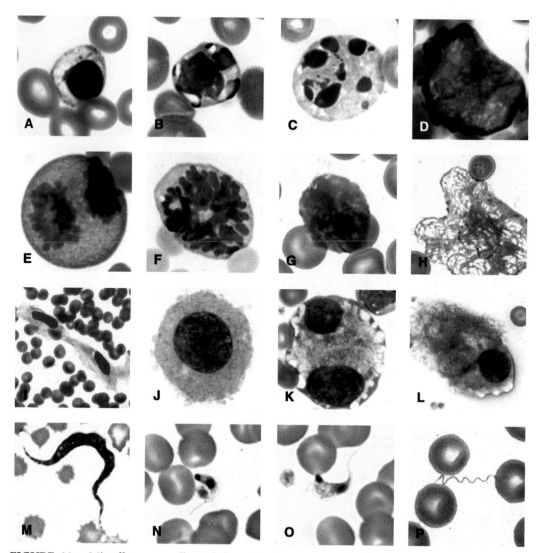

FIGURE 30. Miscellaneous cells and free infectious agents in blood. **A.** Pyknotic cell with condensed chromatin in blood from a dog with a toxic left shift. Wright-Giemsa stain. **B.** Pyknosis and karyorrhexis of a cell in blood from a dog with dirofilariasis. Wright-Giemsa stain. **C.** Pyknosis and karyorrhexis of a cell in blood from a dog with acute monocytic leukemia (AML-M5). Wright-Giemsa stain. **D.** Pyknosis and karyorrhexis of a cell in blood from a cow with leukemic lymphoma. Wright-Giemsa stain. **E.** Mitotic cell in anaphase in blood from a cat with erythroleukemia (AML-M6). Wright-Giemsa stain. **F.** Mitotic cell (presumably lymphoid) in prophase in blood from a horse with equine infectious anemia. Wright-Giemsa stain. **G.** Free nucleus in blood from a dog with CLL. Wright-Giemsa stain. **H.** Free nucleus with distorted netlike structure (basket cell) in blood from a cat. Wright-Giemsa stain. **I.** Two spindle-shaped endothelial cells with elongated nuclei in blood from a cow. These cells were likely dislodged from the vessel wall during blood sample collection. Wright-Giemsa stain. **J.** Dwarf megakaryocyte with single nucleus in blood from a dog with CML. Wright-Giemsa stain. **K.** Dwarf megakaryocyte with two nuclei in blood from a dog with CML. Wright-Giemsa stain. **L.** Dwarf megakaryocyte in blood from a dog with AML-M7. Wright-Giemsa stain. **M.** *Trypanosoma theileri* in blood from a three-day-old female Angus calf. Photograph of a stained blood film from a 1989 ASVCP slide review case submitted by H. Bender, A. Zajak, G. Moore, and G. Saunders. Wright stain. **N.** *Trypanosoma cruzi* in blood from a dog. Photograph of a stained blood film provided by Dr. S.C. Barr. Wright stain. **O.** *Trypanosoma cruzi* in blood from a dog. Photograph of a stained blood film provided by Dr. S.C. Barr. Wright stain. **P.** Spirochete in blood from a North-Central Florida dog that was seronegative for *Borrelia burgdorferi* and five *Leptospira* spp. Wright-Giemsa stain.

■ MEGAKARYOCYTES

Megakaryocytes are multilobulated, platelet-producing giant cells that lie against the outside of vascular sinuses in bone marrow (see the bone marrow section for more details). Cytoplasmic processes of mature megakaryocytes extend into the sinus lumen where they develop into proplatelets and, subsequently, individual platelets. Sometimes whole megakaryocytes enter vascular sinuses, accounting for the rare recognition of these cells in blood films from normal animals.[254] Megakaryocytes are more easily found by examination of blood buffy coat smears. Megakaryocytes reaching blood are quickly trapped in lung capillaries where continued platelet production may occur.

Dwarf megakaryocytes are smaller than normal mature megakaryocytes and have decreased nuclear ploidy, but their cytoplasm generally contains granules and appears similar to that of blood platelets (Figs. 29F, 30J–30L). Dwarf megakaryocytes are common in bone marrow of animals with myeloproliferative disorders but are only rarely seen in blood.

■ PARASITES AND BACTERIA

Parasites and bacteria may be seen in blood which are not associated with blood cells. However, bacterial rods and cocci between cells are usually the result of contaminated stain.

Microfilaria

Potential microfilariae (nematode larvae) include *Dirofilaria immitis* in dogs, cats, and wild canids (Fig. 5D); *Dipetalonema reconditum* in dogs; and *Setaria* species in cattle and horses.[114]

Trypanosoma Species

Various *Trypanosoma* species may be seen in blood (Figs. 30M–30O). These elongated, flagellated protozoa cause important diseases of livestock outside of the United States,[114] but the species seen in cattle (*T. theileri*) in the United States is usually nonpathogenic.[255,256] Many dogs are infected with *T. cruzi* in the United States, but organisms are rarely seen in blood and most cases are subclinical. When present, clinical forms of disease have principally involved heart or neural dysfunctions.[257]

Bacteria

Various bacterial species may be present in blood films. It is important to verify that these are not contaminants, especially during the staining procedure. The presence of phagocytized bacteria within neutrophils indicates that the bacteria are likely of clinical significance. Spirochetes have been seen in blood from dogs with *Borrelia* infections.[175] A species of *Borrelia* different from *B. burgdorferi* has been recognized in the blood of dogs from Florida (Fig. 30P).[258]

BONE MARROW

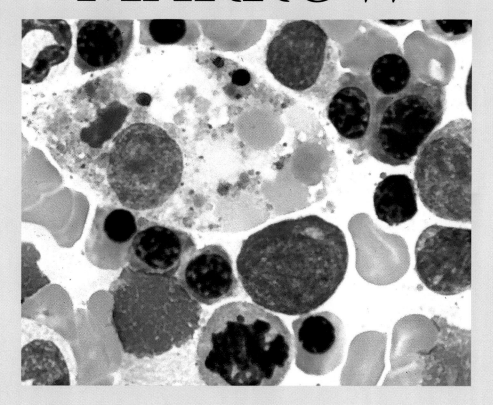

CHAPTER 6

Hematopoiesis

Throughout the adult life of a mammal, all blood cell types are continuously produced from primitive stem cells within extravascular spaces of bone marrow.[259] A totipotent hematopoietic stem cell produces a pluripotent lymphoid stem cell, as well as a pluripotent myeloid stem cell. The pluripotent myeloid stem cell gives rise to a series of increasingly differentiated progenitor cells, with limited self-renewal capabilities, which support the production of all nonlymphoid blood cells. Stem cells and progenitor cells are mononuclear cells that cannot be distinguished morphologically from lymphocytes. When measured in an *in vitro* cell culture assay, progenitor cells are referred to as colony-forming units (CFUs) or burst-forming units (BFUs) if they form multiple subcolonies.[1,259,260] The totipotent hematopoietic stem cell also gives rise to progenitor cells for osteoclasts,[261,262] mast cells,[263] dendritic cells,[264] and Langerhans cells.[265,266]

Blood cell production occurs in the bone marrow of adult animals because of the unique microenvironment present there. The hematopoietic microenvironment is a complex meshwork composed of various stromal cells; accessory cells; glycoprotein growth factors; and extracellular matrix components that profoundly affect hematopoietic stem cell and progenitor cell survival, proliferation, and differentiation. Stromal cells (endothelial cells, fibroblast-like reticular cells, adipocytes, and macrophages) and accessory cells (subsets of lymphocytes and natural killer cells) produce a variety of positive and negative growth factors. Stromal cells also produce components of the extracellular matrix. In addition to providing structural support, the extracellular matrix is important in the binding of hematopoietic cells and soluble growth factors to stromal cells so that optimal proliferation and differentiation can occur.[267–270]

With the exception of macrophages, stromal cells appear to be derived from a common mesenchymal stem cell that is distinctly different from the hematopoietic stem cell. In addition to reticular cells, adipocytes, and endothelial cells, the mesenchymal stem cell also produces osteoblasts and muscle cells.[271–274]

Proliferation of hematopoietic stem cells and progenitor cells cannot occur spontaneously but requires the presence of specific hematopoietic growth factors

(HGFs) that may be produced locally in the bone marrow or produced by peripheral tissues and transported to the marrow through the blood (humoral transport). Some HGFs have been called poietins (erythropoietin and thrombopoietin). Other growth factors have been classified as colony stimulating factors (CSFs) based on *in vitro* culture studies. Finally, some HGFs have been described as interleukins.[259,275]

■ ERYTHROPOIESIS

Rubriblasts are continuously generated from progenitor cells in the extravascular space of the bone marrow. The division of a rubriblast initiates a series of approximately four divisions over a period of 3 or 4 days to produce about 16 metarubricytes, which are no longer capable of division (Fig. 31).[276]

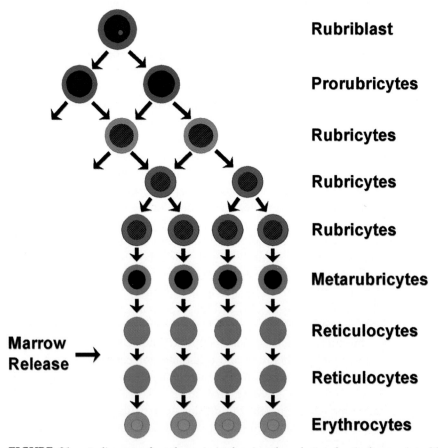

FIGURE 31.   A diagram of erythropoiesis showing the release of reticulocytes into blood as it normally occurs in dogs. (Modified from Meyer DJ, Harvey JW: Veterinary Laboratory Medicine. Interpretation and Diagnosis, 2nd ed. WB Saunders, Philadelphia, PA, 1998, with permission.)

Early precursors have intensely blue cytoplasm when stained with Romanowsky-type blood stains, owing to the presence of many basophilic ribosomes and polyribosomes that are actively synthesizing globin chains and smaller amounts of other proteins. As these cells divide and mature, overall cell size decreases, N:C ratio decreases, nuclear chromatin condensation increases, cytoplasmic basophilia decreases, and hemoglobin progressively accumulates, imparting a red coloration to the cytoplasm. Cells with both red and blue coloration are described as having polychromatophilic cytoplasm. An immature erythrocyte, termed a reticulocyte, is formed following extrusion of the metarubricyte nucleus.

Reticulocyte maturation begins in the bone marrow and is completed in the peripheral blood and spleen in dogs, cats, and pigs.[17] Reticulocytes become progressively more deformable as they mature, a characteristic that facilitates their release from the marrow. Relatively immature aggregate-type reticulocytes are released from dog and pig bone marrow.[17] Reticulocytes are generally not released from bone marrow of normal cats until reticulocytes mature to punctate-type reticulocytes; consequently, few or no aggregate reticulocytes (<0.5%), but up to 10% punctate reticulocytes, are found in blood from normal adult cats.[24] Reticulocytes normally undergo maturation to mature erythrocytes in the bone marrow of horses and ruminants. Reticulocytes may be released into the blood in ruminants in response to anemia, but this rarely occurs in anemic horses.[11]

■ LEUKOPOIESIS

Neutrophils

Neutrophilic cells within the bone marrow can be included in two pools. The proliferation and maturation pool (mitotic pool) includes myeloblasts, promyelocytes, and myelocytes. Approximately four or five divisions occur over several days. During this time, primary (magenta-staining) cytoplasmic granules are produced in late myeloblasts or early promyelocytes and specific (secondary) granules are synthesized within myelocytes. These primary granules have been referred to as azurophilic granules for many years, but they do not really appear blue (azure); rather, they appear magenta (reddish purple) in color. Once nuclear indentation and condensation become apparent, precursor cells are no longer capable of division (Fig. 32). The maturation and storage pool (postmitotic pool) includes metamyelocytes, bands, and segmented neutrophils. Cells within this pool normally undergo maturation and storage for several more days prior to the migration of mature neutrophils through the vascular endothelium and into the circulation.[277]

Eosinophils and Basophils

Eosinophil production in marrow parallels that of neutrophils. The marrow transit time is a week or less, with a significant storage pool of mature eosino-

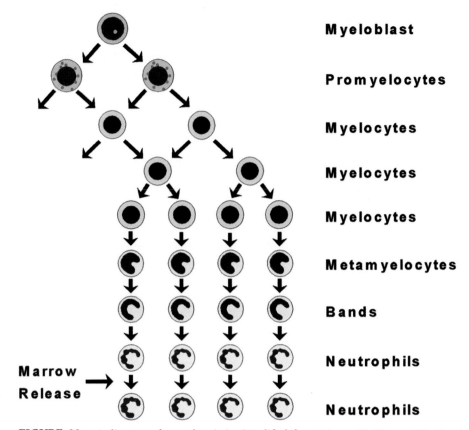

FIGURE 32. A diagram of granulopoiesis. (Modified from Meyer DJ, Harvey JW: Veterinary Laboratory Medicine. Interpretation and Diagnosis, 2nd ed. WB Saunders, Philadelphia, PA, 1998, with permission.)

phils.[278] Basophils and eosinophils appear to share a common marrow progenitor cell that gives rise to precursors specific for each lineage.[279] Eosinophil and basophil precursors become recognizable at the myelocyte stage when their characteristic secondary granules appear. It is unclear whether basophils and mast cells share a common progenitor cell. In contrast to basophils, which mature in the bone marrow, maturation of mast cell progenitors into mast cells occurs in the tissues.[280]

Monocytes

Less time is required to produce monocytes than granulocytes, and there is little marrow reserve of monocytes. Monocytes are not end-stage (finished) cells but enter the tissues to become macrophages.[259]

Lymphocytes

The lymphoid stem cell gives rise to B-lymphocyte progenitor and T/NK progenitor cells, and the T/NK progenitor cell gives rise to T-lymphocyte progenitor and natural killer (NK) progenitor cells. B-lymphocyte progenitors produce B lymphocytes in the marrow in most mammals. B lymphocytes migrate to the cortex in lymph nodes, into follicles in jejunal Peyer's patches, and into follicles of the spleen in mammals.[281]

T-lymphocyte progenitors leave the marrow and migrate to the thymus, where they develop into T lymphocytes under the influence of the thymic microenvironment. After maturation in the thymus, T lymphocytes accumulate within paracortical areas of lymph nodes, periarteriolar lymphoid sheaths of the spleen, and the interfollicular areas of jejunal Peyer's patches in mammals. NK cells are primarily produced and undergo maturation in the bone marrow, but NK progenitor cells are also present in the thymus.[282]

■ THROMBOPOIESIS

Blood platelets in mammals are produced from multinucleated giant cells in bone marrow called megakaryocytes.[283] Beginning with the megakaryoblast, 3 to 5 nuclear reduplications occur without cell division, resulting in 8 to 32 sets of chromosomes in mature megakaryocytes. Individual nuclei can be observed following the first two reduplications (promegakaryocytes), but a large polylobulated nucleus is seen when mature megakaryocytes are formed (Fig. 33). Cell volume increases with each reduplication; consequently, megakaryocytes are much larger than all other marrow cells, except osteoclasts. The cytoplasm in promegakaryocytes is intensely basophilic. There is a progressive decrease in basophilia and increase in granularity as megakaryocytes mature.

Megakaryocytes either lie just outside a vascular sinus or compose part of the wall of a sinus. Cylinders of cytoplasm from megakaryocytes form and extend into sinuses. These beaded-appearing proplatelets eventually fragment into individual platelets within the sinuses and general circulation.[17]

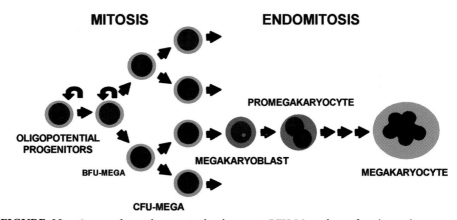

FIGURE 33. Stages of megakaryocyte development. BFU-Mega, burst-forming unit-megakaryocyte; CFU-Mega, colony-forming unit-megakaryocyte. (Modified from Meyer DJ, Harvey JW: Veterinary Laboratory Medicine. Interpretation and Diagnosis, 2nd ed. WB Saunders, Philadelphia, PA, 1998, with permission.)

CHAPTER 7

Bone Marrow Examination

■ REASONS TO EXAMINE BONE MARROW

Bone marrow evaluation is indicated when peripheral blood abnormalities are detected. The most common indications are persistent neutropenia, unexplained thrombocytopenia, poorly regenerative anemia, or a combination thereof. Examples of proliferative abnormalities in which bone marrow examination may be indicated include persistent thrombocytosis or leukocytosis, abnormal blood cell morphology, or the unexplained presence of immature cells in blood (e.g., nucleated erythroid cells in the absence of polychromasia or a neutrophilic left shift in the absence of inflammation).

Bone marrow is sometimes examined to stage neoplastic conditions (lymphomas and mast cell tumors); estimate the adequacy of body iron stores; evaluate lytic bone lesions; and search for occult disease in animals with fever of unknown origin, unexplained weight loss, and unexplained malaise. Bone marrow examination can also be useful in determining the cause of a hyperproteinemia when it occurs secondarily to multiple myeloma, lymphoma, leishmaniasis, and systemic fungal diseases. It may also reveal the cause of a hypercalcemia when associated with lymphoid neoplasms, multiple myeloma, or metastatic neoplasms to bone.

Bone marrow aspirate biopsies are done more frequently than core biopsies in veterinary medicine. Aspirate biopsies are easier, faster, and less expensive to perform than are core biopsies. Bone marrow core biopsies require special needles that cut a solid core of material, which is then placed in fixative, decalcified, embedded, sectioned, stained, and examined microscopically by a pathologist. Core biopsy sections provide a more accurate way of evaluating marrow cellularity and examining for metastatic neoplasia than do aspirate smears, but cell morphology is more difficult to assess.

■ BONE MARROW ASPIRATE TECHNIQUE

There are few contraindications for a bone marrow aspiration biopsy. Restraint, sedation, and anesthesia (when used) generally provide more risks to the patient than the biopsy procedure itself. Postbiopsy hemorrhage is a potential complication in patients with hemostatic diatheses, but it rarely occurs. Hemorrhage may occur after the biopsy of animals with monoclonal hyperglobulinemias, but it is easily controlled by placing a suture in the skin incision and applying pressure over the biopsy site. Postbiopsy infection is also a potential complication, but it is highly unlikely if proper techniques are used.

The usefulness of bone marrow aspirate cytology as a diagnostic aid depends on the proper collection of the bone marrow sample and preparation of high-quality marrow smears. In most cases, only local anesthesia is needed for needle biopsies. Tranquilization is sometimes used in patients that resist positioning by manual restraint. Biopsy sites are prepared by clipping the hair and scrubbing the skin with antiseptic soap preparations. A local anesthetic is injected under the skin and down to the periosteum overlying the site to be biopsied, and a small skin incision is made with a scalpel blade to facilitate passing the needle through the skin. Sterile needles and gloves are always used.

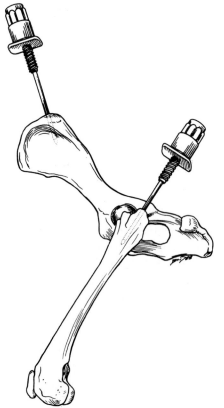

FIGURE 34. Bone marrow biopsy site for the iliac crest and proximal femur. (From Grindem CB: Bone marrow biopsy and evaluation. Vet Clin N Am Small Anim Pract 19:669–696, 1989, with permission.)

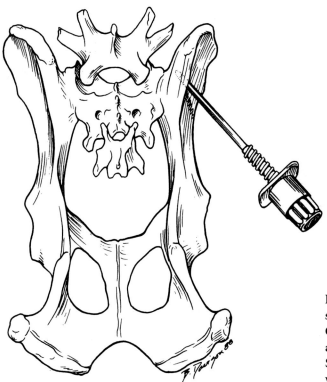

FIGURE 35. Bone marrow biopsy site for the wing of the ilium. (From Grindem CB: Bone marrow biopsy and evaluation. Vet Clin N Am Small Anim Pract 19:669–696, 1989, with permission.)

If general anesthesia is required for other procedures, bone marrow aspiration may be scheduled at the same time to minimize the stress on the animal.

The biopsy needle used to aspirate marrow must have a removable stylet, which remains in place until the marrow cavity is entered to prevent obstruction of the needle lumen with cortical bone. A 16- or 18-gauge needle (Rosenthal, Illinois sternal, or Jamshidi) that is between 1 and 1.5 inches long is satisfactory (Fig. 37A).

Young animals have active (red) marrow throughout most skeletal bones. Active marrow recedes from long bones as adulthood is reached, because the bone marrow space expands faster than the blood volume as the animal grows.[284] Once animals quit growing, blood cell numbers must be maintained, but increased production to accommodate growth is no longer required. As hematopoietic cells disappear, the marrow space is replaced by fat (yellow marrow) and is in a resting state. Hematopoietic cells may expand back into long bones if needed, such as might occur in response to anemia.

Active marrow remains in the flat bones (vertebrae, sternum, ribs, and pelvis) and proximal ends of the humerus and femur in adults.[284] The iliac crest is often used as a site to biopsy marrow in dogs and cats.[284,285] The biopsy needle is positioned so that it enters the greatest prominence of the iliac crest parallel to the long axis of the wing of the ileum (Fig. 34). The wing of the ileum may also be aspirated at the central depression of the wing caudal and ventral to the iliac crest (Fig. 35). For small cats and toy breeds of dogs, in

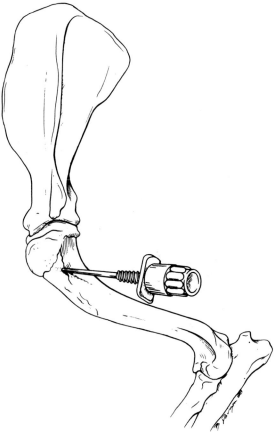

FIGURE 36. Bone marrow biopsy site for the proximal humerus. (From Grindem CB: Bone marrow biopsy and evaluation. Vet Clin N Am Small Anim Pract 19:669–696, 1989, with permission.)

which the ilium is especially thin, marrow may be aspirated from the head of the proximal femur by way of the trochanteric fossa (Fig. 34).[284,285] Aspiration of marrow from the anterior side of the proximal end of the humerus is another popular site, especially in obese patients.[285] The greater tubercle is palpated, and the needle is inserted into the flat area on the craniolateral surface of the proximal humerus distal to the tubercle (Fig. 36). In large dogs, the third, fourth, or fifth sternebra can be biopsied.[284] Biopsies of the sternum have the risk of inadvertent penetration of the thorax and damage to structures in the thoracic cavity. A short biopsy needle (preferably with an adjustable guard) should be used, and care should be taken to remain in the center of these bones to minimize the risk of pneumothorax, uncontrolled hemorrhage, or cardiac laceration. Although there is also some risk to the person collecting sternal biopsies from large animals, the sternum is the preferred site for collecting high-quality biopsies from horses. The dorsal ends of the ribs may be used for bone marrow aspirates in large animals, although the bone is generally difficult to penetrate with the biopsy needle in adults.[286,287] There is also a risk of pneumothorax or uncontrolled hemorrhage when ribs are biopsied.[288] The tuber coxae may be used as a site for bone marrow collection in young horses, but adequate marrow samples cannot usually be obtained from this site in adult horses, because of a lack of active marrow.[287] Biopsies may be taken from other sites if specific lesions are identified using diagnostic imaging.

To enter the marrow space, moderate pressure is applied to the needle (with the stylet locked in place) as the needle is rotated in an alternating clockwise-counterclockwise motion. Once the needle is firmly embedded into the bone, it is usually within the marrow cavity. The stylet is then removed and a 12-mL or 20-mL syringe is attached to the needle. Vigorous negative pressure should be applied by rapidly pulling the plunger back as far as possible. As soon as a few drops of blood appear in the syringe, the negative pressure is released, and the complete assembly is rapidly removed for smear preparation. If marrow does not appear in the syringe, the stylet is replaced, and the needle is repositioned for another aspiration attempt.

If no anticoagulant is used in the syringe, smears must be prepared within seconds after bone marrow collection, because bone marrow clots rapidly. We prefer to collect bone marrow into a syringe that contains several drops of 5% EDTA as an anticoagulant. Although smears need not be made immediately, they should be prepared within minutes after collection, because bone marrow cells (especially granulocytic cells) degenerate rapidly. After mixing the aspirated marrow with the anticoagulant, it is expelled into a petri dish. It is important for accurate bone marrow evaluation that smears contain marrow particles (stroma and associated cells). Marrow particles appear as small white grains in the blood-contaminated aspirate material. They are collected by pipette (Fig. 37B) and placed on one end of a glass slide, which is then held vertically (Fig. 37C). Particles tend to stick to the slide while blood runs off. A second glass slide is placed across the area of particle adherence, perpendicular to the first slide. After marrow spreads between the slides (Fig. 37D), they are pulled apart in the horizontal plane. Resultant smears are rapidly air dried. The same concentrating and smear techniques may be used in marrow that has been collected without an anticoagulant.

Bone marrow aspirate preparations from dead animals are usually of poor quality. Once clots have formed, cells will be lysed during aspiration and smear preparation. If marrow is to be collected from an animal that is to be euthanized, it is recommended that the animal is anesthetized with an intravenous barbiturate for marrow collection and then given the euthanasia solution.

Smears are stained with a Romanowsky-type blood stain such as Wright, Giemsa, or a combination thereof. Satisfactory results can usually be obtained with the Diff-Quik stain, a rapid, modified Wright stain. The appropriate staining time(s) for the stain(s) being used is determined with experience. Thicker smears will require longer staining times. About twice the time is required for staining bone marrow smears compared to blood films. Smears containing marrow particles will have blue-staining material on them, which is visible grossly (Fig. 37E). When examined microscopically, particles contain blood cell precursors and stromal elements (Fig. 37F). Fat is dissolved away during alcohol fixation, but it is represented in particles by the presence of variably sized, unstained circular areas.

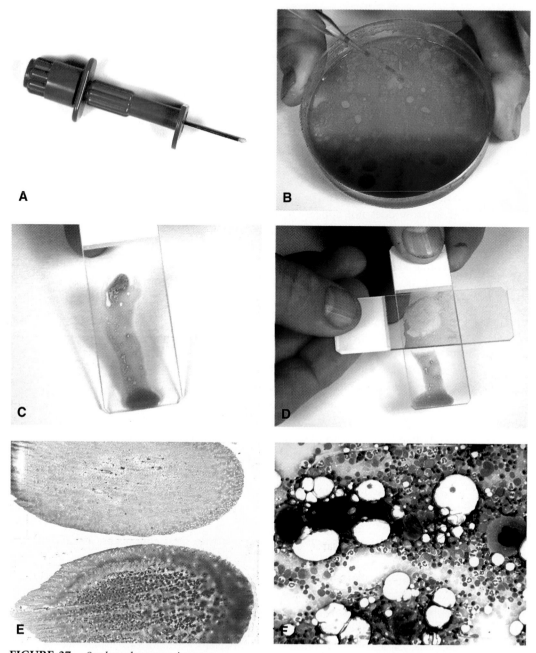

FIGURE 37.   *See legend on opposite page.*

If adequate smears are available, one smear should be stained using the Prussian blue procedure for iron. Additional special stains may be needed to help differentiate the type of leukemia when present.

BONE MARROW CORE BIOPSY TECHNIQUE

Core biopsies are essential if there are repeated dry taps (e.g., failures to collect marrow particles by aspiration). Dry taps may be the result of technical error, but they sometimes occur when the marrow is packed with cells (as when a leukemia is present), and they usually occur when myelofibrosis is present. Dry taps, or poor-quality samples, are common when marrow aspirates are attempted on very young animals, even though the marrow is generally highly cellular. Core biopsy sections provide a more accurate way of evaluating marrow cellularity and examining for myelofibrosis, granulomatous diseases involving bone marrow, and metastatic neoplasia than do aspirate smears.[289]

Preparation of the animal and the biopsy site for a bone marrow core biopsy is the same as that described for an aspirate biopsy. Core biopsies require the use of special needles, which are designed to cut a solid core of material. Eleven- to thirteen-gauge Jamshidi bone marrow biopsy needles that are three to four inches long are used in our veterinary hospital (Fig. 38A). Depending on the species and size of the animal, core biopsies may be taken from the wing of the ilium, head of the humerus, or sternum. Core and aspirate biopsies should be taken from distantly located sites (preferably different bones) to ensure that one biopsy does not result in disruption of the area where the other biopsy is being collected. The collection of two separate sites should also increase the likelihood of identifying a tumor metastasis.[289]

With the stylet locked in place, moderate pressure is applied to the needle as it is rotated in an alternating clockwise-counterclockwise motion. Once the needle is firmly embedded into the bone, the stylet is removed and the needle is advanced using the same clockwise-counterclockwise motion. If possible, the

FIGURE 37.   **Bone marrow aspiration needle, steps in preparing bone marrow aspirate smears, and the gross and microscopic appearance of stained aspirate smears.**   A.   An 18-gauge Illinois bone marrow aspiration needle with stylet in place and adjustable guard to limit the depth of penetration. B.   A bone marrow aspirate collected using EDTA as an anticoagulant was expelled into a petri dish. A pipette was then used to collect particles to be used in preparing marrow smears.   C.   Bone marrow particles collected from a petri dish were expelled onto one end of a glass slide that was then held vertically. Particles tend to stick to the slide while contaminating blood runs off.   D.   A second glass slide was placed across the area of particle adherence, perpendicular to the first slide. The slides were held together, causing bone marrow to spread between them, and then they were rapidly pulled apart in the horizontal plane and air dried.   E.   Two stained bone marrow smears are shown. The scant blue-staining material in the top smear indicates that only a few small marrow particles are present. The abundant blue-staining material in the bottom smear indicates that a large amount of particulate bone marrow is present. Wright-Giemsa stain.   F.   Normal bone marrow aspirate smear from a dog. Variably sized unstained circular areas indicate where fat was dissolved away during alcohol fixation. The large cells present are megakaryocytes. Wright-Giemsa stain.

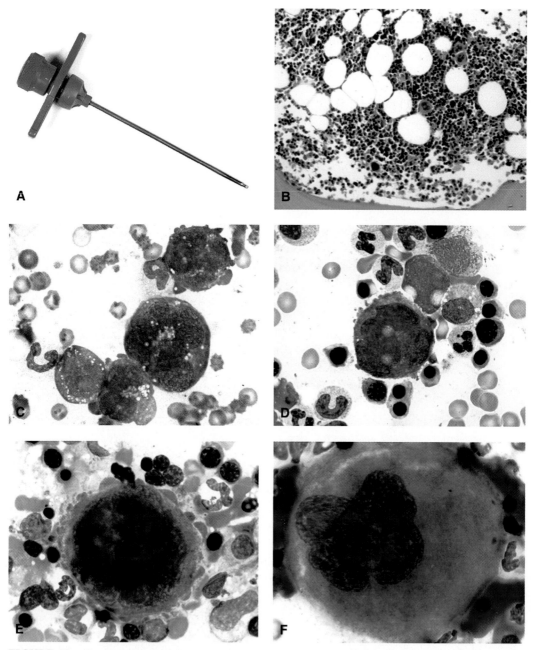

FIGURE 38.   *See legend on opposite page.*

needle should be advanced one inch or more to get sufficient material for evaluation. Once the needle has been advanced to its maximal depth, several 360-degree twists are made and it is withdrawn. The core within the needle is pushed out using a wire that accompanies the needle. This is done by placing the wire in the tip of the needle and forcing the core out of the handle end of the needle. The tip of the needle is tapered, and pushing the core out through the tip would add crush artifacts to the core.

Because core biopsy needles are larger than aspirate biopsy needles, the wing of the ilium is generally too thin in cats to collect a core sample parallel to its long axis, as is typically done in dogs. However, core biopsies may be collected in cats by making two or three perpendicular punch biopsies completely through the most dorsal aspect of the wing of the ilium.

If bone marrow aspirate attempts have resulted in dry taps or poor-quality smears, the core biopsy may be gently rolled across a glass slide using the tip of the needle and stained in the same manner as aspirate smears. These roll preparations are generally of lower quality than aspirate smears. In particular, the number of megakaryocytes and amount of stainable iron present are generally under represented. After one or more roll preparations are made, the core is placed in fixative and submitted to a surgical pathology service where it is decalcified, embedded, sectioned, stained with hematoxylin and eosin (H&E), and possibly other stains, and examined microscopically by a pathologist (Fig. 38B). Fixatives other than formalin are sometimes preferred; consequently, the surgical pathology service should be consulted prior to sample collection. Unstained aspirate smears or other exfoliative cytology preparations should not be mailed in the same package with formalin-fixed tissue, because the formalin vapors will interfere with the staining quality of cells in the cytologic preparations.

FIGURE 38.   Bone marrow core biopsy needle, low-power image of a normal bone marrow core biopsy section, and various stages of megakaryocyte development in aspirate smears.   A. An 11-gauge Jamshidi core bone marrow biopsy needle with stylet in place.   **B.** Low-power image of a normal bone marrow core biopsy from a dog. The bone marrow core biopsy has been fixed, decalcified, sectioned, and stained with hematoxylin and eosin (H&E). Pink-staining trabecular bone is present at the bottom. Variably sized unstained circular areas indicate where fat was dissolved away during fixation. The large cells present are megakaryocytes.   **C.** Megakaryoblast with single nucleus (bottom left), promegakaryocyte with two nuclei (bottom center), promegakaryocyte with four nuclei (top right), and a megakaryocytic cell with six nuclei that may be considered intermediate between a promegakaryocyte and a basophilic megakaryocyte in bone marrow from a dog. Wright-Giemsa stain.   **D.** Promegakaryocyte with four nuclei surrounded by smaller myeloid and erythroid precursors in bone marrow from a dog. Wright-Giemsa stain.   **E.** Basophilic megakaryocyte with blue cytoplasm and multiple fused nuclei in bone marrow from a dog. Wright-Giemsa stain.   **F.** Mature megakaryocyte with magenta granules in the cytoplasm in bone marrow from a dog. Multiple fused nuclei are present. Figures 38C through 38F are taken at the same magnification to demonstrate the enlargement that occurs as megakaryocytes develop. Wright-Giemsa stain.

■ MORPHOLOGIC IDENTIFICATION OF CELLS

This discussion will primarily focus on the morphologic appearance of cells in aspirate smears stained with Wright-Giemsa, but examples of core biopsy sections stained with H&E will also be presented. Marrow particles appear as blue-staining areas in aspirate smears when viewed grossly (Fig. 37E). When examined microscopically, they contain blood cell precursors, vessels, reticular cells, macrophages, and plasma cells (Fig. 37F). Fat is dissolved away during alcohol fixation, but it is represented in particles by the presence of variably sized unstained circular areas. Most particles in normal animals are composed of one third to two thirds cells (Figs. 37F, 38B).

Megakaryocytic Series

Megakaryoblasts are the earliest recognizable cell in this series. They have a single nucleus and deeply basophilic cytoplasm (Fig. 38C). This cell type is not recognized in most normal aspirate smears, because it occurs in small numbers and is difficult to differentiate from other blast cells. Promegakaryocytes, which have two or four nuclei and deeply basophilic cytoplasm, are easily recognized (Figs. 38C, 38D). These cells are much larger than leukocytes or nucleated erythroid precursor cells. Subsequent nuclear reduplications result in progressively larger basophilic megakaryocytes (Fig. 38E). Nuclei in basophilic megakaryocytes are joined into a lobulated mass, making it difficult to count the number of nuclear reduplications that have occurred. The synthesis of magenta-staining cytoplasmic granules imparts a pink color to the cytoplasm characteristic of mature (granular) megakaryocytes (Fig. 38F). Megakaryocytes are gigantic and vary from 50 to 200 μm in diameter, with larger cells having greater nuclear ploidy.

Erythrocytic Series

Morphologic changes that occur as cells of the erythroid series undergo maturation include diminution in size, decrease in N:C ratio, progressive nuclear condensation, and the appearance of red cytoplasmic color as hemoglobin is synthesized and accumulates within the cytoplasm (Fig. 39).

Rubriblasts. The earliest recognizable cell type in the erythroid series is the rubriblast. They are relatively large cells with high N:C ratios and intensely basophilic cytoplasm, resulting from the presence of many polyribosomes. The nucleus of the rubriblast is usually nearly perfectly round and the chromatin is finely granular, containing one or two pale-blue to medium-blue nucleoli (Fig. 40A).

Prorubricytes. When nucleoli are no longer visible and slightly coarser chromatin clumping is present, the cell is classified as a prorubricyte (Fig. 40B). The N:C ratio is generally slightly less than in rubriblasts.

(text continued on page 105)

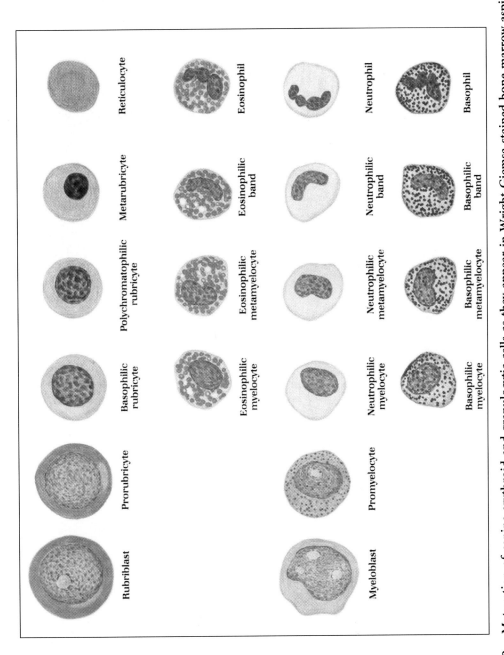

FIGURE 39. Maturation of canine erythroid and granulocytic cells as they appear in Wright-Giemsa-stained bone marrow aspirate smears. Drawing by Dr. Perry Bain. (From Meyer DJ, Harvey JW: Veterinary Laboratory Medicine. Interpretation and Diagnosis, 2nd ed. WB Saunders, Philadelphia, PA, 1998, with permission.)

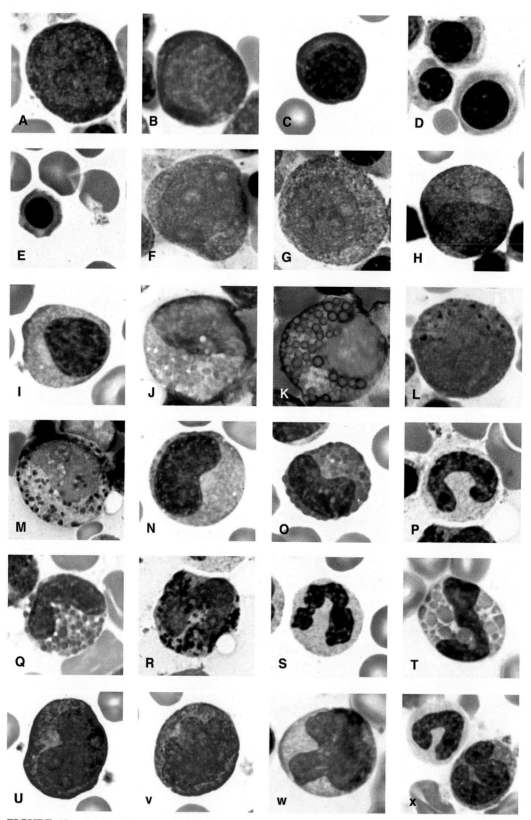

FIGURE 40. *See legend on opposite page.*

Basophilic Rubricytes.   The next cell type in the erythroid series is the basophilic rubricytes. These cells still have blue cytoplasm, but they are smaller than
prorubricytes, have lower N : C ratios, and have nuclear condensation into light
and dark areas, giving the nucleus a cartwheel appearance (Fig. 40C).

Polychromatophilic Rubricytes.   The combined presence of hemoglobin (red)
and ribosomes (blue) account for the reddish blue cytoplasm characteristic of
polychromatophilic rubricytes. They also tend to be smaller than basophilic
rubricytes and have more nuclear condensation (Fig. 40D). A low number of
rubricytes in horses and cats may have red cytoplasm (normochromic rubricytes) similar to mature cells.

Metarubricytes.   The most mature nucleated erythroid cell type is the small
metarubricyte (Fig. 40E). Its nucleus is dark (pyknotic), with few or no clear
areas, and its cytoplasm is usually polychromatophilic but may be normochromic.

**FIGURE 40.   Erythroid, granulocytic, and monocytic precursor cells from bone marrow aspi-
rate smears stained with Wright-Giemsa.   A.**   Rubriblast with intensely basophilic cytoplasm in
bone marrow from a dog. The nucleus has finely clumped chromatin and contains at least two circular
nucleoli.   **B.**   Prorubricyte with intensely basophilic cytoplasm and finely clumped nuclear chromatin in
bone marrow from a cat. Nucleoli are not seen.   **C.**   Basophilic rubricyte with blue-staining cytoplasm
and coarsely clumped nuclear chromatin in bone marrow from a dog.   **D.**   Three polychromatophilic
rubricytes with bluish red (polychromatophilic) cytoplasm and coarsely clumped nuclear chromatin in bone
marrow from a dog.   **E.**   Metarubricyte with polychromatophilic cytoplasm and a pyknotic nucleus (left)
and a polychromatophilic erythrocyte (reticulocyte) formed after nuclear extrusion (right) in bone marrow
from a dog.   **F.**   Myeloblast with blue cytoplasm lacking visible granules in bone marrow from a dog.
The nucleus has finely clumped chromatin and contains three circular nucleoli.   **G.**   Promyelocyte with
blue cytoplasm containing many magenta-staining granules in bone marrow from a dog. The nucleus has
finely clumped chromatin and contains three nucleoli or nuclear rings.   **H.**   Promyelocyte with blue
cytoplasm containing many magenta-staining granules in bone marrow from a dog. The nucleus has finely
clumped chromatin with no nucleoli or nuclear rings visible.   **I.**   Neutrophilic myelocyte with blue
cytoplasm and a round nucleus exhibiting moderately clumped chromatin in bone marrow from a dog.
Neutrophilic granules do not stain.   **J.**   Eosinophilic myelocyte with a round nucleus and large numbers
of eosinophilic granules in the cytoplasm in bone marrow from a dog.   **K.**   Eosinophilic myelocyte from
a horse with a round nucleus and many large round granules in the cytoplasm.   **L.**   Basophilic
myelocyte with a round nucleus and a few purple granules in the cytoplasm in bone marrow from a dog.
M.   Basophilic myelocyte with a round nucleus and a mixture of purple and light-lavender granules in the
cytoplasm in bone marrow from a cat. The light lavender granules overlying the nucleus give it a "moth-
eaten" appearance.   **N.**   Neutrophilic metamyelocyte with blue cytoplasm and a kidney-shaped nucleus
in bone marrow from a dog. Neutrophilic granules do not stain.   **O.**   Eosinophilic metamyelocyte with a
kidney-shaped nucleus and eosinophilic granules in the cytoplasm in bone marrow from a dog.   **P.**
Band neutrophil with light-blue cytoplasm in bone marrow from a dog. Neutrophilic granules do not stain.
Q.   Band eosinophil with eosinophilic granules in the cytoplasm in bone marrow from a dog.   **R.**
Band basophil with purple granules in the cytoplasm in bone marrow from a dog.   **S.**   Mature
neutrophil with light-pink granules in bone marrow from a dog.   **T.**   Mature eosinophil in bone
marrow from a dog.   **U.**   Monoblast with basophilic cytoplasm and kidney-shaped nucleus containing
nucleoli in bone marrow from a dog.   **V.**   Presumptive promonocyte with convoluted nucleus and
basophilic cytoplasm in bone marrow from a dog.   **W.**   Monocyte with convoluted nucleus in bone
marrow from a dog.   **X.**   Monocyte (bottom) and band neutrophil (top) in bone marrow from a dog.
This image is of lower magnification than the other images in this figure.

Polychromatophilic Erythrocytes (Reticulocytes).   When the metarubricyte nucleus is lost, a reticulocyte is formed. Those formed from polychromatophilic metarubricytes will appear as polychromatophilic erythrocytes (Fig. 40E). Continued hemoglobin synthesis and loss of ribosomes result in the formation of mature erythrocytes with red-staining cytoplasm.

Granulocytic Series

Morphologic changes that occur as cells of the granulocytic series undergo maturation include slight diminution in size, decrease in N:C ratio, progressive nuclear condensation, changes in nuclear shape, and the appearance of cytoplasmic granules. The background (i.e., nongranular) cytoplasm color changes from gray-blue to light blue to nearly colorless in the progression from myeloblasts to mature granulocytes (Fig. 39).

Myeloblasts.   The first recognizable cells in the granulocytic series are called myeloblasts. Type I myeloblasts appear as large round cells with round to oval nuclei, which are generally centrally located in the cell. The N:C ratio is high (>1.5) and the nuclear outline is usually regular and smooth (Fig. 40F). Nuclear chromatin is finely stippled, containing one or more nucleoli or nucleolar rings. The cytoplasm is generally moderately basophilic (gray-blue in color) and not as dark as that in rubriblasts. Primary granules begin to form in late myeloblasts; consequently, some of these cells may contain a few (<15) small, magenta-staining granules in the cytoplasm. Such cells may be classified as type II myeloblasts.[236]

Promyelocytes (Progranulocytes).   Once large numbers of magenta-staining, primary granules are visible within the cytoplasm, the cell is classified as a promyelocyte or progranulocyte. Although nucleoli or nucleolar rings may be seen in some promyelocytes (Fig. 40G), others exhibit no evidence of nucleolar structures (Fig. 40H). Promyelocytes may be somewhat larger than myeloblasts because of their more abundant cytoplasm.

Myelocytes.   Primary, magenta-staining granules characteristic of promyelocytes are no longer visualized in myelocytes, and secondary granules that characterize neutrophils, eosinophils, and basophils appear at this stage. Myelocytes still have round nuclei, but they are generally smaller with more nuclear condensation and have lighter-blue cytoplasm than promyelocytes. It is difficult to visualize the secondary granules within neutrophilic myelocytes because of their neutral staining characteristics (Fig. 40I). Eosinophilic myelocytes and basophilic myelocytes are identified by their characteristic granules (Figs. 40J–40M). Eosinophil granules are generally round, except in the cat, where they are rod-shaped. Cat basophilic myelocytes are also distinctive, having a mixture of dark-purple and light-lavender round to oval granules that typically fill the cytoplasm (Fig. 40M).

Metamyelocytes.   Once nuclear indentation and condensation become readily apparent, precursor cells are no longer capable of division. Precursors with kidney-shaped nuclei are called metamyelocytes (Figs. 40N, 40O). Nuclei with slight indentations extending less than 25% into the nucleus are still classified as myelocytes. Like myelocytes, the granules may be neutrophilic, eosinophilic, or basophilic in staining characteristics.

Band Cells. Cells with thinner rod-shaped nuclei with parallel sides are called bands (Figs. 40P–40R). No area of the nucleus has a diameter less than two-thirds the diameter of any other area of the nucleus. Band cell nuclei twist to conform to the space within the cytoplasm, and horseshoe or s-shaped nuclei are common.

Segmented Granulocytes. The final stage in granulocyte development is the segmented or mature granulocyte. The nuclear membrane is no longer smooth and the nuclear width becomes irregular and segments into two or more lobes in these cells (Fig. 40S). The nuclear chromatin is moderately to densely clumped and the background cytoplasm is often colorless but may appear faintly blue or faintly pink in neutrophils. Nuclei of eosinophils and basophils are generally less segmented than are the nuclei of neutrophils, and specific granules can be identified in their cytoplasm (Fig. 40T).

Monocytic Series

The monocytic series consists of monoblasts, promonocytes, and monocytes. They account for a small percentage of total marrow cells and cannot be reliably differentiated from early granulocytic cells, except for promyelocytes, which have numerous magenta-staining granules. Monoblasts resemble myeloblasts, except that their nuclear shape is irregularly round to convoluted in appearance (Fig. 40U). Promonocytes are similar in appearance to myelocytes and metamyelocytes (Fig. 40V). Monocytes in bone marrow are identical to those seen in peripheral blood (Figs. 40W, 40X).

Macrophages

Macrophages are large cells with abundant cytoplasm and nuclei that are round to oval in shape with finely clumped chromatin (Fig. 42A). The cytoplasm of macrophages generally contains vacuoles and phagocytized material such as pyknotic nuclear debris, hemosiderin, and, rarely, erythrocytes and leukocytes. Hemosiderin in macrophages appears gray to black when stained with routine blood stains. Although nucleated erythrocyte precursors develop around central macrophages in the marrow, these erythroblastic islets are rarely seen in aspirate smears (Figs. 42B, 42C) because they are easily disrupted during aspiration and smear preparation.

Lymphocytes

Lymphopoiesis normally occurs in bone marrow; consequently, low numbers of lymphoblasts and prolymphocytes may be present, but they are difficult to

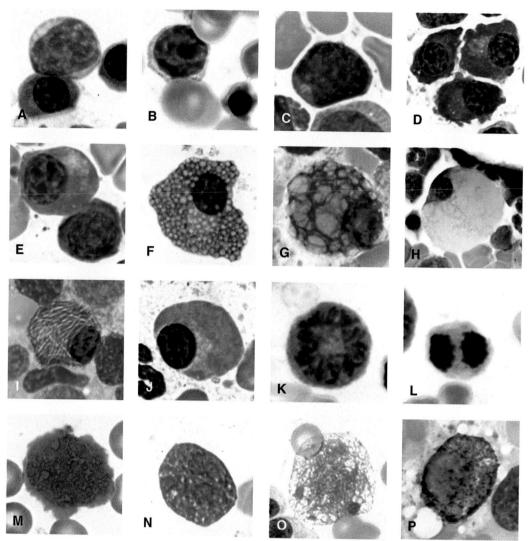

FIGURE 41. **Lymphocytes, plasma cells, mitotic cells, free nuclei, and a mast cell from bone marrow aspirate smears stained with Wright-Giemsa.**   **A.** A small lymphocyte (top) and a polychromatophilic rubricyte (bottom) in bone marrow from a horse.   **B.** A small lymphocyte (top left) and metarubricyte (bottom right) in bone marrow from a dog.   **C.** A prolymphocyte or reactive lymphocyte in bone marrow from a dog.   **D.** Three plasma cells with voluminous deeply basophilic cytoplasm, eccentric nuclei, and pale Golgi zones in their cytoplasm in bone marrow from a dog. The nuclei exhibit coarse chromatin clumping in a mosaic pattern. This image is of lower magnification than the other images in this figure.   **E.** A plasma cell (top) and basophilic rubricyte (bottom) in bone marrow from a dog.   **F.** A plasma cell containing large numbers of small bluish inclusions (Russell bodies) within the cytoplasm in bone marrow from a dog.   **G.** A plasma cell containing large bluish inclusions (Russell bodies) within the cytoplasm in bone marrow from a dog.   **H.** A plasma cell with cytoplasm filled with turquoise-staining material in bone marrow from a dog.   **I.** A plasma cell with cytoplasm filled with blue-staining needlelike inclusions in bone marrow from a dog.   **J.** A plasma cell with reddish cytoplasm in bone marrow from a dog with multiple myeloma. Many plasma cells stained similarly in the bone marrow of this animal.   **K.** Large mitotic cell in the bone marrow of a dog.   **L.** Mitotic cell in the bone marrow of a dog. Based on size and cytoplasmic color, this is probably a

(Continued)

differentiate from rubriblasts and prorubricytes. Most marrow lymphocytes are small, with morphology identical to that seen in blood (Figs. 41A, 41B), although reactive lymphocytes may also be present (Fig. 41C).

Plasma Cells

Plasma cells are larger, have a lower N : C ratio, and have greater cytoplasmic basophilia than resting lymphocytes (Figs. 41D, 41E). The presence of a prominent Golgi apparatus may create a pale perinuclear area (Golgi zone) in the cytoplasm. They typically have eccentrically located nuclei with coarse chromatin clumping in a mosaic pattern. Plasma cells may rarely contain pinkish or bluish inclusions (Russell bodies) within the cytoplasm (Figs. 41F–41I). These inclusions are composed of dilated rough endoplasmic reticulum containing immunoglobulin and other glycoproteins.[11,290] This appears to result from a defect in processing or transport of these proteins.[290] Plasma cells filled with Russell bodies have been called Mott's cells. The cytoplasm of some plasma cells stains reddish, especially at the periphery of the cell. These plasma cells have been called flame cells (Fig. 41J).[291,292]

Osteoclasts

Osteoclasts are multinucleated giant cells that phagocytize bone. When observed in histologic sections, they lie next to bony surfaces (Fig. 42D). Osteoclasts may be confused with megakaryocytes; however, the nuclei present in osteoclasts are clearly separate (Fig. 42E), in contrast to the fused nuclear material present in megakaryocytes. The cytoplasm stains blue and often contains variably sized magenta-staining granular material associated with the removal and digestion of bone (Fig. 42F). Osteoclasts are rarely seen in marrow aspirates from adult animals, but they may be present in disorders in which lysis of bone is increased, such as the hypercalcemia of malignancy.[293] Osteoclasts are consistently found in aspirates from young growing animals in which bone remodeling is active.

Osteoblasts

Osteoblasts are relatively large cells with eccentric nuclei and foamy basophilic cytoplasm (Figs. 43A, 43B). A clear area (Golgi zone) may be visible in the central part of the cytoplasm. Superficially, osteoblasts appear similar to plasma cells, but they are larger and have less-condensed nuclear chromatin. Osteoblast nuclei are round to oval in shape, have reticular chromatin, and may have one

---

polychromatophilic rubricyte.   **M.**   Reddish staining material is a free nucleus. The blue inclusions are nucleoli.   **N.**   Reddish staining material is a free nucleus with some open spaces. The blue inclusions are nucleoli.   **O.**   Reddish staining material is a free nucleus in which the chromatin is dispersed in a lacelike manner. This appearance has been called a basket cell even though it has no cytoplasm.   **P.** Mast cell with round eccentric nucleus (left part of cell) and purple granules in the cytoplasm in bone marrow from a dog.

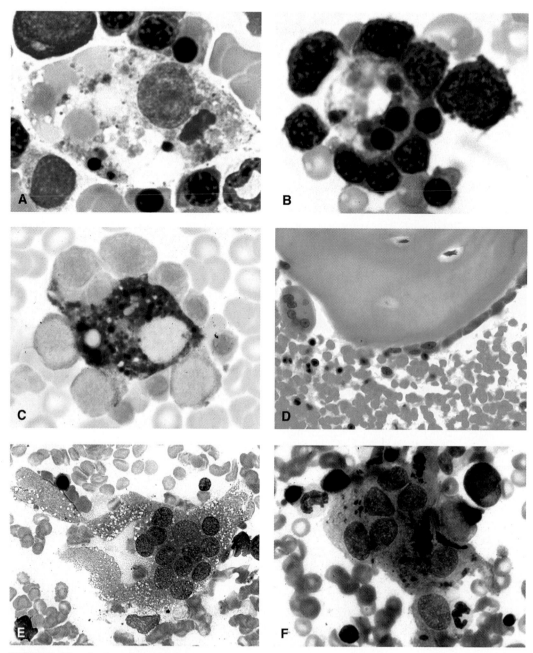

FIGURE 42. *See legend on opposite page.*

or two nucleoli. Osteoblasts generally occur in groups lining trabecular surfaces (Fig. 42D) and tend to remain in small groups when present in aspirate smears (Figs. 43A, 43B).

Mitotic Figures

The bone marrow is actively producing new blood cells at all times, but mitosis itself is a brief part of the cell cycle. Consequently, mitotic cells normally account for less than 2% of all nucleated cells in bone marrow (Figs. 41K, 41L). The origin of some mitotic cells may be identified by the characteristics of the cytoplasm, for example, presence of granules or hemoglobin (Figs. 41L, 43C).

Miscellaneous Cells and Free Nuclei

Vascular and connective tissue cells are usually ruptured during aspiration and smear preparation, although low numbers of intact cells may occasionally be seen (Figs. 43D, 43E). Stromal cells are more obvious in aplastic bone marrow aspirates in which normal blood cell precursors are markedly reduced or absent (Fig. 43F). Ruptured stromal cells account for some of the free nuclei found in bone marrow smears (Figs. 41M–41O). Free nuclei also come from various other bone marrow cells, especially in smears made from clotted marrow, in thin smears, or in thin areas of smears where excess forces have destroyed the cells. Free nuclei from metarubricytes have been called hematogones. The term "basket cell" has been used to refer to free nuclei in which the chromatin is dispersed in a lacelike manner (Fig. 41O).

Adipocytes vary in size and number in bone marrow. Although normal marrow contains many adipocytes, these cells readily rupture during sample collection and smear preparation. Adipocytes appear as large vacuoles in marrow particles after the fat has been removed during smear fixation (Figs. 38F, 43F).

FIGURE 42.   Bone marrow macrophages with phagocytized material surrounded by developing erythroid cells (erythroblastic islets) and osteoclasts.   A. Macrophage with erythrophagocytosis in bone marrow from a dog. The cytoplasm also contains nuclear debris and gray-staining material consistent with hemosiderin. Wright-Giemsa stain.   **B.** Erythroblastic island in bone marrow aspirate from a cat. A central macrophage with phagocytized material is surrounded by developing nucleated erythroid cells. Pale spots in some erythrocytes are Heinz bodies. Wright-Giemsa stain.   **C.** Erythroblastic island in bone marrow aspirate from a dog. A central macrophage with phagocytized red-staining nuclear material is surrounded by developing nucleated erythroid cells. The cytoplasm of the macrophage stains dark blue, indicating the presence of large amounts of hemosiderin. Prussian blue stain.   **D.** Osteoclast (multinucleated cell on left) and osteoblasts (line of adjacent cells on right) along trabecular bone in a core bone marrow biopsy from a dog with generalized marrow hypoplasia secondary to severe chronic ehrlichiosis. H&E stain.   **E.** Multinucleated osteoclast in bone marrow aspirate from a dog. Wright-Giemsa stain.   **F.** Multinucleated osteoclast in bone marrow aspirate from a dog. The magenta-staining granular material in the cytoplasm results from the phagocytosis and digestion of bone. Wright-Giemsa stain.

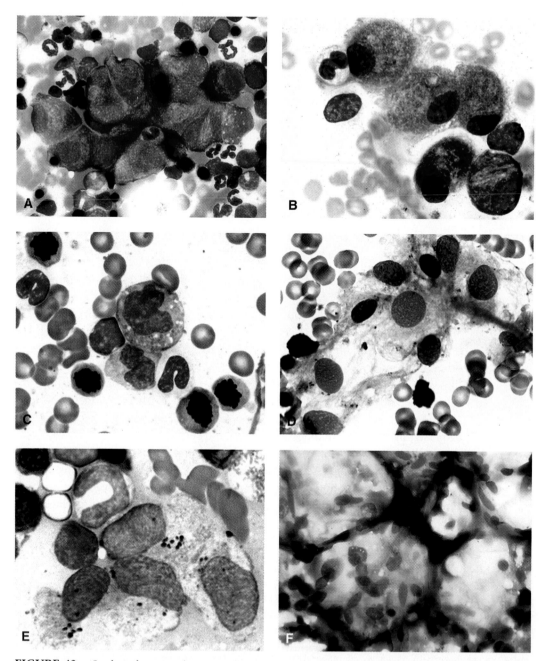

FIGURE 43.   *See legend on opposite page.*

Mast cell precursors are produced in the bone marrow, but mature mast cells are rarely seen in normal bone marrow.[196] Mast cells are round cells with round nuclei. They typically have large numbers of purple granules in the cytoplasm (Fig. 41P).

ORGANIZED APPROACH TO BONE MARROW EVALUATION

Smears and core biopsy sections should be scanned with low-power objectives to gain an appreciation of the overall cellularity and determine the adequacy of megakaryocyte numbers. Normal marrow appears heterogenous. If some or all of the marrow smear or core section appears homogenous, an abnormal population of cells is probably present. Regional infiltrates of neoplastic cells are more easily appreciated in core sections than in aspirate smears.

As a general rule, erythroid precursors are smaller, have more nearly spherical nuclei with more condensed nuclear chromatin, and have darker cytoplasm than do granulocyte precursors at similar maturation stages. Consequently, smaller and darker cells, observed by scanning marrow smears at low power, are usually erythroid precursors (unless lymphocytes are increased in numbers), and the larger, paler cells are usually granulocyte precursors. Identification of specific cell types is more difficult in core biopsy sections compared to aspirate smears; consequently, sections may be stained with Giemsa and PAS, in addition to H&E, in an attempt to identify cell types present.

Complete 500 cell differential cell counts from several normal domestic animal species are given (Table 3) to provide information concerning the normal distribution of cells. The time required to perform such counts (up to 1 hour) precludes their use in clinical practice. Either a modified differential count may be performed or mental estimates concerning the distribution of cells may be done. Because veterinary students and residents are trained in our laboratory and information from our cases may be published, we routinely perform a modified differential as shown in Appendix 1. Others may categorize cells into groups and use the values to calculate an erythroid maturation index (EMI) and myeloid maturation index (MMI).[81] Trained professionals, who regularly examine bone marrow aspirate smears, typically examine the bone

FIGURE 43. Osteoblasts, mitotic rubricytes, and stromal cells in bone marrow aspirate smears stained with Wright-Giemsa. **A.** Large clump of osteoblasts with eccentric nuclei and voluminous cytoplasm in bone marrow from a dog. **B.** Five osteoblasts with eccentric nuclei and voluminous cytoplasm in bone marrow from a dog. **C.** Four mitotic polychromatophilic erythroid cells are present in bone marrow from a dog 6 hours after an intravenous vincristine treatment. The largest cell in the center is an eosinophilic metamyelocyte. **D.** Spindle-shaped stromal cells with "wispy" cytoplasm in bone marrow from a dog. **E.** Four spindle-shaped stromal cells with elongated nuclei and cytoplasmic granules in bone marrow from a dog. **F.** Residual stroma with three plasma cells (below and left of center) in bone marrow from a dog with aplastic anemia secondary to severe chronic ehrlichiosis. Variably sized unstained circular areas indicate where fat was dissolved away during alcohol fixation. The black-staining material is hemosiderin.

TABLE 3	Bone Marrow Differential Cell Counts in Some Domestic Animal Species			
CELL TYPE	DOGS (n=6)	CATS (n=7)[a]	HORSES (n=4)[a]	CATTLE (n=3)[a]
Myeloblast	0.4–1.1	0–0.4	0.3–1.5	0–0.2
Promyelocyte	1.1–2.3	0–3.0	1.0–1.9	0–1.4
Neutrophilic myelocyte	3.1–6.1	0.6–8.0	1.9–3.2	2.8–3.4
Neutrophilic metamyelocyte	5.3–8.8	4.4–13.2	2.1–7.3	2.8–6.2
Neutrophilic band	12.7–17.2	12.8–16.6	6.8–14.7	4.6–8.4
Neutrophil	13.8–24.2	6.8–22.0	9.6–21.0	11.2–22.6
Total eosinophilic cells	1.8–5.6	0.8–3.2	2.8–6.8	2.8–3.8
Total basophilic cells	0–0.8	0–0.4	0–1.5	0–1.0
Rubriblast	0.2–1.1	0–0.8	0.6–1.1	0–0.2
Prorubricyte	0.9–2.2	0–1.6	1.0–2.0	0.4–1.2
Basophilic rubricyte	3.7–10.0	1.6–6.2	4.5–11.1	4.8–8.4
Polychromatophilic rubricyte	15.5–25.1	8.6–23.2	14.7–26.0	23.0–36.4
Metarubricyte	9.2–16.4	1.0–10.4	11.4–19.7	9.2–16.8
M:E ratio	0.9–1.76	1.21–2.16	0.52–1.45	0.61–0.97
Lymphocytes	1.7–4.9	11.6–21.6	1.8–6.7	3.6–6.0
Plasma cells	0.6–2.4	0.2–1.8	0.2–1.8	0.2–1.2
Monocytes	0.4–2.0	0.2–1.6	0–1.0	0.4–2.2
Macrophages	0–0.4	0–0.2	0	0–0.8

[a] Values for cats, horses, and cattle from Jain 1993,[11] n = number of animals evaluated.

marrow in a systematic manner, make a number of judgments based on their knowledge of the normal appearance of bone marrow, and record their finding in narrative form as presented here.

Cellularity

The cellularity of bone marrow is estimated by examining the proportion of cells versus fat present in particles (Figs. 44A, 44B). If the particles are composed of more than 75% cells, the marrow is interpreted as hypercellular (Figs. 44C, 44D), and if the particles are composed of more than 75% fat, the marrow is interpreted as hypocellular (Figs. 44E, 44F). Unfortunately, the cellularity of the marrow is not uniform. Some marrow particles may have normal or high cellularity and others may have low cellularity on the same smear, because of patchy differences in cellularity (Figs. 45A–45C). Obviously, the more particles one can evaluate, the more likely it will be that the estimate of the overall marrow cellularity will be accurate. If few or no particles are present on smears, it is not possible to accurately estimate the marrow cellularity.

The overall cellularity of bone marrow decreases with age.[294,295] The marrow is highly cellular in young growing animals where cells must be produced not only to compensate for normal cell turnover but also in response to growth of the cardiovascular system. Marrow cellularity decreases with age, because the ratio of bone marrow space to blood volume increases.

Marrow can become hypercellular when one or more cell types exhibit increased proliferation in response to peripheral needs, such as occurs in response to anemia (erythroid hyperplasia) or purulent inflammation (granulocytic hyperplasia). The marrow may also become hypercellular secondary to dysplastic or neoplastic proliferations of marrow cells or from infiltration of neoplastic cells from peripheral tissues (e.g., a metastatic lymphoma). Defects in either progenitor cells or the bone marrow microenvironment necessary for their survival and proliferation can result in hypocellular marrow, as will be presented in a subsequent section.

Megakaryocytes

The frequency and morphology of megakaryocytes should be evaluated by scanning the preparation at low power. Most large particles should have several associated megakaryocytes (Fig. 45D), and normally a majority of megakaryocytes are of the granular, mature type. Megakaryocytes are not evenly distributed in bone marrow; consequently, it is not possible to have definitive guidelines for estimates of megakaryocyte numbers in bone marrow aspirate smears. If only a few megakaryocytes are seen examining several particles, the numbers are probably low. If 10 to 20 are seen per field using the 10x objective, the numbers are likely increased.[285] Abnormal megakaryocyte morphology (e.g., increased numbers of promegakaryocytes or the presence of dwarf megakaryocytes) should be noted when present.

Erythroid Cells

The maturation and morphology of the erythroid series should be evaluated to determine if it is complete (frequent polychromatophilic erythrocytes should be present) and orderly. There is generally a progressive increase in numbers with each stage of development, from low numbers of rubriblasts (generally less than 1%) to high numbers of polychromatophilic rubricytes, which may account for one quarter of all nucleated cells in the bone marrow.[11] Metarubricytes are numerous but generally not as numerous as polychromatophilic rubricytes.

Rubriblasts and prorubricytes usually do not exceed 5% of all nucleated cells. If the proportion of these immature cells is increased, this finding should be noted. An increase in mature as well as immature cells of the erythroid series is expected in response to anemia. If immature erythroid cells are increased and later stages are not, it suggests a proliferative abnormality is present. Additional abnormal morphologic findings that should be recorded when present include megaloblastic cells, frequent binucleated cells, and pleomorphic nuclei.

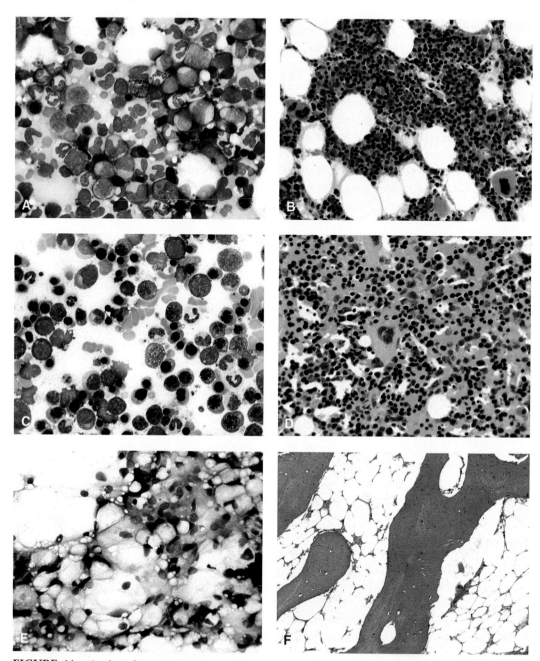

FIGURE 44.   *See legend on opposite page.*

Because reticulocytes are rarely released into blood in response to anemia in horses, reticulocyte counts can be done in bone marrow aspirates from horses to assist in the differential diagnosis of anemia. Greater than 5% reticulocytes suggests a regenerative response to anemia.[287]

Granulocytic Cells

The distribution of granulocytic cells should be evaluated to determine whether the series is complete (i.e., a normal number of mature granulocytes are present) and orderly. There is generally a progressive increase in numbers with each stage of development, from low numbers of myeloblasts (often less than 1%) to high numbers of mature neutrophils, which may account for nearly one quarter of all nucleated cells in the bone marrow.[11] Myeloblasts and promyelocytes generally do not exceed 5% of all nucleated cells. If the proportion of these immature cells is increased, this finding should be noted. An increase in mature as well as immature cells of the myeloid series is expected in inflammatory disorders resulting in granulocytic hyperplasia. If immature granulocytic cells are increased and later stages are not, it indicates either that more mature cells have been depleted in the marrow granulocyte pool, as occurs in acute inflammation, or that a proliferative abnormality is present.[286] Morphologic abnormalities such as large cell size and vacuolated cytoplasm should be reported when present.

Total eosinophilic cells generally account for less than 6% of all nucleated cells in the marrow, with basophilic precursors usually accounting for less than 1% of all nucleated cells. Increased representation of eosinophilic or basophilic series should be recorded. An increase in one or both of these cell lines is usually associated with inflammatory conditions that result in increased numbers of eosinophils or basophils in blood and/or tissues. They may also be increased in association with some myeloproliferative disorders.

FIGURE 44. Normal, increased, and decreased overall cellularity in bone marrow aspirate smears and core biopsy sections.   A. Normal overall cellularity in a bone marrow aspirate smear from a horse; however, no megakaryocytes are visible in this field. The unstained circular areas represent adipocytes dissolved away during alcohol fixation. Wright-Giemsa stain.   B. Normal overall cellularity in a bone marrow section from a core biopsy collected from the same horse as the aspirate shown in Figure 44A. The unstained circular areas represent adipocytes dissolved away during fixation. Low magnification with H&E stain.   C. Increased cellularity, primarily resulting from erythroid hyperplasia, in a bone marrow aspirate smear from a horse with hemolytic anemia that may have been secondary to a lymphoid neoplasm. The M:E ratio was 0.16. Wright-Giemsa stain.   D. Increased cellularity in a bone marrow section from a core biopsy collected from the same horse as the aspirate shown in Figure 44C. The large cell near the center is a megakaryocyte. Clear areas indicate a small amount of fat was present. Low magnification with H&E stain.   E. Low cellularity in a bone marrow aspirate smear, consisting primarily of stromal cells and fat, from a cat with an aplastic anemia following chemotherapy for an ocular lymphoma. Wright-Giemsa stain.   F. Low cellularity in a bone marrow core biopsy section collected from the same cat as the aspirate shown in Figure 44E. The red-staining material is trabecular bone. Low magnification with H&E stain.

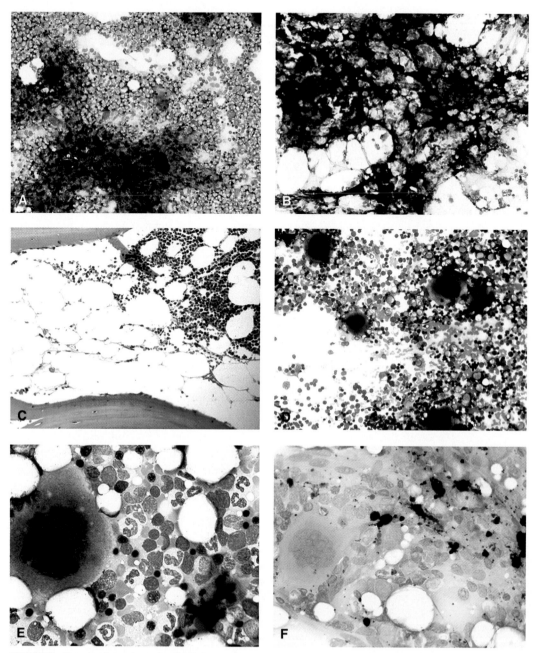

FIGURE 45.   *See legend on opposite page.*

TABLE 4	Normal Myeloid to Erythroid Ratios in Some Domestic Animal Species	
SPECIES	RANGE	MEAN
Dog	0.75–2.53	1.25
Cat	1.21–2.16	1.63
Horse	0.50–1.50	0.93
Cattle	0.31–1.85	0.71
Sheep	0.77–1.68	1.09
Pig	0.73–2.81	1.77

Values from Jain 1993.[11]

Myeloid to Erythroid Ratio

A myeloid to erythroid (M : E) ratio (also referred to as a granulocytic to erythroid ratio) is calculated by examining 500 cells and dividing the number of granulocytic cells, including mature granulocytes, by the number of nucleated erythroid cells. Alternately, this ratio may be estimated by experienced professionals. Normal M : E ratios in some domestic animals are given in Table 4. Dilution of a bone marrow aspirate with blood can result in a falsely high M : E ratio, especially if a substantial neutrophilia is present in blood.

Lymphocytes

Specific comments should be made about the number and morphology of lymphocytes. Small lymphocytes generally account for less than 10% of all nucleated cells in normal animals, but they may reach 14% in some healthy dogs[81,296] and 20% in some healthy cats.[11,295] Low numbers of lymphoblasts and prolymphocytes may be present, but they are difficult to differentiate from rubriblasts and prorubricytes. Increased numbers of mature lymphocytes may be seen in animals with chronic lymphocytic leukemias and in disorders with cell-mediated immune responses.[297] Although highly unlikely, increased num-

---

FIGURE 45. Variable cellularity in bone marrow and the appearance of megakaryocytes and hemosiderin in marrow particles. **A.** High cellularity of a particle present in a bone marrow aspirate smear from dog with ehrlichiosis. Wright-Giemsa stain. **B.** Low cellularity in a different particle present in the same bone marrow aspirate smear as shown in Figure 45A. Wright-Giemsa stain. **C.** Variable cellularity in a section from a bone marrow core biopsy collected from the same dog as the aspirate particles shown in Figures 45A and 45B. H&E stain. **D.** Five megakaryocytes are visible in a bone marrow aspirate particle from a dog. Wright-Giemsa stain. **E.** Bone marrow from a dog with hemosiderin visible as black globules in the bottom right. A mature megakaryocyte is present at the left edge. Wright-Giemsa stain. **F.** Bone marrow aspirate from a dog with hemosiderin visible as blue-staining material. A mature megakaryocyte is present at the left edge. Prussian blue stain.

bers of small lymphocytes may also be present in a smear if a bone marrow lymphoid follicle is aspirated. Lymphoid follicles occur in both normal and diseased animals.[298,299]

Increased numbers of prolymphocytes and/or lymphoblasts suggest the presence of either acute lymphoblastic leukemia or a metastatic lymphoma. Glucocorticoid treatment results in the movement of recirculating lymphocytes from blood to bone marrow,[300,301] but the percentage of lymphocytes in the marrow does not appear to increase,[300,302] possibly because glucocorticoids can concomitantly decrease the population of proliferating lymphocytes normally present within the marrow.[300]

Plasma Cells

Plasma cells tend to be concentrated within particles on bone marrow smears. This uneven distribution prevents accurate counting. They are generally present in low numbers (<2% of all nucleated cells). When plasma cells exceed 3% of total nucleated cells, they are considered to be increased. In addition to multiple myeloma, increased numbers of plasma cells can occur in bone marrow in disorders in which immune stimulation is present (e.g., ehrlichiosis or leishmaniasis) and is associated with myelodysplasia in dogs.[303]

Mononuclear Phagocytes

Monocytes and their precursors comprise a small portion (<3%) of bone marrow cells. They are difficult to differentiate from early granulocytic cells. Increased numbers of monocyte precursors may be present in response to inflammatory conditions, but the occurrence of high numbers of monoblasts indicates that a myeloproliferative disorder is present.

Macrophages generally do not exceed 1% of total nucleated cells present in the bone marrow of normal animals. Prominent phagocytosis of nucleated and/or anucleated erythrocytes by macrophages may occur in association with primary or secondary immune-mediated anemias,[304] malignant histiocytosis, the hemophagocytic syndrome,[305] and acquired and congenital dyserythropoiesis.[43,306,307] Prominent leukophagocytosis is rare but may be seen in association with immune-mediated neutropenia[308] and when increased marrow apoptosis is present, as occurs in myeloproliferative disorders.[309] Macrophages may contain phagocytized cellular debris in response to marrow necrosis.[310,311] Macrophages can phagocytize damaged or dead cells not coated with antibody or complement because of the presence of scavenger receptors on their surfaces that are capable of recognizing altered carbohydrate and/or phospholipid moieties.[312]

Macrophages may be increased in the bone marrow in both inflammatory and neoplastic (malignant histiocytosis) conditions. Infectious agents may be present within macrophages in conditions such as leishmaniasis, histoplasmosis, cytauxzoonosis, and ehrlichiosis.

Other Cells Types

Comments should always be made concerning the cell types listed above, if only to report that they are present in normal numbers with normal morphology. Comments are generally only made concerning cell types listed below when they are present in increased numbers.

Mitotic figures are increased when the proportion of cells undergoing replication in the bone marrow is increased. Mitotic figures may be somewhat increased in myeloid or erythroid hyperplasia, but they are more consistently increased in acute myelocytic and acute lymphoblastic leukemias. Dramatically increased numbers of mitotic erythroid cells occur within the first few hours after the administration of vincristine (Fig. 43C)[313] and increased numbers of mitotic figures have been reported in animals with congenital dyserythropoiesis.[43,100]

Osteoclasts and osteoblasts are commonly seen in bone marrow aspirates of young growing animals but rarely seen in normal adult animals. Increased numbers of osteoclasts and osteoblasts may be seen in adult animals when bone remodeling is increased, such as in disorders of calcium metabolism and in association with osteogenic sarcoma.

Mast cells are rarely seen in bone marrow from normal domestic animals[196] but may occur in dogs with aplastic anemia of various etiologies.[314] They may also be present in some inflammatory conditions. The administration of interleukin-3 and interleukin-6 together, but neither factor alone, results in marrow mast cell development in rats.[315] Mast cells may occur in the marrow of animals with metastatic mast cell tumors. Bone marrow involvement is especially likely in noncutaneous systemic mastocytosis.[316-319]

Increased numbers of reticular stromal cells suggests that stromal hyperplasia and/or myelofibrosis is present. A core biopsy is essential to confirm these suspicions.

Metastatic cells from nonhematopoietic sarcomas or carcinomas are rarely recognized in bone marrow biopsies but should be reported when present.

Stainable Iron

Hemosiderin appears gray to black when stained with routine blood stains. It may be seen within macrophages or as free material from ruptured macrophages (Fig. 45E). The amount of hemosiderin present is routinely evaluated as the amount of stainable iron observed using the Prussian blue reaction. Stainable iron is easily found in normal marrow aspirates from most domestic mammals, as long as particles are present (Fig. 45F). It is decreased or absent in iron-deficient animals (Fig. 46A), including dogs with polycythemia,[298] and may be increased in association with all anemias (Fig. 46B), except those resulting from hemorrhage. Bone marrow iron increases in horses with age; consequently, normal old horses can have marked amounts of stainable iron present in the marrow (Fig. 46C). Likewise, the amount of stainable iron tends to

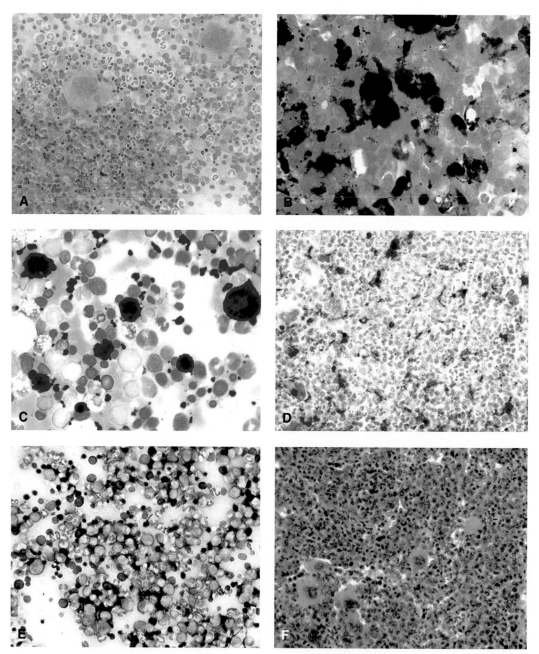

FIGURE 46. *See legend on opposite page.*

increase in canine bone marrow with age.[81] Normal cat bone marrow does not exhibit stainable iron, so its absence cannot be used to confirm a diagnosis of iron deficiency. The presence of stainable iron is considered an abnormal finding in cats and may be detected in some animals with myeloproliferative disorders (Figs. 46D–46F) or hemolytic anemias, or after blood transfusions.[131,297]

Interpretation

The final step in evaluating a bone marrow aspirate is to provide an interpretation of the cytologic findings in light of the history, clinical findings, CBC, and results from other diagnostic tests and procedures. For example, a high M:E ratio could indicate the presence of either increased granulocytic cells or decreased erythroid cells. Examination of CBC results from blood collected at the same time, as well as an estimate of the overall cellularity, usually allows the correct interpretation to be made. Bone marrow examination generally provides information concerning the pathogenesis of abnormalities recognized in blood and sometimes a specific diagnosis can be made.

FIGURE 46. Lack of stainable iron in bone marrow from a dog with iron-deficiency anemia and increased stainable iron in bone marrow from a dog with hemolytic anemia, an aged horse, and a cat with myelodysplastic syndrome (MDS).   **A.** Lack of stainable iron (hemosiderin) in a bone marrow aspirate from a dog with chronic iron-deficiency anemia. Two megakaryocytes are visible in the upper portion of the image. Prussian blue stain.   **B.** Increased stainable iron (blue-staining material) in a bone marrow aspirate from a dog with a hemolytic anemia. Prussian blue stain.   **C.** A large amount of stainable iron (blue-staining material) is present in a bone marrow aspirate from a normal aged horse. Prussian blue stain.   **D.** Prominent stainable iron (blue-staining material) in a hypercellular postmortem bone marrow section collected from a cat with MDS. Several megakaryocytes are present along the edge of the image. Prussian blue stain.   **E.** Generalized hypercellularity in an aspirate smear of bone marrow from the same cat with MDS as presented in Figure 46D. A left shift in both granulocytic and erythroid series is present. Wright-Giemsa stain.   **F.** Generalized hypercellularity in a postmortem bone marrow section from the same cat with MDS as presented in Figures 46D and 46E. Several megakaryocytes are present in the left corner and central area of the image. H&E stain.

CHAPTER 8

Disorders of Bone Marrow

■ GENERALIZED INCREASES IN HEMATOPOIETIC CELLS

The marrow is highly cellular in young growing animals where cells must be produced not only to compensate for normal cell turnover but also in response to growth of the cardiovascular system. Marrow cellularity decreases with age, because the ratio of bone marrow space to blood volume increases.

Marrow can become hypercellular when one or more cells exhibit increased proliferation in response to peripheral needs or demands. For example, both erythrocytic and granulocytic cell lines may be increased in autoimmune hemolytic anemia in dogs in which animals often exhibit a regenerative anemia, with accompanying leukocytosis and left shift.[320] Megakaryocytic hyperplasia can also occur if immune-mediated thrombocytopenia is present. Although rare, generalized marrow hyperplasia may occur in response to cytopenias in blood resulting from hypersplenism.[69,321] Generalized hypercellular marrow may be present in some animals with myelodysplastic disorders, but abnormalities in cell morphology and/or distributions are present (Figs. 46E, 46F). Primary erythrocytosis (polycythemia vera) may sometimes exhibit a generalized marrow hyperplasia.[298,322]

■ GENERALIZED DECREASES IN HEMATOPOIETIC CELLS

Hypocellular/Aplastic Bone Marrow

When more than 75% of the marrow sample from an adult animal is composed of fat, it is considered to be hypocellular. When all hematopoietic cell types, erythrocytic, granulocytic, and megakaryocytic, are markedly reduced or absent, the marrow is said to be aplastic and anemic animals with generalized marrow aplasia are reported to have aplastic anemia (Figs. 47A, 47B). Stromal cells (adipocytes, reticular cells, endothelial cells, and macrophages), plasma cells, and some lymphocytes are still present in aplastic bone marrow samples (Fig. 47C). Macrophages typically contain increased amounts of hemosiderin,

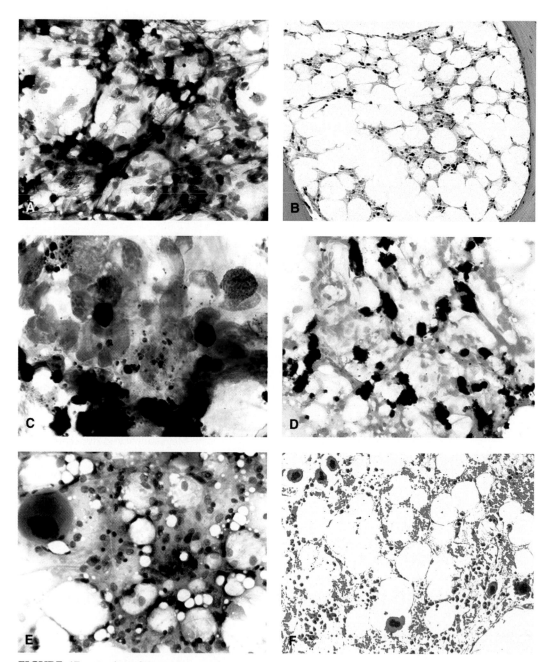

FIGURE 47. *See legend on opposite page.*

because storage iron is not utilized for erythrocyte production (Figs. 47C, 47D). Mast cells may also be present in moderate numbers in aplastic bone marrow samples in dogs (Fig 47C).[314] The peripheral blood is characterized by nonregenerative anemia, neutropenia, and thrombocytopenia.

When only one cell line is reduced or absent, more restrictive terms, such as granulocytic hypoplasia or erythroid aplasia are used to describe the abnormalities present. Hypocellular or aplastic bone marrow may result from insufficient numbers of stem cells, abnormalities in the hematopoietic microenvironment, or abnormal humoral or cellular control of hematopoiesis. These factors are interrelated, and the exact defect in a given disorder is usually unknown.

Many drugs have been incriminated in the production of aplastic anemia in humans.[323] Drug-induced causes of aplastic anemia or generalized marrow hypoplasia in animals include estrogen toxicity in dogs,[324–326] phenylbutazone toxicity in dogs[326,327] and possibly a horse,[328] trimethoprim-sulfadiazine administration in dogs,[326,329] bracken fern poisoning in cattle and sheep,[330,331] trichloroethylene-extracted soybean meal in cattle,[332] albendazole toxicity in dogs and cats,[333] griseofulvin toxicity in cats,[334,335] various cancer chemotherapeutic agents,[321,336–338] and radiation.[339–341] Thiacetarsamide,[342] meclofenamic acid,[326] and quinidine[326] have also been incriminated as potential causes of aplastic anemia in dogs.

Exogenous estrogen injections can result in aplastic anemia in dogs, as can high levels of endogenous estrogens produced by Sertoli cell, interstitial cell, and granulosa cell tumors.[343–346] Functional cystic ovaries also have the potential of inducing myelotoxicity in dogs.[347] Ferrets have induced ovulations and may remain in estrus for long periods of time when not bred. This prolonged exposure to high endogenous estrogen concentrations can result in aplastic anemia.[348,349]

Parvovirus infections can cause erythroid hypoplasia, as well as myeloid hypoplasia in canine pups,[350,351] but animals may not become anemic because of the long life spans of erythrocytes. Thrombocytopenia is mild or absent, because megakaryocytes are still present in the bone marrow (Figs. 47E, 47F). Either affected pups die acutely or the bone marrow returns rapidly to normal

FIGURE 47. Hypocellular bone marrow aspirate smears and core biopsy sections from dogs. A. Generalized hypocellularity in an aspirate smear of bone marrow from a dog with estrogen-induced aplastic anemia. Stromal cells and fat predominate. The circular purple objects are mast cells and the black globular material is hemosiderin. Wright-Giemsa stain.   **B.** Generalized hypocellularity in a section from a bone marrow core biopsy collected from a dog with an idiopathic aplastic anemia. H&E stain.   **C.** Purple-staining mast cells (top) and brown to black-staining hemosiderin in the same aspirate smear of bone marrow collected from a dog with estrogen-induced aplastic anemia as presented in Figure 47A. Wright-Giemsa stain.   **D.** Blue-staining hemosiderin in an aspirate smear of bone marrow from the same dog with estrogen-induced aplastic anemia as presented in Figures 47A and 47C. Prussian blue stain. **E.** Hypocellular bone marrow aspirate smear from a leukopenic dog with acute parvovirus infection. Stromal cells and fat predominate, but a megakaryocyte is present (upper left). Wright-Giemsa stain.   **F.** Hypocellular section from a bone marrow core biopsy collected from the same leukopenic dog with acute parvovirus infection as presented in Figure 47E. Although granulocytic and erythroid precursors are markedly reduced, normal numbers of megakaryocytes remain. H&E stain.

before anemia can develop. In contrast to its effects in pups, parvovirus is reported to have a minimal effect on erythroid progenitors in adult dogs.[352] Only myeloid hypoplasia was reported during histologic examination of bone marrow from parvovirus infected viremic cats.[353,354]

Although some degree of marrow hypoplasia and/or dysplasia often occurs in cats with feline leukemia virus (FeLV) infections,[355] true aplastic anemia is not a well-documented sequela.[356] Hypocellular bone marrow has been reported in experimental cats co-infected with FeLV and feline parvovirus.[357]

Dogs with acute *Ehrlichia canis* infections may spontaneously recover or develop chronic disease that generally exhibits some degree of marrow hypoplasia. Although rare, aplastic anemia may develop in association with severe chronic ehrlichiosis in dogs.[358,359]

Hypocellular bone marrow has been reported in a dog with splenomegaly and marked extramedullary hematopoiesis, which returned to normal after splenectomy.[84] It was speculated that the spleen might have produced cellular or humoral inhibitors of hematopoiesis in bone marrow.

Congenital aplastic anemia, renal abnormalities, and skin lesions have been reported in newborn foals whose mothers were treated for equine protozoal myeloencephalitis with sulfonamides, pyrimethamine, folic acid, and vitamin E during pregnancy.[360] Aplastic anemia in a 14-day-old Holstein calf may have also developed *in utero*, although the calf was treated for diarrhea with sulfamethazine 5 days before examination.[361] An *in utero* toxic insult was suspected in a 9-week-old Clydesdale foal with aplastic anemia.[362] Generalized bone marrow hypoplasia, with myeloid and megakaryocytic hypoplasia more prominent than erythroid hypoplasia, has been reported in eight young standardbred horses sired by the same stallion.[363] Genetic defects involving the marrow microenvironment, one or more growth factors, or pluripotent stem cells were suggested as possible causes.

Idiopathic aplastic anemia has also been reported in dogs[314,321,364,365] and horses.[288,362,366] One case of erythroid and myeloid aplasia, with normal megakaryocyte numbers, has been reported in a horse, the etiology of which was unknown.[367]

A primary immune-mediated reaction directed against hematopoietic precursor cells has been proposed as a cause of aplastic anemia in dogs.[314] This possibility is supported by evidence that some cases of aplastic anemia in humans are mediated by a T-lymphocyte immune reaction against hematopoietic stem cells.[323,368] Interferons (especially interferon-γ) have antiproliferative effects on hematopoietic progenitor cells and have been postulated to be mediators of hematopoietic suppression in people with aplastic anemia.[315]

Necrosis

Two forms of cell death, necrosis and apoptosis, are recognized. Necrosis refers to a form of cell death and degeneration secondary to the inability of mitochondria to generate sufficient energy in the form of ATP. Cells swell and burst after losing their ability to regulate osmotic balance. A variable inflammatory response occurs secondary to the release of intracellular contents. In contrast, mitochondria function normally in cells undergoing apoptosis (physiologic cell death). The nuclear chromatin condenses, the nucleus rounds up into a single dense sphere (pyknosis) or fragments into multiple dense spheres (karyorrhexis), and the cell shrinks by as much as 30%. Soon after the process is begun, the cell is recognized and phagocytized by macrophages, probably while still alive. Cytoplasmic contents are not shed externally; therefore, there is no spillage of proinflammatory mediators.[369]

Necrosis may be caused by direct damage to the hematopoietic cells or by ischemia that results from injury or disruption of the microcirculation. Necrosis may be recognized antemortem (Fig. 48A), but it is most often recognized when histologic samples are examined postmortem (Figs. 48B, 48C), because it is a transient event that often has a focal distribution.

The appearance of necrosis varies depending on the time course and cause.[370] When histologic sections are examined, initial lesions exhibit altered staining of hematopoietic cells with indistinct cellular outlines.[298] Hemorrhage may also be present if vessels are injured.[370] Later, the areas of necrosis become hypocellular as the cells lyse and are replaced by amorphous granular eosinophilic debris. This stage of necrosis must be differentiated from fibrin, edema, and collection artifact. A Fraser-Lendrum stain for fibrin can be helpful in this regard.[298] Macrophages, many of which contain phagocytized cellular debris, occur in increased numbers. Myelofibrosis occurs subsequently to necrosis, similar to the healing process that occurs in other damaged tissues.[370,371]

Aspirate smears from necrotic marrow may be confused with smears resulting from poor-quality sample collection and staining techniques. Marrow particles may appear elongated and "stringy." [310] The background appears granular and is bluish to purple in color. Cells remaining are difficult to classify because of morphologic changes caused by degeneration (Fig. 48A). Nuclei appear smudged and cytoplasmic margins are usually ill defined. When visible, the cytoplasm is basophilic and sometimes vacuolated.[371,372] Often only free nuclei or nuclear fragments are seen. Macrophages with phagocytized debris are commonly observed.[310,311]

Disorders that have been reported in association with marrow necrosis in animals include septicemia and/or endotoxemia;[310,321] neoplasia (Fig. 48C); [68,298,373] disseminated intravascular coagulation;[83,321,374] experimental drug administration;[310,375] and bovine viral diarrhea[376] and estrogen toxicity,[310,371] acute parvovirus infection,[377] systemic lupus erythematosus,[311] and ehrlichiosis[310] in dogs. The cause of bone marrow necrosis may not be identified.[371,378,379]

Myelofibrosis

Myelofibrosis is suspected when repeated marrow aspiration attempts are unsuccessful or a poor-quality aspirate sample is obtained that contains some spindle-shaped cells (Fig. 48D). A definitive diagnosis can only be made by the examination of histologic sections of bone marrow.

Fibrous tissue consists of variable amounts of actively proliferating fibro-

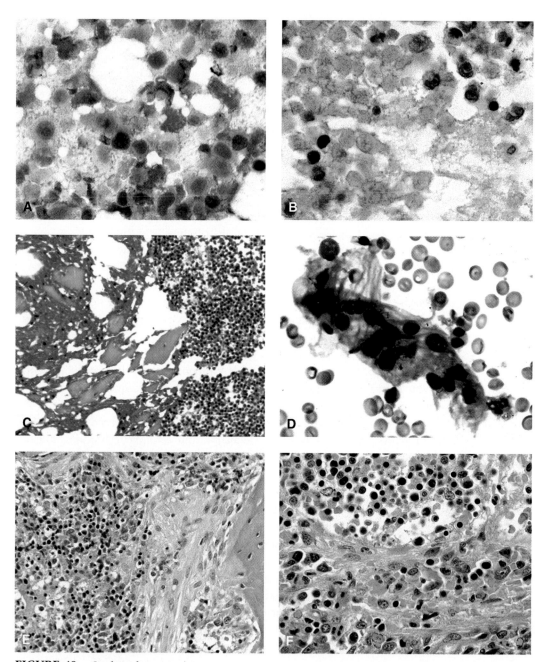

FIGURE 48. *See legend on opposite page.*

blasts, reticulin fibers, and dense collagenous connective tissue.[298] The term myelofibrosis is used when there is an apparent excess of collagen and/or reticulin in bone marrow that is produced by activated and/or proliferating marrow reticular cells.[380] When myelofibrosis is extensive, it is recognized in sections stained with H&E (Figs. 48E, 48F, 49A). In these instances, marrow sections contain little or no fat. Low levels of myelofibrosis may only be recognized using special stains, such as Masson's trichrome stain for collagen (Fig. 49B) and Gomori's stain or Manuel's stain for reticulin.[299,380] Hematopoietic cells may be present in linear arrangements, separated by palely eosinophilic extracellular collagenous material (Fig. 48F). Areas of marked myelofibrosis consist of fibroblasts and extracellular matrix, with no remaining hematopoietic cells (Fig. 49C).

Myelofibrosis appears to be a sequela to marrow injury, including necrosis, vascular damage, inflammation, and neoplasia. It is postulated that these disorders result in the direct or indirect production of growth factors capable of stimulating fibroblasts.[83]

Prominent myelofibrosis has been documented in animals with marrow necrosis,[374] myeloproliferative disorders,[131,299,381,382] lymphoproliferative disorders,[374] and nonmarrow origin neoplasia,[374] and in dogs with inherited pyruvate kinase deficiency.[72,386] It has also been recorded as a result of unknown causes.[83,374,380,383–385] Myelofibrosis has been described in a family of poodles with laboratory and clinical findings similar to pyruvate kinase deficiency,[387] and definitive studies were not performed to eliminate the possibility that these animals had this deficiency as well. Extremely high-pharmacologic doses of recombinant human erythropoietin elicited both marked erythropoiesis and myelofibrosis in experimental dogs, suggesting a possible explanation for the myelofibrosis that accompanies pyruvate kinase deficiency in dogs.[388]

FIGURE 48. Necrosis and fibrosis in bone marrow. **A.** Necrosis in an antemortem bone marrow aspirate smear from a FeLV-negative, pancytopenic cat. The background appears granular and bluish to purple in color and the remaining cells are impossible to classify, because of degenerative changes. Wright-Giemsa stain. **B.** Necrosis in a postmortem bone marrow section from the same cat presented in Figure 48A. The circular pink areas represent necrotic cells in which the nucleus is no longer visible. Most remaining cells with visible nuclei appear to be granulocytic cells. H&E stain. **C.** Low-power image of necrosis in a postmortem bone marrow section from a dog with ALL. An area of necrosis (dark pink), containing iatrogenic trabecular bone fragments (light pink), is located at the left and an infiltrate of leukemic cells is located at the right. H&E stain. **D.** A cluster of stromal cells is present in a smear prepared from a bone marrow aspirate attempt from a dog with a nonregenerative anemia. The presence of a few stromal cells in an unsuccessful attempt to collect bone marrow particles by aspiration suggested the possibility of fibrosis, which was confirmed by core biopsy and histopathology. Wright-Giemsa stain. **E.** Myelofibrosis in a bone marrow section from a core biopsy collected from a dog with MDS. Reticular cells and collagen are readily visible at the top and to the right next to the darker pink trabecular bone. Hematopoietic cells (primarily erythroid precursors) are concentrated to the left. H&E stain. **F.** Myelofibrosis in a bone marrow section from a core biopsy collected from a dog with a poorly regenerative anemia. Hematopoietic cells are present in linear arrangements, separated by pale eosinophilic extracellular collagenous material, at the bottom of the field. H&E stain.

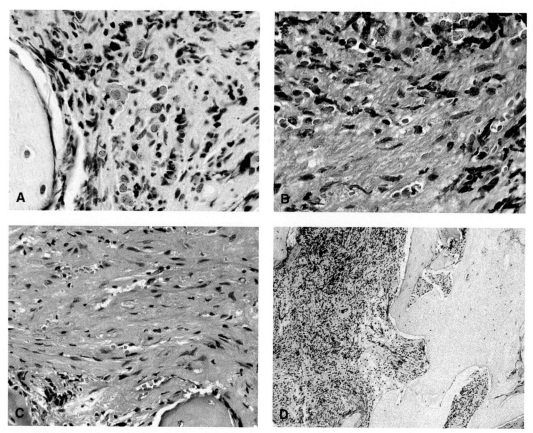

FIGURE 49.   Fibrosis and osteosclerosis in bone marrow.   A.   Myelofibrosis in a postmortem bone marrow section from a cat with chronic lymphocytic leukemia (CLL). Trabecular bone is located at the left edge. Reticular cells and collagen dominate the field although some hematopoietic precursors are present. The orange globular material is hemosiderin. H&E stain.   **B.**   Myelofibrosis in a postmortem bone marrow section from the same cat as presented in Figure 48A. Reticular cells and collagen (turquoise fibers) dominate the field although some hematopoietic precursors are present. The orange globular material is hemosiderin. Masson's trichrome stain.   **C.**   Marked myelofibrosis, consisting of fibroblasts and extracellular matrix with no remaining hematopoietic cells, in a bone marrow section from a core biopsy collected from a dog with a metastatic carcinoma. Trabecular bone is located at bottom right. Tumor cells are not present in this field. H&E stain.   **D.**   Low-power image of fibrosis and osteosclerosis in a bone marrow core biopsy section from a cat with CLL. The cat was FeLV-negative and FIV-negative. Thickened trabecular bone is located at the right edge of the field. H&E stain.

With the exception of the dogs with inherited hemolytic anemias, animals with myelofibrosis typically have nonregenerative anemia. Blood leukocyte counts and platelet counts are often normal or increased in idiopathic cases of myelofibrosis, but may be decreased.[385] Multiple cytopenias are more likely to occur in animals with concomitant myeloproliferative disorders.

Generalized Osteosclerosis/Hyperostosis

Osteosclerosis refers to a thickening of trabecular (spongy) bone (Fig. 49D) and hyperostosis refers to a widening of cortical (compact) bone from apposition of osseous tissue at endosteal and/or periosteal surfaces. Osteopetrosis is a form of osteosclerosis resulting from decreased bone resorption secondary to decreased numbers and/or abnormal function of osteoclasts.[389] As a result of osteosclerosis, and sometimes hyperostosis, the space available for hematopoiesis decreases. The remaining marrow space may appear hypocellular or exhibit fibrosis. Anemia occurs more often than thrombocytopenia or leukopenia. A variety of inherited, metabolic, inflammatory, and neoplastic disorders have been reported to cause generalized osteosclerosis in humans.[389]

Generalized osteosclerosis/hyperostosis is suspected when increased difficulty is encountered in the manual advancement of biopsy needles into bone, and marrow aspirates cannot be obtained. Osteosclerosis can potentially be recognized using core biopsies, but the presence of increased bone relative to marrow space may simply be reflective of the area of bone the needle has entered. Antemortem diagnosis of generalized osteosclerosis and/or hyperostosis is usually made using diagnostic imaging.

Osteopetrosis has been described in dogs, cats, and horses with mild to severe nonregenerative anemia.[390–393] Thrombocytopenia and neutropenia are less likely to be present.[390,391] Osteopetrosis has been described as a congenital disorder in calves, but hematologic findings were not given.[394]

Osteosclerosis and myelofibrosis have been described in a dog with erythroid hypoplasia.[395] Osteosclerosis and nonregenerative anemia have been reported in cats infected with FeLV, although it was suggested that these disorders occurred independently.[396] Osteosclerosis and myelofibrosis occur in dogs with erythrocyte pyruvate kinase deficiency and in poodles with clinical and laboratory findings similar to those in documented cases of pyruvate kinase deficiency.[72,386,387] The anemia in dogs with pyruvate kinase deficiency is regenerative, although the magnitude of the reticulocyte count may be lower as the marrow pathology becomes more severe.[72,386]

■ ABNORMALITIES OF THE ERYTHROID SERIES

Erythroid Hyperplasia

Erythroid hyperplasia is reported when the bone marrow cellularity is normal or increased, the absolute neutrophil count is normal or increased, and the M:E ratio is low (Figs. 50A–50C). If the marrow is hypocellular and/or the absolute neutrophil count is low, a low M:E ratio indicates granulocytic hypoplasia is present.

Approximately 4 days are required from the time an experimental animal is made anemic by phlebotomy and a peak reticulocyte response occurs in blood, because this is the time required for reticulocytes to be produced following stimulation of erythroid progenitor cells by erythropoietin.[22,397,398] Early

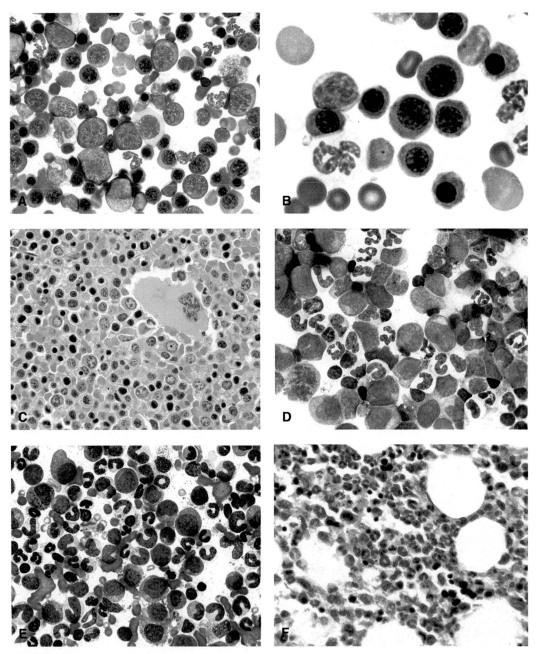

FIGURE 50. *See legend on opposite page.*

erythroid precursors can increase in bone marrow within 12 hours after eryth-ropoietin stimulation,[399] but several days are probably required after hemor-rhage or hemolysis has occurred before erythroid hyperplasia is prominent enough to result in a low M:E ratio. Bone marrow examination is generally not needed in anemic animals with an absolute reticulocytosis unless other cytope-nias are also present.

Horses rarely release reticulocytes from the bone marrow even when an increased production of erythrocytes occurs. Consequently, bone marrow evalu-ation is often needed to determine whether an appropriate response to anemia is present in a horse. If the marrow cellularity is normal or increased and the neutrophil count is normal or increased, an M:E ratio below 0.5 suggests a regenerative response to anemia is present (Figs. 50A–50C).[287]

Erythroid hyperplasia may be effective (increasing hematocrit and/or reti-culocytosis) or ineffective. Effective erythroid hyperplasia occurs in response to hemolytic or blood-loss anemia. It also occurs in response to primary or secondary erythrocytosis (polycythemia),[322,400–403] although the M:E ratio is of-ten within the reference range. Rubriblasts and prorubricytes are usually in-creased slightly in animals with effective erythroid hyperplasia; however, the predominant nucleated erythroid cells remain rubricytes and metarubricytes.[81] Many polychromatophilic erythrocytes (reticulocytes) should be present in bone marrow aspirates when the erythroid hyperplasia is effective (Fig. 50B). A reticulocyte count may be done in the bone marrow aspirate to assist in this assessment. Bone marrow reticulocyte counts above 5% provide evidence for an effective regenerative response in horses.[287]

Ineffective erythroid hyperplasia may occur in severe iron deficiency, folate deficiency, certain myeloproliferative and myelodysplastic disorders,[9,17,101,102,404] congenital dyserythropoiesis,[43,100] and in dogs with nonregenerative immune-mediated hemolytic anemia in which the immune response is directed at meta-rubricytes and/or reticulocytes.[304,405] Erythroid hypoplasia occurs when the im-mune response is directed at earlier stages of erythroid development.[405,406]

FIGURE 50.   Erythroid hyperplasia and erythroid hypoplasia in bone marrow aspirate smears and core biopsy sections.   A. Erythroid hyperplasia in an aspirate smear of bone marrow from a horse with immune-mediated hemolytic anemia. The large cells with dark-blue cytoplasm are early erythroid precursors. Wright-Giemsa stain.   **B.** Higher magnification showing erythroid hyperplasia in an aspirate smear of bone marrow from the same horse as presented in Figure 50A. Increased numbers of polychro-matophilic erythrocytes (reticulocytes) indicate that the erythroid response is effective. Wright-Giemsa stain. **C.** Erythroid hyperplasia in a bone marrow section from a core biopsy collected from the same horse as presented in Figures 50A and 50B. A large mature megakaryocyte is present near the center of the image. H&E stain.   **D.** Selective erythroid aplasia in an aspirate smear of bone marrow from a Coombs'-positive, 8-month-old Maltese dog. Small lymphocytes accounted for 15% of all nucleated cells. Wright-Giemsa stain.   **E.** Selective erythroid aplasia in an aspirate smear of bone marrow from a cat given chloramphenicol at a high therapeutic dosage for 9 days. Wright-Giemsa stain.   **F.** Moderate erythroid hypoplasia in a bone marrow section from a core biopsy collected from a horse with a chronic polyarthritis. Nucleated erythroid precursors have round nuclei and appear darker than granulocytic precursors. H&E stain.

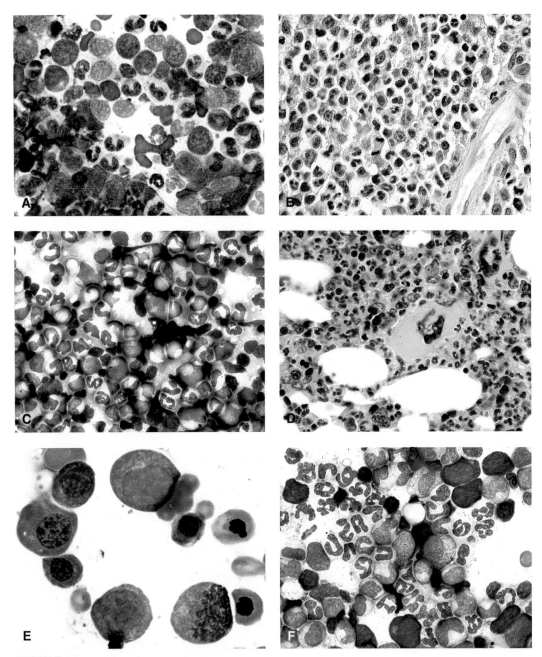

FIGURE 51.   *See legend on opposite page.*

Selective Erythroid Hypoplasia or Aplasia

Erythroid hypoplasia is reported when the bone marrow cellularity is normal or decreased, the absolute neutrophil count is normal or decreased, and the M:E ratio is high (Figs. 50D–50F). If the marrow is hypercellular and/or the absolute neutrophil count is high, a high M:E ratio indicates granulocytic hyperplasia is present.

Selective erythroid aplasia (pure red cell aplasia) occurs as either a congenital or acquired disorder in people.[407] Acquired erythroid aplasia is often associated with abnormalities of the immune system. Erythroid aplasia may also occur secondary to disorders such as B-19 parvovirus infection, lymphoid malignancies, and drug or chemical toxicities.[408]

Acquired erythroid hypoplasia or aplasia occurs in dogs (Fig. 50D).[409,410] Some cases have immune-mediated etiologies based on positive responses to immunosuppressive therapy and the presence of antibodies that inhibit CFU-E development in marrow cultures.[409] Acquired, immune-mediated erythroid aplasia has also been reported in FeLV-negative cats.[297] In addition to a lack of erythroid precursors, a mature lymphocytosis (up to 45% of all nucleated cells) was present in most of the marrow samples.

Erythroid hypoplasia or dysplasia is reported to be a rare sequela to vaccination against parvovirus in dogs.[411] High doses of chloramphenicol cause reversible erythroid hypoplasia in some dogs[412] and erythroid aplasia in cats (Fig. 50E).[413] Erythroid aplasia together with megakaryocytic aplasia and neutrophilic hyperplasia is present in early estrogen toxicity in dogs.[69,336] A dog has been reported to have congenital erythroid aplasia based on histopathologic examination of bone marrow at necropsy, but the M:E ratio was normal when aspirate smears were examined several days prior to euthanasia.[414] Transient erythroid hypoplasia apparently occurs at regular intervals in gray collie dogs with inherited cyclic hematopoiesis, but it does not cause anemia because it is of short duration, followed by a period of erythroid hyperplasia.[415–417]

Selective erythroid hypoplasia or aplasia occurs in cats infected with FeLV subgroup C but not in cats infected only with subgroups A or B (Figs. 51A,

FIGURE 51.   Erythroid hypoplasia, erythroid dysplasia, and maturation arrest of erythroid cells in bone marrow.   A. Marked erythroid hypoplasia in an aspirate smear of bone marrow from a FeLV-positive cat. There was also a left shift in granulocytic cells with some giantism noted. Wright-Giemsa stain.   **B.** Erythroid and megakaryocytic hypoplasia in a bone marrow biopsy section collected from the same cat as presented in Figure 51A. H&E stain.   **C.** Mild erythroid hypoplasia and granulocytic hyperplasia in an aspirate smear of bone marrow from a dog with the anemia of inflammatory disease. Black-staining material near the center of the image is hemosiderin. Wright-Giemsa stain.   **D.** Erythroid hypoplasia and increased hemosiderin (orange-staining material) in a bone marrow section from a core biopsy collected from a dog with the anemia of inflammatory disease. Two mature megakaryocytes are present. H&E stain.   **E.** Dyserythropoiesis in an aspirate smear of bone marrow from a horse with MDS. A megaloblastic rubricyte is present at the far left, and a macrocytic metarubricyte with peanut-shaped nucleus is present at the right center. A mitotic figure is present near the bottom right. Wright-Giemsa stain.   **F.** Erythroid maturation arrest in an aspirate smear of bone marrow from a dog with systemic lupus erythematosus that included a Coombs'-positive nonregenerative anemia. Most erythroid cells present were rubriblasts or prorubricytes. Wright-Giemsa stain.

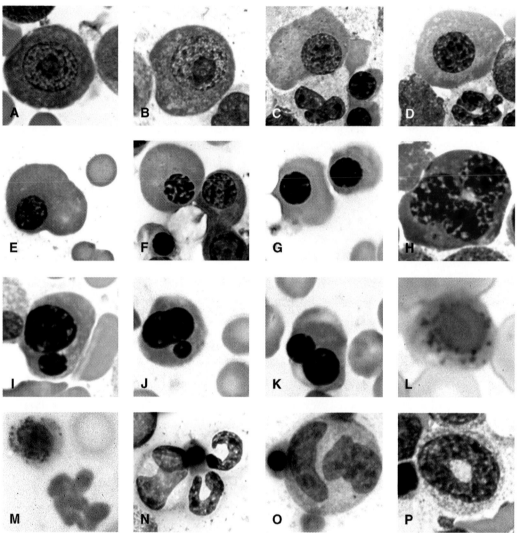

FIGURE 52. Dysplastic erythroid and neutrophilic cells in bone marrow aspirate smears Wright-Giemsa stain except as indicated. **A.** Megaloblastic erythroid precursor in an aspirate smear of bone marrow from a cat with erythroleukemia (AML-M6). **B.** Megaloblastic erythroid precursor in an aspirate smear of bone marrow from a cat with AML-M2. **C.** Megaloblastic erythroid precursor in an aspirate smear of bone marrow from a FeLV-positive cat with MDS. **D.** Megaloblastic erythroid precursor in an aspirate smear of bone marrow from the same cat with AML-M2 as presented in Figure 52B. **E.** Macrocytic polychromatophilic rubricyte in an aspirate smear of bone marrow from a cat with MDS. **F.** Macrocytic polychromatophilic rubricyte (top left) in an aspirate smear of bone marrow from a horse with MDS. **G.** Macrocytic orthochromatic metarubricyte (*left*) in an aspirate smear of bone marrow from the same horse with MDS as presented in Figure 52F. **H.** Trinucleated polychromatophilic rubricyte in an aspirate smear of bone marrow from a dog with lymphoma and mild dyserythropoiesis. Prior chemotherapy was not listed in the medical record. **I.** Lobulated polychromatophilic rubricyte in an aspirate smear of bone marrow from the same dog with mild dyserythropoiesis as presented in Figure 52H. **J.** Lobulated polychromatophilic metarubricyte in an aspirate smear of bone marrow from a dog 1 day after treatment with vincristine. **K.** Lobulated polychromatophilic metarubricyte in an aspirate smear of bone marrow from the same vincristine-treated dog as presented in Figure 52J. **L.** Iron-positive metarubricyte (sideroblast) in an aspirate smear of bone marrow from a dog

(Continued)

51B).[418] When some erythroid cells remain, an apparent maturation arrest may be present with an increased ratio of rubriblasts and prorubricytes relative to rubricytes and metarubricytes. Although both myeloid and erythroid progenitor cells are infected with the virus, only erythroid progenitor cell numbers are decreased in cat marrow. Studies suggest that CFU-E numbers are markedly decreased because the virus results in an impairment of the differentiation of BFU-E into CFU-E.[418]

Marked erythroid hypoplasia has been reported in dogs, cats, and horses given recombinant human erythropoietin.[419–421] Antibodies made against this human recombinant glycoprotein apparently cross-react with the animals' endogenous erythropoietin.

Erythroid production is reduced in chronic renal disease[81] and endocrine deficiencies (hypopituitarism, hypoadrenocorticism, hypothyroidism, and hypoandrogenism) but often not enough to result in an M:E ratio in the marrow that is increased above the reference range. Dogs with idiopathic myelofibrosis often have an associated erythroid hypoplasia.[81]

A mild to moderate nonregenerative anemia often accompanies chronic inflammatory and neoplastic disorders. The cause of this anemia of inflammatory disease (anemia of chronic disease) is multifactorial and only partially understood. Abnormalities that can contribute to the anemia include the production of inflammatory mediators that directly or indirectly inhibit erythropoiesis, decreased serum iron, shortened erythrocyte life spans, and blunted erythropoietin response to the anemia.[422,423] The M:E ratio is typically high in clinical cases of the anemia of inflammatory disease in dogs (Figs. 51C, 51D),[81] not only because of deficient erythropoiesis but also because of concomitant granulocytic hyperplasia.[423]

Dyserythropoiesis

The term "dyserythropoiesis" is used to refer to various disorders in which abnormal erythrocyte maturation and/or morphology is associated with ineffective erythropoiesis. Erythroid abnormalities that may be present include megaloblastic cells, abnormal nuclear shapes, premature nuclear pyknosis, nuclear fragmentation, multinucleated cells, internuclear chromatin bridging, nuclear and cytoplasmic asynchrony, maturation arrest, and siderotic inclusions.

Megaloblastic erythroid cells are larger than normal with a more stranded arrangement of chromatin and abundant parachromatin, giving a pronounced light and dark pattern to the nucleus (Figs. 51E, 52A–52D). The cytoplasm is

---

receiving chloramphenicol therapy. Blue granules in the cytoplasm indicate the presence of iron. Prussian blue stain.   **M.**   Iron positive metarubricyte (upper left) in an aspirate smear of bone marrow from a dog receiving chloramphenicol therapy. Because the iron-positive granules circle the nucleus, it may be called a ringed sideroblast. Prussian blue stain.   **N.**   Giant band neutrophil (left) in an aspirate smear of bone marrow from the same cat with MDS as presented in Figure 52N. Two normal-sized band neutrophils (right) are also present.   **O.**   Giant binucleated granulocytic precursor in bone marrow from a cat with MDS.   **P.**   Doughnut-shaped neutrophil precursor in an aspirate smear of bone marrow from an FIV-infected leukopenic cat.

generally abundant and hemoglobin synthesis may be present at earlier stages of development than is typically seen (e.g., nuclear and cytoplasmic asynchrony).[52] Rubricytes and metarubricytes may be macrocytic without prominent nuclear abnormalities (Figs. 52E–52G). These morphologic abnormalities are most often seen in animals with myeloproliferative disorders.[11,101,102,404,424,425] Megaloblastic erythropoiesis occurs most commonly in ill cats with FeLV infections but has also been reported in cats with feline immunodeficiency virus (FIV) infections.[426] Megaloblastic erythroid cells have been reported in the marrow of cats with natural and experimentally induced folate deficiency[181,427] and in dogs with prolonged anticonvulsant drug therapy.[52] Finally, some miniature and toy poodles exhibit macrocytosis without anemia and variable megaloblastic abnormalities in the bone marrow with normal serum folate and B_{12} values.[428,429]

Multinucleated erythroid cells (Fig. 52H) have been reported in animals with myeloproliferative disorders[11,303,404,425,430] and in animals with acquired and congenital dyserythropoiesis.[100,307] Nuclear lobulations, pyknosis, and/or fragmentation may occur in animals with myeloproliferative disorders and[101,426] acquired and congenital dyserythropoiesis[43,100,307] and following treatment with certain chemotherapeutic drugs such as vincristine (Figs. 52I–52K).[313] Internuclear chromatin bridging has been reported in cattle with congenital dyserythropoiesis.[100]

Maturation arrests at various stages of erythroid development, with a resultant lack of polychromatophilic erythrocytes, may occur in acquired myeloproliferative disorders[431] and in congenital dyserythropoiesis,[100] as well as in some immune-mediated disorders (Fig. 51F).[405,406] Asynchrony of nuclear and cytoplasmic maturation in which hemoglobinization precedes nuclear maturation may occur in acquired myeloproliferative disorders as well as in congenital dyserythropoiesis.[17,100] Iron-positive basophilic stippling has been reported in rubricytes and metarubricytes (sideroblasts) from animals with myeloproliferative disorders,[58,101,303,432] a dog with idiopathic dyserythropoiesis,[306] and a dog given chloramphenicol therapy (Figs. 52L, 52M).[433]

◼ ABNORMALITIES OF THE GRANULOCYTIC SERIES

Granulocytic Hyperplasia

Granulocytic hyperplasia is reported when the bone marrow cellularity is normal or increased, the hematocrit is normal or increased, and the M:E ratio is high. If the marrow is hypocellular and/or the hematocrit is low, a high M:E ratio suggests that erythroid hypoplasia is present. Because neutrophilic cells are usually much more numerous than eosinophilic or basophilic cells in bone marrow, the term "granulocytic hyperplasia" generally indicates the presence of neutrophilic hyperplasia. Eosinophilic and/or basophilic hyperplasia may accompany neutrophilic hyperplasia, but they rarely account for increased M:E ratios on their own.

Neutrophilic Hyperplasia

Neutrophilic hyperplasia may be effective or ineffective. Effective neutrophilic hyperplasia results in neutrophilia, with or without a left shift. It occurs in response to various hematopoietic growth factors, with granulocyte-colony stimulating factor (G-CSF) being most important.[423] Several days are required from the time of growth factor stimulation until hyperplasia is prominent enough to increase the M:E ratio outside the reference range.[423] The proportions of myeloblasts and promyelocytes are generally not increased out of proportion to more mature neutrophilic cells in animals with neutrophilic hyperplasia, but they may sometimes be increased with early and/or intense stimulation with growth factors.[81,315,406,423,434] Myeloblasts did not exceed 6% of all nucleated cells in cats with myeloid hyperplasia.[238] The proportion of mature granulocytes in marrow may be decreased, because cytokines such as G-CSF, interleukin-1, and tumor necrosis factor (either directly or indirectly) result in increased release of neutrophils from the marrow.[315,423]

Neutrophilic hyperplasia occurs most frequently in response to bacterial infections, but may also occur in response to immune-mediated inflammatory disorders, necrosis, chemical and drug toxicities, and malignancy (Figs. 53A, 53B).[1,17,435] The natural release or injection of recombinant G-CSF or granulocyte/macrophage-colony stimulating factor (GM-CSF) result in neutrophilia in blood and neutrophilic hyperplasia in the bone marrow.[436–438] Extreme neutrophilic hyperplasia in bone marrow and neutrophilia in blood has been reported as a paraneoplastic syndrome in dogs and cats with tumors that produce hematopoietic growth factors.[434,439,440]

Neutrophilic hyperplasia may be present in animals with inherited hematologic disorders.[441,442] Marked neutrophilia with or without a modest left shift is usually present in dogs and cattle with deficiencies in β_2 integrin adhesion molecules.[443,444] Granulocyte hyperplasia also follows cyclic episodes of neutrophilic hypoplasia in gray collie dogs with cyclic hematopoiesis.[445,446]

Marked neutrophilic hyperplasia and concomitant erythroid and megakaryocytic aplasia occur during the first 3 weeks after the injection of a toxic dose of estrogen in dogs (Fig. 53C).[336] This is followed by generalized hypoplasia or aplasia and death or slow recovery.

Neutrophilic hyperplasia is present in animals with chronic myelocytic leukemia. The percentage of immature neutrophilic cells is increased, but the percentage of myeloblasts does not exceed 30% of all nucleated cells. Dysplastic changes are also typically present in one or more marrow cell lines.[131,132,447–449]

Ineffective neutrophilic hyperplasia refers to the occurrence of a persistent neutropenia with neutrophilic hyperplasia in the bone marrow (Fig. 53D). Increased numbers of immature granulocyte precursors and decreased numbers of mature neutrophils are typically present within the marrow. Ineffective neutrophilic hyperplasia frequently occurs in myelodysplastic disorders and acute myelocytic leukemias.[131,431] It is especially common in neutropenic cats with FeLV and/or FIV infections.[426,431,450,451]

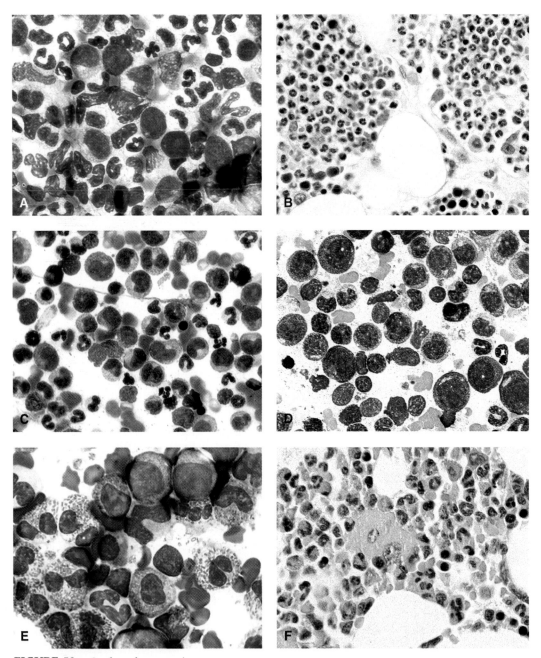

FIGURE 53.   *See legend on opposite page.*

Neutropenia has been reported in dogs treated with anticonvulsants that had neutrophilic hyperplasia and orderly maturation in the marrow, suggesting a peripheral destruction of neutrophils.[452]

Immune-mediated neutropenia may result in secondary neutrophilic hyperplasia in response to the premature removal of blood neutrophils. A dog with neutropenia, thrombocytopenia, and neutrophilic and megakaryocytic hyperplasia in the bone marrow, which rapidly responded to glucocorticoid therapy, appeared to have been an immune-mediated disorder.[453]

Eosinophilic Hyperplasia

Eosinophilic hyperplasia is generally present in bone marrow when eosinophilia is present in blood (Figs. 53E, 53F, 54A)[11] Eosinophilia may accompany parasitic diseases, especially those caused by nematodes and flukes. It is more likely to be present when intestinal nematodes are migrating within the body than when they are only located within the intestine. Eosinophilia may occur in association with inflammatory conditions of organs that normally contain numerous mast cells, such as the skin, lung, intestine, and uterus. It may be present in animals with IgE-mediated allergic hypersensitivity reactions such as fleabite allergies and feline asthma. Although not usually present, eosinophilia may occur in animals with mast cell tumors and, rarely, in animals with other tumor types.[454–456]

Eosinophilia occurs in some animals with eosinophilic granulomas, and it is consistently present in animals with the hypereosinophilic syndrome, a heterogenous group of disorders that can be difficult to differentiate from eosinophilic leukemia.[186,457–460] The maturation is orderly in hypereosinophilic syndrome. Prominent eosinophilic left shifts in bone marrow, blood, and organ infiltrates are more likely to occur in animals with eosinophilic leukemia.[184–186] Eosinophilia has been reported in animals with CML.[130,131,184,449,461]

Increased numbers of eosinophils may be present in bone marrow samples from animals with myelodysplastic disorders and acute myeloid leukemia (AML), even in the absence of peripheral eosinophilia.[236,238]

FIGURE 53.   Neutrophilic and eosinophilic hyperplasia in bone marrow aspirate smears and core bone marrow biopsy sections.   A.   Neutrophilic hyperplasia in an aspirate smear of bone marrow from a dog with neutrophilia and nonregenerative anemia secondary to a bacterial endocarditis. The black globular material near the bottom right is hemosiderin. Wright-Giemsa stain.   **B.**   Neutrophilic hyperplasia and erythroid hypoplasia in a bone marrow section from a core biopsy collected from a cat with marked mature neutrophilia and nonregenerative anemia, for which a cause was not determined. H&E stain.   **C.**   Neutrophilic hyperplasia and erythroid hypoplasia in an aspirate smear of bone marrow from a dog 13 days after an estradiol cypionate (ECP) injection for mismating. Wright-Giemsa stain.   **D.** Ineffective neutrophilic hyperplasia and erythroid hypoplasia in an aspirate smear of bone marrow from a persistently leukopenic, FIV-infected cat. Fewer band and mature neutrophils were present than normal. Wright-Giemsa stain.   **E.**   Eosinophilic hyperplasia in an aspirate smear of bone marrow from a cat with marked eosinophilia, probably associated with a hypereosinophilic syndrome. Wright-Giemsa stain.   **F.** Eosinophilic hyperplasia in a bone marrow core biopsy section collected from a cat with lymphocytic-plasmacytic gastritis and eosinophilia in the peripheral blood. H&E stain.

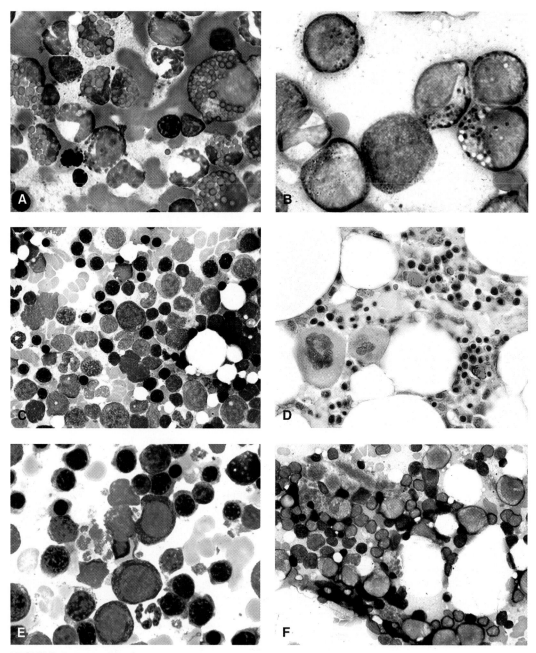

FIGURE 54.   *See legend on opposite page.*

Basophilic Hyperplasia

Basophilic hyperplasia is generally present in bone marrow when basophilia is present in blood.[11,462] Basophilia is usually associated with the same types of disorders that result in eosinophilia. It is most commonly seen in dogs and cats with dirofilariasis.[463,464] Basophilia may occur in some dogs and cats with systemic mastocytosis.[318,319,455,465,466] Basophilia has been reported in dogs with lymphomatoid granulomatosis[467] and in a dog with thrombocythemia.[247,468] A marked basophilic left shift is present in blood and bone marrow of dogs with basophilic leukemia,[189,190,469] and increased numbers of basophilic precursors may rarely be present in the bone marrow of cats with myeloproliferative disorders (Fig. 54B).[236,238]

Granulocytic Hypoplasia

Granulocytic hypoplasia is reported when the bone marrow cellularity is normal or decreased, the hematocrit is normal or increased, and the M:E ratio is low. If the marrow is hypercellular and/or the hematocrit is low, a low M:E ratio indicates erythroid hyperplasia is present. Because neutrophilic cells are normally much more numerous than eosinophilic or basophilic cells in bone marrow, the term "granulocytic hypoplasia" indicates that neutrophilic hypoplasia is present (Figs. 54C–54E). Eosinophilic hypoplasia and/or basophilic hypoplasia may accompany neutrophilic hypoplasia, but few basophil precursors are normally present in bone marrow, making an interpretation of basophilic hypoplasia difficult.

FIGURE 54.   Eosinophilic and basophilic hyperplasia, granulocytic hypoplasia, and granulocyte maturation arrest in bone marrow.   A.   Eosinophilic hyperplasia in an aspirate smear of bone marrow from a horse with an abdominal mast cell tumor and marked eosinophilia in peripheral blood. Some of the granules in the eosinophilic myelocytes stain bluish red. Wright-Giemsa stain.   **B.**   Basophilic hyperplasia in an aspirate smear of bone marrow from a cat with AML-M2. Four basophilic myelocytes (one upper left, three right center) are present. A type II myeloblast is present at bottom center and a promyelocyte is present at bottom left. Wright-Giemsa stain.   **C.**   Granulocytic hypoplasia of unknown etiology in an aspirate smear of bone marrow from a FeLV-negative, FIV-negative, neutropenic cat with normal hematocrit and platelet count. Wright-Giemsa stain.   **D.**   Granulocytic hypoplasia in a bone marrow section from a core biopsy collected from a dog 6 days after therapy with vincristine, L-asparaginase, and prednisone was begun for a mediastinal tumor. Two megakaryocytes and many erythroid precursors are present. The orange-staining globular material is hemosiderin. H&E stain.   **E.**   Granulocytic hypoplasia of unknown etiology in an aspirate smear of bone marrow from a FeLV-negative cat with severe neutropenia. The hematocrit and platelet counts were normal. Most cells present are nucleated erythrocyte precursors. Wright-Giemsa stain.   **F.**   Maturation arrest of granulocytes in an aspirate smear of bone marrow from a severely neutropenic cat that had been treated with griseofulvin and prednisone for skin lesions. Increased numbers of small lymphocytes are also present. Slight neutrophilia and normal bone marrow cytology were present 3 days later, following cessation of drug treatments. Wright-Giemsa stain.

Selective Neutrophilic Hypoplasia or Aplasia

Selective neutrophilic hypoplasia may be immune mediated, drug induced (which may be secondary immune-mediated disorder), inherited, or idiopathic in people.[336,470–472] Cytotoxic drugs used to treat immune-mediated diseases and cancer typically result in generalized marrow injury, but in some cases, injury to the neutrophilic series is more severe than injury to the erythroid or megakaryocytic series. Azathioprine can produce neutropenia resulting from selective neutrophilic hypoplasia in some cats.[473] Experimental studies in cats have also demonstrated that doxorubicin can produce neutropenia without anemia or thrombocytopenia at times, but the investigators did not examine bone marrow to determine whether selective neutrophilic hypoplasia was present.[42]

Many drugs have been reported to cause neutropenia in people, and neutrophilic hypoplasia is commonly present in bone marrow.[470,471] Griseofulvin is a fungistatic antibiotic that has been reported to cause neutropenia in cats with dermatophyte infections but not in experimental cats without dermatophyte infections (Fig. 54F).[334,474] FIV-infected cats appear to have an increased risk of developing griseofulvin-induced toxicity.[475] In these cases, bone marrow evaluation has revealed evidence of neutrophilic hypoplasia. Methimazole treatment has been reported to cause neutropenia in hyperthyroid cats, but bone marrow findings were not given.[476] Transient methimazole-induced generalized marrow aplasia has been reported in humans.[477]

Neutropenia has been reported in animals given recombinant G-CSF from another species.[478] This phenomenon apparently occurs because the recipient develops antibodies that react not only against the foreign recombinant protein but also against the recipient's endogenous G-CSF. Marked neutrophilic hypoplasia occurred when canine recombinant G-CSF was injected into rabbits[478] but not when recombinant human G-CSF was injected into dogs.[479] In the latter instance, the authors speculated that the antibody was bound to G-CSF on the surface of circulating neutrophils, resulting in an immune-mediated premature destruction of these cells.

Neutrophilic hypoplasia occurs in the bone marrow of neutropenic cats and dogs with parvovirus infections.[351,353,354,377] Parvovirus infections in pups can also cause a severe erythroid hypoplasia, but animals usually do not become anemic because of the long life spans of erythrocytes.[350]

Transient neutrophilic hypoplasia in the marrow and resultant transient neutropenia in blood occurs at 12- to 14-day intervals in gray collie dogs with inherited cyclic hematopoiesis.[417,446,480] When examined early in the neutropenic phase, myeloblasts and promyelocytes are present, but later stages of neutrophil development are absent and the M:E ratio is low.[417] Over the next few days, later maturation stages increase until the neutrophilic series is complete, the M:E ratio is high, and the number of neutrophils in blood is normal or increased.[417,480] Overall marrow cellularity is fairly constant, because the oscillations of granulopoiesis and erythropoiesis occur in a reciprocal manner.[480] A similar repetitive pattern of neutrophilic hypoplasia, followed by neutrophilic hyperplasia, has been described in cats with FeLV-induced cyclic hematopoiesis.[481] Cyclic neutropenia has been produced experimentally in dogs using continuous low-dose cyclophosphamide treatment, but bone marrow was not examined.[482]

Familial neutropenia and thrombocytopenia have been reported in eight horses with severe neutrophilic hypoplasia/aplasia and megakaryocytic hypoplasia.[363] Erythroid maturation was orderly, but some degree of erythroid hypoplasia was believed to be present in half of the horses.

Dysgranulopoiesis

The term "dysgranulopoiesis" is used to refer to various disorders in which abnormal granulocyte maturation and/or morphology is present (Figs. 52N–52P, 54F, 55A–55F). Dysgranulopoiesis is often associated with ineffective granulopoiesis, resulting in a neutropenia in peripheral blood. Neutrophilic abnormalities that may be present in bone marrow include increased numbers (5% to 29%) of myeloblasts, maturation arrest in the neutrophilic series at the myelocyte-metamyelocyte stage, giant metamyelocytes, band and mature neutrophils, multinucleated cells, abnormal granulation such as large primary granules or granules surrounded by vacuoles, hyposegmented neutrophils (pseudo-Pelger-Huet), hypersegmented neutrophils, and neutrophils with bizarre nuclear shapes.[58,101,131,303,404,430,431] Dysgranulopoiesis frequently occurs in myelodysplastic disorders and acute myelocytic leukemias. It is especially common in cats with FeLV and/or FIV infections.[426,431,450,451] Dysgranulopoiesis in the form of occasional giant metamyelocytes and band neutrophils may be seen in cats with myeloid hyperplasia unrelated to myeloproliferative disorders.[238]

Experimental studies have shown that lithium treatment causes a neutropenia in cats as a result of a neutrophilic maturation arrest in the bone marrow.[483] Unfortunately, investigators did not provide an M:E ratio or comment on marrow cellularity. Maturation arrests in both neutrophilic and erythroid series have been reported in bone marrow of neutropenic, anemic dogs treated with a cephalosporin antibiotic.[98] Dysgranulopoiesis and mild erythroid hypoplasia have been reported in the marrow of cats given valacyclovir, an antiviral drug designed for the treatment of herpes virus infections.[484]

Giant schnauzer dogs with an inherited malabsorption of cobalamin may have neutropenia with hypersegmented neutrophils in blood and megaloblastic changes in the bone marrow neutrophilic cell line.[180,485]

The early recovery stage from neutrophilic hypoplasia can exhibit some of the morphologic abnormalities reported in animals with dysgranulopoiesis.[11] When neutrophils begin to proliferate after a period of neutrophilic aplasia, myeloblasts and promyelocytes are predominant early, followed progressively by the appearance of the later stages of development.[417,446,481] When examined prior to the production of mature neutrophils, the appearance of a maturation arrest is present. Overwhelming sepsis with a compensatory premature release of mature neutrophils can also give the impression of a maturation arrest.

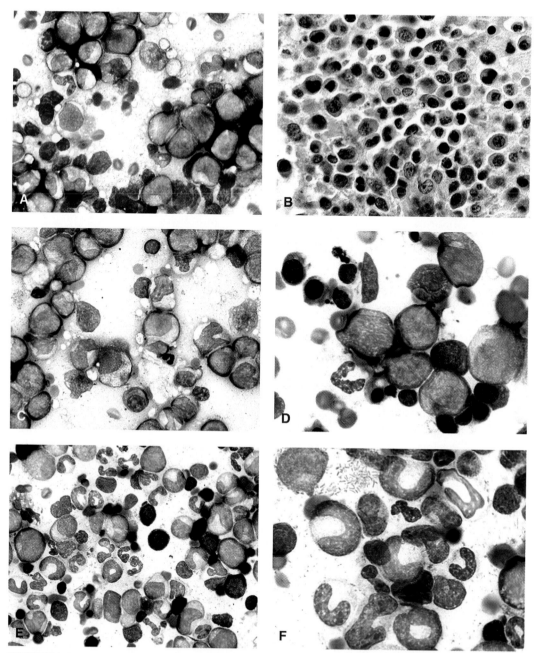

FIGURE 55. *See legend on opposite page.*

ABNORMALITIES OF MEGAKARYOCYTES

Megakaryocytic Hyperplasia

Megakaryocyte number, ploidy, and size increase in bone marrow within a few days following thrombocytopenia that results from premature destruction or utilization of platelets in blood (Figs. 56A, 56B).[486,487] Although other growth factors have synergistic effects, these changes are largely the result of increased thrombopoietin, which also accelerates the rate of megakaryocyte maturation. Most megakaryocytes are mature in animals with megakaryocytic hyperplasia, but increased numbers of promegakaryocytes and basophilic megakaryocytes are often recognized. Thrombocytopenic disorders in which megakaryocytic hyperplasia is expected include primary and secondary immune-mediated thrombocytopenia, ongoing intravascular coagulation, hypersplenism, and vascular injury.[488–492] Various viral, rickettsial, bacterial, protozoal, and fungal agents[493–496] and therapeutic drugs[98,452,497–499] result in platelet destruction (often immune mediated) or utilization and subsequent megakaryocytic hyperplasia (Fig. 56E). *Ehrlichia canis* infection is a common cause of thrombocytopenia in dogs. Although generalized marrow hypoplasia occurs in severe chronic ehrlichiosis, megakaryocytic hyperplasia is present early in the disease when immune-mediated platelet destruction largely accounts for the thrombocytopenia.[494,500]

Megakaryocytic hyperplasia also occurs in association with thrombocythemia, a myeloproliferative disorder that is characterized by persistent, markedly increased ($>1 \times 10^6/\mu L$) platelet counts in the absence of iron deficiency, an underlying inflammatory condition, or another myeloproliferative disorder that might account for the high platelet count.[247,468,501–505] Megakaryocyte morphology generally appears normal when examined by light microscopy (Figs. 56C, 56D), but dwarf megakaryocytes (small mature megakaryocytes with decreased ploidy) may be present.[247]

FIGURE 55.   Dysgranulopoiesis with maturation arrest and giant precursors cells.   A. Maturation arrest in neutrophil development at the myelocyte-metamyelocyte stage in an aspirate smear of bone marrow from a neutropenic dog with MDS. No mature neutrophils and only one band neutrophil are present. Erythroid precursors are absent in this field. The M:E ratio was 19. Wright-Giemsa stain.   **B.** Maturation arrest in neutrophil development at the myelocyte-metamyelocyte stage in a bone marrow section from a core biopsy collected from the same neutropenic dog as presented in Figure 55A. H&E stain. **C.** Maturation arrest in neutrophil development at the myelocyte-metamyelocyte stage in an aspirate smear of bone marrow from a FeLV-negative, neutropenic cat with MDS. Erythroid precursors are absent in this field. Wright-Giemsa stain.   **D.** Increased numbers of myeloblasts (six largest cells) in an aspirate smear of bone marrow from a horse with MDS. Myeloblasts accounted for 9% of all nucleated cells and 28% of granulocytic cells in the bone marrow. Wright-Giemsa stain.   **E.** Giant band neutrophils in an aspirate smear of bone marrow from a cat with MDS. Wright-Giemsa stain.   **F.** Giant band neutrophils in an aspirate smear of bone marrow from the same cat with MDS as presented in Figure 55E. Wright-Giemsa stain.

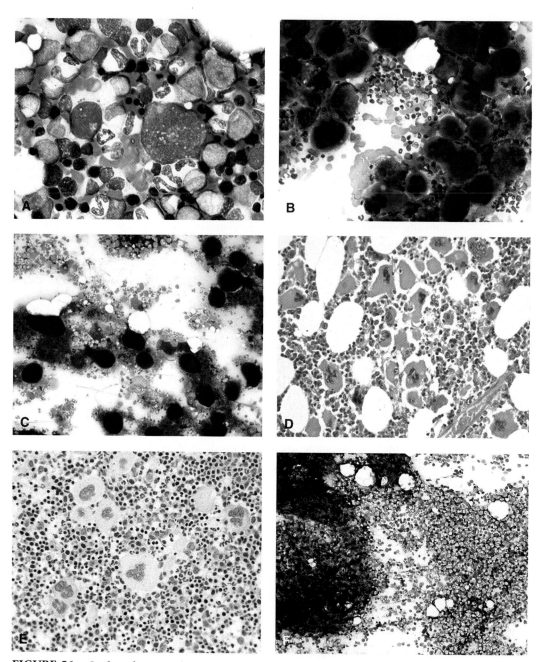

FIGURE 56. *See legend on opposite page.*

Selective Megakaryocytic Hypoplasia or Aplasia

Selective amegakaryocytic thrombocytopenia is a rare syndrome in people, in which it occurs as a congenital defect or an acquired defect in adults.[506] Idiopathic amegakaryocytic thrombocytopenia is also rare in adult dogs and cats, in which it is presumed to be immune mediated (Fig. 56F).[490,507–509] It has been reported in a quarter-horse foal with associated immune-mediated hemolytic anemia.[510] Familial neutropenia and thrombocytopenia have been reported in eight horses with severe neutrophilic hypoplasia/aplasia and megakaryocytic hypoplasia.[363]

Various drugs may induce thrombocytopenia as result of marrow suppression. Usually, marrow suppression is generalized, but megakaryocytes may be specifically decreased.[497] For example, dapsone treatment has been associated with amegakaryocytic thrombocytopenia in a dog[511] and megakaryocytic and/or erythroid hypoplasia were reported to occur in cats treated with ribavirin, a broad-spectrum antiviral agent.[512]

Dysmegakaryocytopoiesis

Dysmegakaryocytopoiesis refers to the presence of maturation and/or morphologic abnormalities in megakaryocytic cells. Apparent maturation arrests with early stages (e.g., promegakaryocytes) predominating may not be reflective of a dysplastic process but rather may result from immune-mediated reactions against megakaryocyte antigens (Fig. 56A).[513] Dysplastic abnormalities that may be present in bone marrow include asynchronous maturation resulting in the formation of dwarf granular megakaryocytes with single or multiple nuclei and large megakaryocytes with nuclear abnormalities including hypolobulation, hyperlobulation, or multiple round nuclei (Figs. 57A–57C).[431] Megakaryocytic dysplasia may occur following drug administrations[512] but most frequently occurs in myelodysplastic disorders and acute myelocytic leukemias.[131,303,425,431,514]

FIGURE 56. **Variations in megakaryocyte numbers and morphology in bone marrow.** **A.** Lack of mature megakaryocytes in an aspirate smear of bone marrow from a dog with immune-mediated thrombocytopenia. Most megakaryocyte precursors present were promegakaryocytes (binucleated cell at left), but some basophilic megakaryocytes (large cell at right) were observed. Wright-Giemsa stain. **B.** Marked megakaryocytic hyperplasia in an aspirate smear of bone marrow from the same dog with immune-mediated thrombocytopenia as presented in Figure 56A. This aspirate was taken 1 week after prednisone therapy was begun and photographed at lower magnification. Wright-Giemsa stain. **C.** Megakaryocytic hyperplasia in an aspirate smear of bone marrow from a cat with thrombocythemia and a platelet count of $1.4 \times 10^6/\mu L$. Wright-Giemsa stain. **D.** Megakaryocytic hyperplasia in a bone marrow section from the same cat with thrombocythemia as presented in Figure 56C. H&E stain. **E.** Megakaryocytic hyperplasia in a bone marrow section from a core biopsy collected from a thrombocytopenic dog with disseminated intravascular coagulation that developed 1.5 weeks after treatment for occult heartworm disease. H&E stain. **F.** Megakaryocyte aplasia in a hypercellular aspirate smear of bone marrow from a thrombocytopenic cat with associated immune-mediated hemolytic anemia. Only one megakaryocyte was seen when multiple smears were scanned. Megakaryocytes were not seen in sections of bone marrow collected at necropsy. Wright-Giemsa stain.

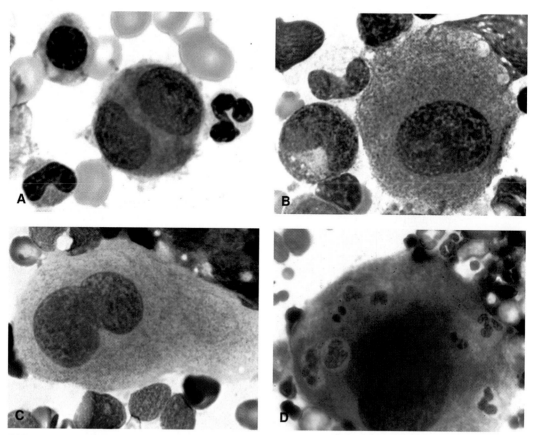

FIGURE 57. Dwarf megakaryocytes and megakaryocytic emperipolesis in bone marrow aspirate smears. Wright-Giemsa stain.   **A.** Binucleated dwarf megakaryocyte in an aspirate smear of bone marrow from a dog with CML. Magenta-staining granules in the cytoplasm and lack of intense basophilia indicate that it is not a promegakaryocyte.   **B.** Dwarf megakaryocyte in an aspirate smear of bone marrow from a FeLV-positive, thrombocytopenic cat with MDS. Large numbers of magenta-staining granules are present in the cytoplasm as is expected for mature megakaryocytes, but the cell has a single nucleus and is much smaller than normal.   **C.** Binucleated dwarf megakaryocyte in an aspirate smear of bone marrow from a dog with AML-M7.   **D.** Megakaryocytic emperipolesis in an aspirate smear of bone marrow from the same cat with thrombocythemia as presented in Figures 56C and 56D.

Emperipolesis

Megakaryocytic emperipolesis refers to the movement of blood cells (neutrophils, erythrocytes, and lymphocytes) within megakaryocytes (Fig. 57D). Emperipolesis differs from phagocytosis in that entering cells temporarily exist within the cell. The mechanism and significance of this finding remain to be defined. Increased emperipolesis has been reported in humans with various conditions including active blood loss, carcinomas, myeloproliferative disorders, and reactive thrombocytosis.[515,516] Emperipolesis occurs at low levels in young rats but is common in aged rats, and the incidence is markedly increased in animals with hyperplastic bone marrow secondary to chronic suppurative or neoplastic lesions.[517] Increased emperipolesis has been produced experimentally in animals in which thrombopoiesis is increased by phlebotomy,[518] interleukin-6 injections,[519] vincristine treatment,[520] and lipopolysaccharide (LPS) injections.[521] Studies with LPS indicate that emperipolesis is at least partly dependent on interactions between adhesion molecules on leukocytes and megakaryocytes.[521] Internalization of *Histoplasma capsulatum* organisms within megakaryocytes has also been reported.[522]

ABNORMALITIES OF MONONUCLEAR PHAGOCYTES

Monocytic Hyperplasia

Monocyte precursors are normally present in low numbers in the bone marrow, and they are difficult to differentiate from neutrophilic precursors based on morphology alone. Consequently, mild monocytic hyperplasia is difficult to recognize, and monocytic hypoplasia is not recognized at all. Monocytic hyperplasia may be appreciated in inflammatory conditions with increased monocyte production and in certain myelodysplastic and myeloproliferative disorders.[183] Monocyte precursors are markedly increased in two forms of AML. When myeloblasts as well as monoblasts are increased, the term "acute myelomonocytic leukemia" (AML-M4) may be used. When only monoblasts are increased, the disorder is classified as acute monocytic leukemia (AML-M5).[236]

Reactive Macrophage Hyperplasia

Macrophage hyperplasia occurs in the bone marrow in response to a variety of systemic viral, bacterial, fungal, and protozoal infectious agents (Fig. 58A).[523] Organisms that may be visualized in bone marrow macrophages include *Mycobacterium* spp.,[171,524] *Histoplasma capsulatum* (Fig. 58B),[522,525–527] *Leishmania donovani*, (Figs. 58C, 58D),[528–530] *Cytauxzoon felis* (Figs. 59A–59D),[116,531] and *Phialemonium obovatum*.[532]

Macrophages may be increased in marrow and contain phagocytized cellular debris in response to marrow necrosis[370,372] or increased apoptosis, as may occur in dyserythropoiesis[307] or myeloproliferative disorders (Figs. 60A, 60B).[303,309] Increased numbers of vacuolated macrophages may be seen in some inherited lipid storage diseases (Fig. 60C).[224,533,534]

Phagocytosis of Blood Cells and Their Precursors

Phagocytosis of blood cells is rare in bone marrow of normal animals and generally only involves mature erythrocytes. Phagocytosis of blood precursor cells is considered abnormal and implies increased cell destruction or death

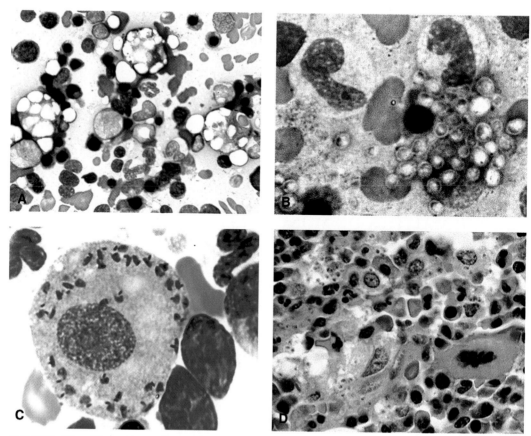

FIGURE 58.   Macrophage hyperplasia, histoplasmosis, and leishmaniasis in bone marrow.
A.   Increased numbers of vacuolated macrophages in bone marrow from an anemic cat with erythroid hyperplasia but minimal increase in blood reticulocyte numbers. Wright-Giemsa stain.   **B.**   Macrophage (right) containing many *Histoplasma capsulatum* organisms in an aspirate smear of bone marrow from a cat with disseminated histoplasmosis. Free organisms (left bottom) may have come from damage to this cell or other macrophages present. Wright-Giemsa stain.   **C.**   Macrophage containing many *Leishmania donovani* organisms in an aspirate smear of bone marrow from a dog with disseminated leishmaniasis. These protozoal organisms are identified by a distinctive bar-shaped kinetoplast in the cytoplasm which stains similar to the nucleus. Wright-Giemsa stain.   **D.**   Macrophages containing *Leishmania donovani* organisms (dark dots) in a bone marrow section from a core biopsy collected from a dog with disseminated leishmaniasis. A megakaryocyte is present at the right side. H&E stain.

within the marrow (Figs. 60D–60F). Increased phagocytosis of blood cells and/ or their precursors—primarily erythroid cells—may be observed in primary or secondary immune-mediated disorders.[70] However, increased phagocytosis of blood cells and/or their precursors may also be observed secondary to various infectious and neoplastic diseases.[305,377,535,536] This finding apparently results from the production of inflammatory cytokines such as γ-interferon, tumor

(text continued on page 157)

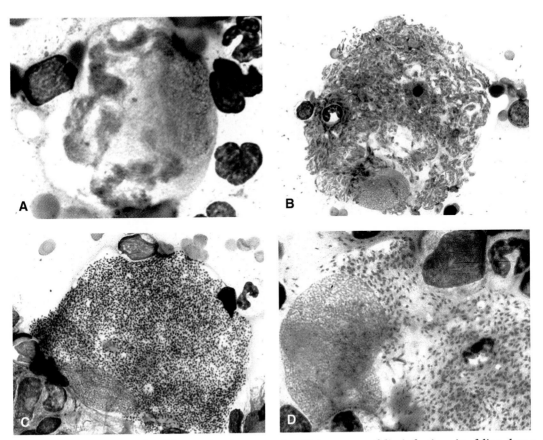

FIGURE 59. Stages of schizont development in *Cytauxzoon felis* infection in feline bone marrow aspirate smears. **Wright-Giemsa stain.**   **A.** Early *Cytauxzoon felis* schizont development within a macrophage in an aspirate smear of bone marrow from a cat with cytauxzoonosis. The "ribbons" of darker blue material with reddish inclusions represent protoplasm of the infectious agent. The macrophage nucleus is eccentrically located on the right side of the cell.   **B.** Intermediate *Cytauxzoon felis* schizont development within a macrophage in an aspirate smear of bone marrow from a cat with cytauxzoonosis shown at a much lower magnification than in Figure 59A. Separation of nuclear and cytoplasmic material has occurred. The nucleus of the macrophage is eccentrically located at the bottom edge of the cell. **C.** Mature *Cytauxzoon felis* schizont within a macrophage in an aspirate smear of bone marrow from a cat with cytauxzoonosis shown at the same magnification as in Figure 59B. Nuclei of hundreds of individual merozoites appear as small dots. The nucleus of the macrophage is eccentrically located at the bottom left edge of the cell.   **D.** Free *Cytauxzoon felis* merozoites (elongated magenta-staining nuclei with wisps of pale-blue cytoplasm) in an aspirate smear of bone marrow from a cat with cytauxzoonosis shown at considerably higher magnification than in Figure 59C. The nucleus of a ruptured macrophage that likely released the merozoites is located at the left of the field.

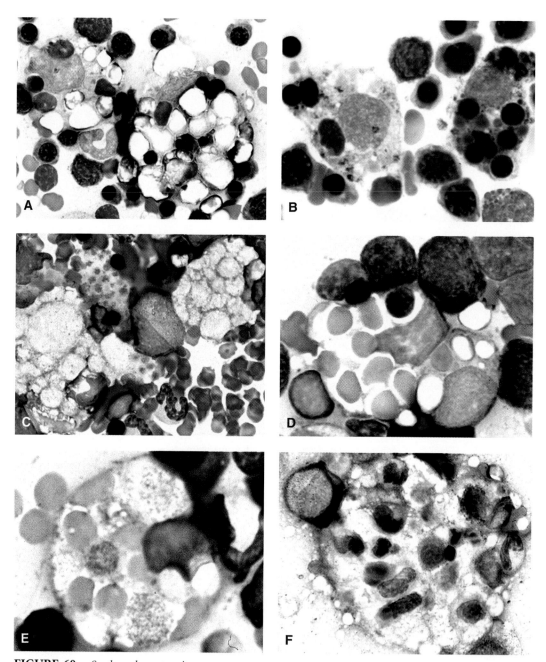

FIGURE 60.   *See legend on opposite page.*

necrosis factor-α, and/or interleukin-1 which, either directly, or indirectly through the production of growth factors such as macrophage-CSF (M-CSF) and GM-CSF, stimulate the production and phagocytic activity of macrophages.[305,523,537]

A hemophagocytic syndrome (hematophagic histiocytosis) has been characterized in humans and animals in which there are cytopenias in blood associated with an increased number of benign-appearing macrophages in bone marrow (a minimum of 2% of all nucleated cells), spleen, lymph nodes, and/or liver that have phagocytized blood cells and/or their precursors. Schistocytes and activated monocytes may also be present in blood.[305,535,538–540]

Malignant Histiocytosis

The term "histiocyte" is used to describe cells of both the monocyte/macrophage series and the Langerhans cell/dendritic cell series.[540] The term "malignant histiocytosis" refers to a malignant neoplasm of macrophages (Figs. 61A–61F). A more descriptive term would be "malignant macrophage histiocytosis."[540] Macrophages present in this disorder exhibit criteria of malignancy not seen in reactive histiocytic disorders. Malignant histiocytes exhibit moderate to marked anisocytosis and anisokaryosis, with moderate to abundant lightly basophilic vacuolated cytoplasm. Nuclei are round, oval, or reniform with prominent nucleoli. Bizarre mitotic figures and multinucleated giant cells may be present. Phagocytosis of blood cells, especially erythrocytes, is common with resultant presence of hemosiderin (Fig. 61B).[321,541–545]

Bernese mountain dogs have a predilection for malignant histiocytosis. Infiltrates are generally prominent in the lungs and hilar lymph nodes, but other lymph nodes, spleen, liver, bone marrow, and central nervous system may be involved.[541,546] In other breeds of dogs and other species of animals, neoplastic infiltrates are most commonly found in spleen, liver, bone marrow, and lymph nodes.[542,544,545,547,548]

In Bernese mountain dogs, malignant histiocytosis must be differentiated from a nonneoplastic disorder termed "systemic histiocytosis," which primarily involves skin and peripheral lymph nodes.[549] Lesions consist of perivascular infiltrates of large histiocytes, as well as minor populations of lymphocytes, neutrophils, and eosinophils. Infiltrates may occur in other organs, including

FIGURE 60. Vacuolated macrophages and phagocytosis of erythrocytes, leukocytes, and platelets in bone marrow aspirate smears. Wright-Giemsa stain.   **A.** Two large macrophages filled with phagocytized cellular material and vacuoles in an aspirate smear of bone marrow from the same cat as presented in Figure 58A.   **B.** Two macrophages with phagocytized cellular material (primarily nuclei) in an aspirate smear of bone marrow from a dog with mild nonregenerative anemia and erythroid hyperplasia in the bone marrow.   **C.** Two vacuolated macrophages in an aspirate smear of bone marrow from a cat with inherited Niemann-Pick type C disease. Photograph of a stained bone marrow smear from a 1993 ASVCP slide review case submitted by Drs. D.E. Brown and M.A. Thrall.   **D.** Macrophage with phagocytized erythrocytes (left) and a nucleus in an aspirate smear of bone marrow from the same cat presented in Figures 58A and 60A.   **E.** Macrophage with phagocytized erythrocytes and platelets in an aspirate smear of bone marrow from a cat with cytauxzoonosis.   **F.** Macrophage with phagocytized leukocytes in an aspirate smear of bone marrow from a leukopenic cat with MDS.

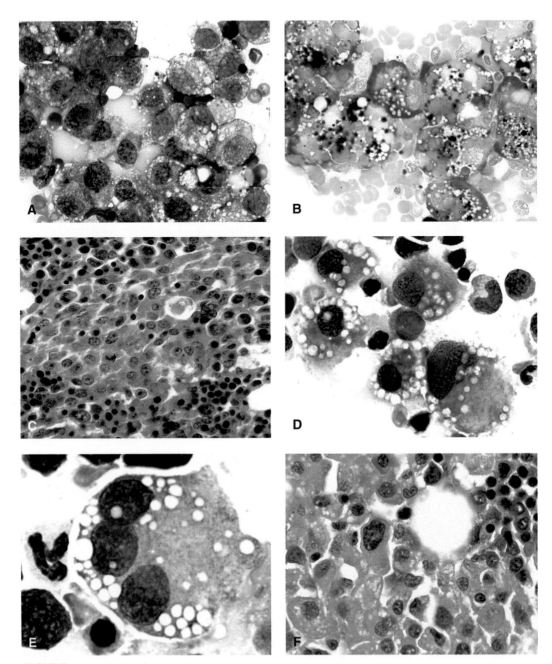

FIGURE 61. *See legend on opposite page.*

bone marrow, in which infiltration is typically sparse, blending almost imperceptibly into surrounding hematopoietic tissue in histologic sections.[549]

◼ INFLAMMATORY DISORDERS OF BONE MARROW

Inflammatory disorders of bone marrow are seldom recognized, because inflammatory cells, including neutrophils, eosinophils, monocytes, macrophages, lymphocytes, and plasma cells, are normally present in bone marrow, making recognition of inflammation difficult in aspirate smears. Increased numbers of neutrophils, eosinophils, and monocytes in bone marrow usually represent increased production to meet peripheral demands, rather than inflammation within the marrow. Core biopsies are generally needed to make a diagnosis of inflammation in the bone marrow, but it is rarely diagnosed because the multifocal distributions of the lesions are easily missed using a small biopsy needle. Recognition of inflammation within the marrow is increased if biopsies are collected from lesions identified using diagnostic imaging techniques. Inflammation in bone marrow has been classified into the various categories discussed below.[550]

Acute Inflammation

Lesions are characterized by circumscribed infiltrates of mature neutrophils (Fig. 62A). Some of these microabscesses have necrotic material in their centers. Vascular dilatation, fibrin exudate, and hemorrhage may also be present. Acute inflammation is generally associated with bacterial infection.[550–552]

FIGURE 61.   Malignant histiocytosis in canine bone marrow aspirate smears and core biopsy sections.   A.   Macrophage proliferation with moderate anisocytosis and anisokaryosis in an aspirate smear of bone marrow from a dog with malignant histiocytosis. Phagocytized erythrocytes are present in two cells at top left. The cytoplasm contains some gray-black material consistent with hemosiderin. Wright-Giemsa stain.   **B.**   Macrophage proliferation with cells containing large amounts of hemosiderin (diffuse and granular blue-staining cytoplasm) in an aspirate smear of bone marrow from the same dog with malignant histiocytosis as presented in Figure 61A. Prussian blue stain.   **C.**   Macrophage proliferation with moderate anisocytosis and anisokaryosis (center of the image) in a bone marrow section from a core biopsy collected from the same dog with malignant histiocytosis as presented in Figures 61A and 61B. Erythroid precursors predominate in the top left corner and along the bottom of the image. H&E stain.   **D.**   Macrophage proliferation with marked anisocytosis and anisokaryosis in an aspirate smear of bone marrow from a dog with malignant histiocytosis. The cytoplasm of each cell contains prominent vacuolation. Cell at left center contains a phagocytized erythrocyte. Wright-Giemsa stain.   **E.**   A large trinucleated macrophage with prominent cytoplasmic vacuolation in an aspirate smear of bone marrow from the same dog with malignant histiocytosis as presented in Figure 61D. Wright-Giemsa stain.   **F.**   Macrophage proliferation with marked anisocytosis and anisokaryosis in a bone marrow section from a core biopsy collected from the same dog with malignant histiocytosis as presented in Figures. 61D and 61E. The cytoplasm of each cell contains prominent vacuolation. A cluster of erythroid precursors is located in the upper right corner. H&E stain.

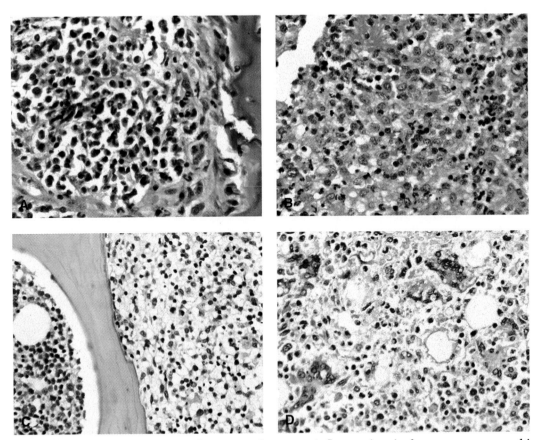

FIGURE 62.   Granulomatous and pyogranulomatous inflammation in bone marrow core biopsy sections.   A.   Focal area of neutrophilic inflammation (microabscess) in a postmortem bone marrow section from a dog with pyogranulomatous inflammation of unknown etiology. Trabecular bone is located at the right edge of the image. H&E stain.   **B.**   Pyogranulomatous inflammation in a postmortem bone marrow section from the same dog as presented in Figure 62A. Macrophages and neutrophils are distributed throughout the image. H&E stain.   **C.**   Granulomatous inflammation in a postmortem bone marrow section from a horse with widely disseminated granulomatous inflammation. A herpesvirus of unknown classification was observed by electron microscopy. The area to the right of the trabecular bone contains primarily macrophages, and the area to the left contains primarily normal marrow elements. H&E stain.   **D.**   Granulomatous inflammation in a postmortem bone marrow section from the same horse as presented in Figure 62C. Macrophages, neutrophils, and several multinucleated giant cells are distributed throughout the image. H&E stain.

Fibrinous Inflammation

Fibrin exudation without accompanying inflammatory cells has been called fibrinous inflammation. Fibrin, which typically appears as small tangled pink fibrils in bone marrow sections stained with H&E, must be differentiated from edema and necrotic debris, which appear as pink homogenous material. Special stains may be used to identify fibrin. Fibrinous inflammation has been recognized in animals with disseminated intravascular coagulation and systemic vasculitis.[550]

Chronic Inflammation/Hyperplasia

Chronic inflammation consists of proliferations or infiltrations of plasma cells, lymphocytes, and/or mast cells. Proliferations of plasma cells and/or lymphocytes have been reported in the bone marrow of dogs with chronic renal disease and in dogs with myelofibrosis.[550]

Chronic Granulomatous Inflammation

Macrophage infiltrates characterize chronic granulomatous inflammation (Figs. 62B, 62C). Both diffuse macrophage infiltrates and focal granulomas have been described.[550] Diffuse infiltrates are included in the section on macrophage hyperplasia in this text. A granuloma is a site of chronic inflammation characterized by the presence of various monocytic cells (monocytes, macrophages, epithelioid cells, and multinucleated giant cells) arranged in compact masses (Fig. 62D). Fibrosis and variable numbers of neutrophils and eosinophils may also be present. When neutrophilic inflammation is also prominent, the term pyogranulomatous inflammation is used (Figs. 62A, 62B). Multifocal granulomatous or pyogranulomatous inflammation involving bone marrow occurs in animals, especially in association with mycobacteriosis and fungal infections such as coccidiomycosis, aspergillosis, blastomycosis, cryptococcosis, histoplasmosis, and *Phialemonium obovatum* infections.[532,551,553,554] German shepherd dogs appear to be more susceptible to systemic *Aspergillus* and *Phialemonium* infections than other dog breeds.[532] The specific etiology cannot always be determined.[555]

CHAPTER 9

HEMATOPOIETIC NEOPLASMS

Hematopoietic neoplasms arise from bone marrow, lymph nodes, spleen, or thymus. They are classified as either lymphoproliferative disorders or myeloproliferative disorders. The term "leukemia" is used when neoplastic cells are seen in blood and/or bone marrow. An exception is the neoplastic proliferation of plasma cells in bone marrow (multiple myeloma), which is not referred to as a leukemia. Leukocyte counts may be low, normal, or high in animals with leukemias. The term "acute" is used to describe leukemias in which a predominance of blast cells occurs in the bone marrow, and the term "chronic" is used for leukemias in which there is a predominance of well-differentiated cells in blood and bone marrow. The progression of disease is usually rapid (weeks to months) in acute leukemias and slow (months to years) in chronic leukemias.

Precursor cells for mast cell tumors and malignant histiocytosis arise from bone marrow,[280,556] but these neoplasms usually develop from more mature cells in the peripheral tissues. Consequently, they are typically not included with myeloproliferative disorders, even though it is possible that some cases of noncutaneous systemic mastocytosis and some cases of malignant histiocytosis might qualify as hematopoietic neoplasms.

■ LYMPHOPROLIFERATIVE DISORDERS

The term "lymphoma" denotes a solid tumor(s) of neoplastic lymphocytes located outside the bone marrow. The term "lymphoid leukemia" indicates a neoplastic condition of lymphocytes present in bone marrow and/or blood that is not associated with a solid tumor(s). Lymphoid leukemias are further classified as acute or chronic depending on the maturity of the cells involved. When neoplastic cells are present in the blood of an animal with a lymphoma, the terms "lymphoma with leukemia" or "lymphosarcoma cell leukemia" have been used, but the former term is preferred. A metastasis from bone marrow to lymphoid tissues and from lymphoid tissues to bone marrow is common. Consequently, it may be difficult to differentiate a true leukemia from a lymphoma with leukemia in animals with advanced stages of disease.

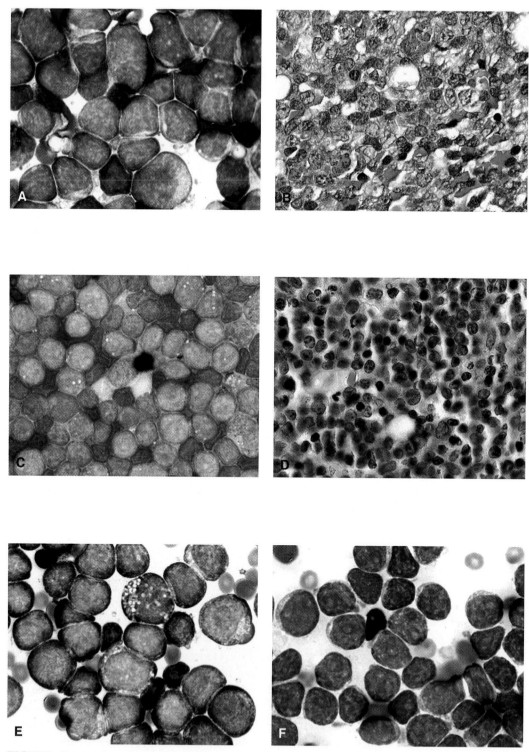

FIGURE 63. *See legend on opposite page.*

Acute Lymphoblastic Leukemia

Neoplastic lymphoblasts and/or prolymphocytes are present in bone marrow of animals with acute lymphoblastic leukemia (ALL) (Figs. 63A–63F). Neoplastic cells are also usually present in blood (Figs. 24F, 24G, 25A), with or without an absolute lymphocytosis. Pancytopenia, with ALL diagnosed by bone marrow biopsy, has been reported in horses.[228] Neoplastic lymphocytes present in ALL exhibit decreased nuclear chromatin condensation and increased cytoplasmic basophilia compared to normal blood lymphocytes.[226,557] Nucleoli may or may not be seen in these neoplastic cells and, when present, may be difficult to visualize. Other abnormalities, including increased anisocytosis, anisokaryosis, and nuclear pleomorphism, may also be present. Lymphoblasts are generally difficult to differentiate from blast cells of other hematopoietic lineages without the use of special stains and/or surface markers. Compared to myeloblasts, lymphoblasts tend to exhibit more-condensed chromatin and less-prominent nucleoli.[558]

Most cases of ALL in cats have the T-lymphocyte phenotype, and most are FeLV positive,[557] but FIV positive, FeLV negative cats with ALL have been reported.[426,559,560] Dogs with ALL may be of the T-lymphocyte, B-lymphocyte, NK-cell, or null-cell phenotypes.[211,561]

Chronic Lymphocytic Leukemia

Chronic lymphocytic leukemia (CLL) is reported most often in old animals. The nuclear chromatin is more condensed in CLL than in ALL. Lymphocytosis, involving normal-appearing lymphocytes, is consistently present in blood (Figs. 23C, 23D).[207,557,562] In contrast with ALL, most cats with CLL are FeLV negative.[557]

T-lymphocyte, B-lymphocyte, and large granular lymphocyte (LGL) types of CLL have been identified.[207,208,210,211,215,561,562] T-lymphocyte and B-lymphocyte types of CLL have normal-appearing, small to medium-sized lymphocytes with scant amounts of light-blue cytoplasm. Dogs with B-lymphocyte type CLL often have an accompanying monoclonal gammopathy that is most often of the IgM

FIGURE 63. Acute lymphoblastic leukemia (ALL) in bone marrow aspirate smears and core biopsy sections. A. Lymphoblasts with dark-blue cytoplasm and indistinct nucleoli in an aspirate smear of bone marrow from a dog with ALL. Wright-Giemsa stain. **B.** Lymphoblasts in a bone marrow section from a core biopsy collected from the same dog with ALL as presented in Figure 63A. The orange material present is hemosiderin. H&E stain. **C.** Lymphoblasts with dark-blue cytoplasm and indistinct nucleoli in an aspirate smear of bone marrow from a different dog with ALL from the one shown in Figures 63A and 63B. Lymphoblasts were not visible in blood from this animal. Wright-Giemsa stain. **D.** Lymphoblasts in a bone marrow section from a core biopsy collected from the same dog with ALL as presented in Figure 63C. The orange material present is hemosiderin. H&E stain. **E.** Lymphoblasts with dark-blue cytoplasm and indistinct nucleoli in an aspirate smear of bone marrow from a cat with ALL. A minority of neoplastic cells had cytoplasmic vacuoles. Wright-Giemsa stain. **F.** Lymphoblasts, often with visible nucleoli, in a roll preparation from a core biopsy from a horse with ALL. Wright-Giemsa stain.

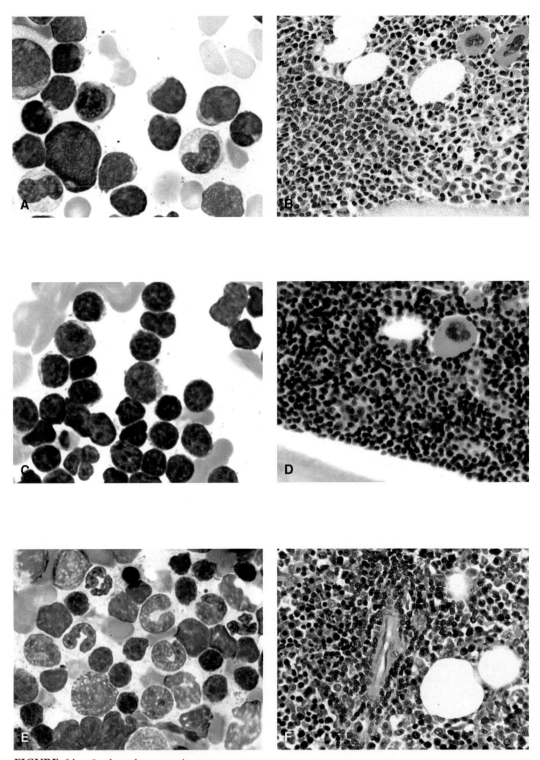

FIGURE 64. *See legend on opposite page.*

type.[558,562,563] An IgG monoclonal gammopathy has also been reported in a horse with CLL.[207]

Lymphocytes present in the LGL type of CLL have red- or purple-staining (generally focal) granules within light-blue cytoplasm (Fig. 23E). These cells also have condensed nuclear chromatin, but they are generally larger, with more cytoplasm and lower N:C ratios, than cells present in non-LGL types of CLL.[208,210,215] Although most dogs with LGL leukemia behave like CLL and progress slowly over several years, some dogs with LGL leukemia behave like an aggressive form of ALL (Fig. 23F).[211,214] Nearly all dogs with the LGL form of CLL have neoplastic T lymphocytes, but dogs with the LGL form of ALL may be of either the T-lymphocyte or the NK-cell types.[211]

Bone marrow examination of animals with CLL often reveals increased numbers of normal-appearing lymphocytes (Figs. 64A–64E); however, the extent of infiltration is generally less than that seen in ALL. Bone marrow may contain some normal lymphoid follicles, consisting primarily of normal-appearing lymphocytes (Fig. 64F), which must be differentiated from a neoplastic lymphoid infiltrate. B-lymphocyte type CLL appears to originate in the bone marrow. In contrast, T-lymphocyte development requires processing by the thymus and T-lymphocyte CLL appears to develop outside the marrow (e.g., the spleen) with secondary marrow infiltration.[211] Special surface marker tests are usually needed to identify the cell type involved, although the coexistence of a monoclonal gammopathy with CLL indicates B-lymphocyte type neoplasia.[211,561]

Lymphomas

Lymphomas are solid tumors of neoplastic lymphocytes that develop outside the bone marrow. They may be classified by the anatomic site involved (e.g., alimentary, thymic, cutaneous, multicentric), by cell morphology in lymph nodes (e.g., centroblastic, lymphoblastic, immunoblastic), and by cell type (e.g., B-lymphocyte, T-lymphocyte, LGL).[191,557,558,564–567]

FIGURE 64.   Chronic lymphocytic leukemia (CLL) in bone marrow aspirate smears and core biopsy sections compared to a lymphoid follicle.   A.   Infiltrate of small lymphocytes with condensed nuclear chromatin and minimal cytoplasm in an aspirate smear of bone marrow from a dog with CLL. Wright-Giemsa stain.   **B.**   Infiltrate of small lymphocytes (especially in the left half of the image) in a bone marrow section from a core biopsy collected from the same dog with CLL as presented in Figure 64A. Two megakaryocytes are present in the upper right corner. H&E stain.   **C.**   Infiltrate of small lymphocytes with condensed nuclear chromatin and minimal cytoplasm in an aspirate smear of bone marrow from a dog with CLL. A monoclonal hyperglobulinemia also present in this dog indicated that these cells are B lymphocytes. Wright-Giemsa stain.   **D.**   Marked infiltrate of small lymphocytes in a bone marrow section from a core biopsy collected from the same dog with CLL as presented in Figure 64C. Cortical bone is located at lower left and a megakaryocyte is present at upper right. H&E stain.   **E.** Infiltrate of normal-appearing small lymphocytes in an aspirate smear of bone marrow from a cat with CLL. Wright-Giemsa stain.   **F.**   A small lymphoid follicle around a longitudinal section of a vessel (left of center) in a bone marrow section from a core biopsy collected from a dog. H&E stain.

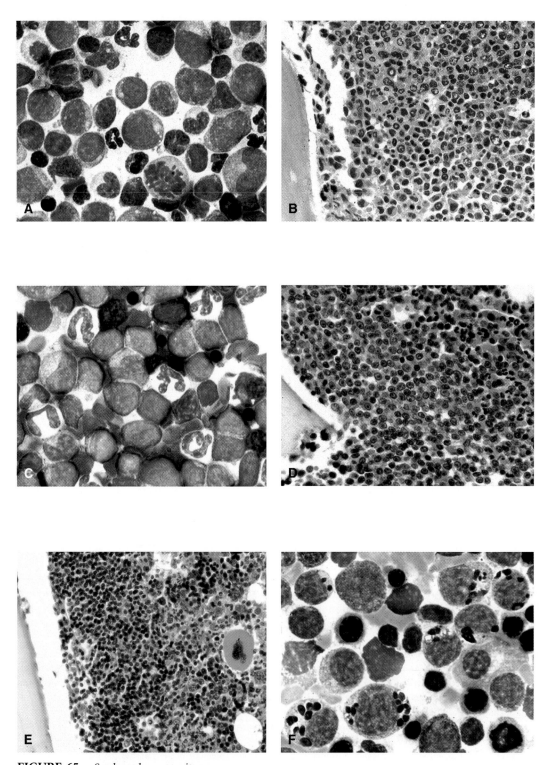

FIGURE 65. *See legend on opposite page.*

Based on abnormal morphology, neoplastic cells are recognized in the blood of about one quarter to one half of the animals presenting with a lymphoma.[230,557,568,569] In the remaining cases, neoplastic lymphocytes may be absent from blood or may not have sufficiently abnormal morphology to be recognized. Bone marrow infiltrates may sometimes be recognized in animals even when neoplastic cells are not appreciated in blood (Figs. 65A–65E).[230,569,570] Core biopsies offer the advantage that small aggregates of lymphoid cells that would be dispersed during bone marrow aspiration and smear preparation can be recognized (Figs. 65D, 65E). Lymphoid infiltrates in the bone marrow of dogs with lymphomas are most often paratrabecular in location.[570] Focal infiltrates must be differentiated from benign lymphoid follicles, which have well-defined borders and are composed primarily of small mature lymphocytes (Fig. 64F). Neoplastic aggregates are generally larger, with poorly defined borders, and cells within these aggregates are often large and immature in appearance.[570]

Lymphomas involving LGLs have been primarily reported in cats, where they generally occur as intestinal lymphomas that metastasize to various other organs including the spleen, liver, lymph nodes, blood, and bone marrow (Fig. 65F).[217–219,571] Some authors have classified these neoplasms as globule leukocyte tumors or granulated round cell tumors.[572,573] Their granules are generally much larger than those seen in normal LGLs in blood. They appear blue, red, or purple with Wright-Giemsa stain but may not stain well with Diff-Quik stain.[217] In some cases, the granules appear eosinophilic in H&E-stained sections, but in other cases, they are difficult to identify with H&E. The neoplastic cells may originate from intraepithelial lymphocytes and most, but not all, of these tumors appear to be composed of cytotoxic T lymphocytes.[218]

Two cases of LGL lymphoma have been reported in horses.[216,574] Neoplastic cells were recognized in the blood of one case and in the bone marrow of the other case.

FIGURE 65. Metastatic lymphoma in bone marrow aspirate smears and core biopsy sections. A. Infiltrate of variably sized lymphoblasts in an aspirate smear of bone marrow from a dog with metastatic lymphoma. A mitotic cell is present at bottom center. Wright-Giemsa stain.   **B.** Diffuse infiltrate of variably sized lymphoblasts in a bone marrow section from a core biopsy from the same dog with metastatic lymphoma as presented in Figure 65A. Cortical bone is located along the left edge of the image. H&E stain.   **C.** Infiltrate of variably sized lymphoblasts in an aspirate smear of bone marrow from a dog with metastatic lymphoma. The lymphoblasts have round nuclei and scant amounts of cytoplasm. Wright-Giemsa stain.   **D.** Focal infiltrate of lymphoblasts near cortical bone (lower left) in a bone marrow section from a core biopsy from the same dog with metastatic lymphoma as presented in Figure 65C. H&E stain.   **E.** Focal infiltrate of lymphocytes near cortical bone (left) in a bone marrow section from a core biopsy from a dog with metastatic lymphoma. H&E stain.   **F.** Infiltrate of large granular lymphocytes in an aspirate smear of bone marrow from a cat with metastatic lymphoma involving large granular lymphocytes. The granules in these cells are larger than those seen in the granular lymphocytes that normally circulate in blood. Wright-Giemsa stain.

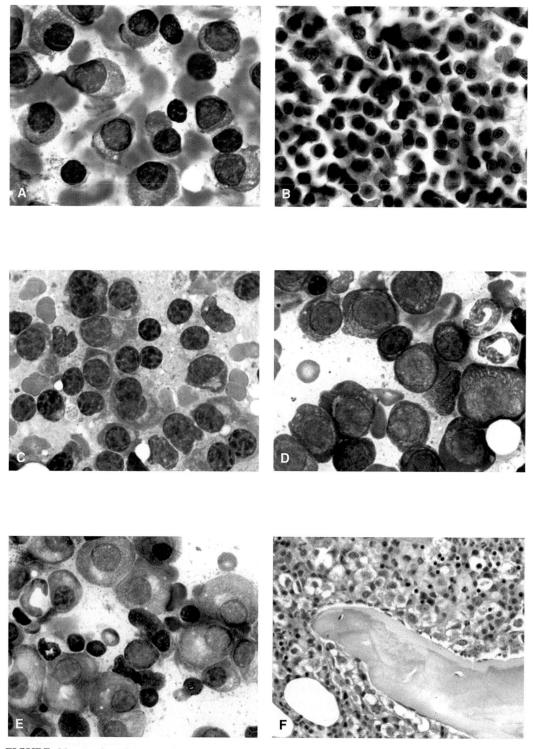

FIGURE 66. *See legend on opposite page.*

Multiple Myeloma and Other Immunoproliferative Neoplasms

Any cell type in the normal B-lymphocyte maturation pathway may become neoplastic and produce an immunoglobulin. The nature of a lymphoproliferative disorder is determined by the stage at which B-lymphocyte maturation is arrested.

Multiple Myeloma. Multiple myeloma (plasma cell myeloma) is a B-lymphocyte tumor of bone marrow that is manifested as a proliferation of plasma cells.[567,575–582] A monoclonal IgG or IgA immunoglobulin is usually secreted by the tumor, resulting in a monoclonal hyperglobulinemia, which is recognized using serum protein electrophoresis.[577] The type of immunoglobulin produced can be identified using immunoelectrophoresis and quantified using methods such as single radial immunodiffusion. Rarely, multiple myeloma secretes no measurable monoclonal protein,[583,584] produces biclonal proteins,[585,586] or produces only a component of an immunoglobulin molecule (light chains or heavy chains).[587,588] Focal lytic or diffuse osteoporotic bone lesions are often recognized using survey radiography, and a Bence-Jones proteinuria (immunoglobulin light chains in urine) may be present. Plasma cell infiltrates may be found in other tissues including the spleen, liver, lymph nodes, and kidneys.

Increased numbers of plasma cells are usually identified in routine bone marrow biopsies of animals with multiple myeloma (Figs. 66A–66F, 67A–67C). In some cases, it is necessary to biopsy lytic bone lesions to demonstrate the plasma cell infiltrates. The morphology of the neoplastic cells present can vary from normal-appearing mature plasma cells to large immature pleomorphic plasma cells with diffuse chromatin, abundant cytoplasm, and increased mitotic index. Multiple nuclei may be present. The cytoplasm generally appears light blue to dark blue when Romanowsky-type blood stains are used, but in rare instances, the cytoplasm of the neoplastic cells is filled with Russell bodies (Mott's cells), or the cytoplasm stains red (flame cells), especially at the periphery of the cell.[291,292] The appearance of the flame cells may depend on the blood stain used (Figs. 67A, 67B).

FIGURE 66. **Multiple myeloma in bone marrow aspirate smears and core biopsy sections.** **A.** Infiltrate of plasma cells with basophilic cytoplasm and eccentric nuclei in an aspirate smear of bone marrow from a dog with multiple myeloma. Wright-Giemsa stain. **B.** Infiltrate of plasma cells with eccentric nuclei, exhibiting coarsely clumped chromatin in a characteristic mosaic pattern, in a section of bone marrow collected as a core biopsy from the same dog with multiple myeloma as shown in Figure 41J. H&E stain. **C.** Infiltrate of plasma cells with eccentric nuclei and basophilic cytoplasm containing pale Golgi zones in an aspirate smear of bone marrow from a cat with multiple myeloma. Nuclear chromatin is coarsely clumped in a characteristic mosaic pattern. Two binucleated plasma cells are present. Wright-Giemsa stain. **D.** Infiltrate of plasmacytoblasts with intensely basophilic cytoplasm and eccentric nuclei in an aspirate smear of bone marrow from a dog with multiple myeloma. Wright-Giemsa stain. **E.** Infiltrate of plasma cells with eccentric nuclei and abundant basophilic cytoplasm containing pale Golgi zones in an aspirate smear of bone marrow from a dog with multiple myeloma. Wright-Giemsa stain. **F.** Infiltrate of plasma cells with abundant cytoplasm near trabecular bone in a section of bone marrow collected as a core biopsy from the same dog with multiple myeloma as presented in Figure 66E. H&E stain.

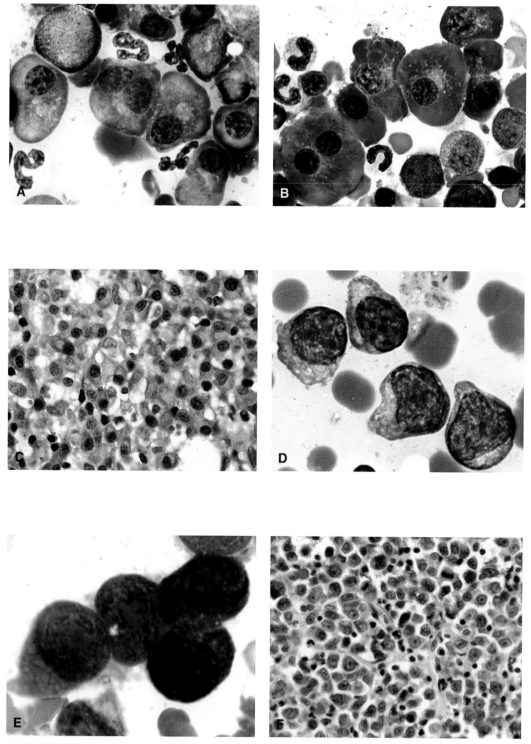

FIGURE 67.   *See legend on opposite page.*

Plasmacytoma.   In addition to the metastasis of multiple myeloma from bone marrow, extramedullary plasma cell tumors (plasmacytomas) may arise as primary tumors of soft tissues. They occur most frequently as solitary tumors in the skin or mouth of dogs and cats but have also been reported in various gastrointestinal sites.[589-595] They rarely have an associated monoclonal or biclonal hyperglobulinemia[593,595-597] and rarely metastasize to distant sites.[593,598]

Other B-Lymphocyte Neoplasms.   Other B-lymphocyte neoplasms, including multicentric lymphomas (Figs. 67E, 67F), B-lymphocyte CLL (discussed previously), and primary macroglobulinemia may produce monoclonal hyperglobulinemias.[576] Lytic bone lesions are generally absent in these disorders, even when bone marrow infiltrates are present. In humans, primary (Waldenstrom) macroglobulinemia is characterized as a lymphoplasmacytic neoplasm that produces an IgM monoclonal protein. The marrow aspirate is often of low cellularity, but the core biopsy is generally hypercellular and diffusely infiltrated with lymphocytes, plasmacytoid lymphocytes, and some plasma cells.[599] This syndrome is rarely reported in animals (Fig. 67D).[576,600,601] The spleen, liver, and lymphoid tissues may have neoplastic infiltrates rather than bone marrow.[581]

■ MYELOPROLIFERATIVE DISORDERS

Myeloproliferative disorders are characterized by the purposeless proliferation of one or more of the nonlymphoid marrow cell lines (granulocytic, monocytic, erythrocytic, or megakaryocytic).[131,183,236,238,431,602] Myeloproliferative disorders are generally considered to be benign or malignant neoplastic diseases, but many hematologists also consider the hypercellular myelodysplastic syndrome (MDS) to be a myeloproliferative disorder because MDS has been shown to be clonal and may precede the development of AML in humans and ani-

---

FIGURE 67.   Immunoglobulin-secreting tumors in bone marrow aspirate smears and core biopsy sections.   A.   Infiltrate of plasma cells with eccentric nuclei and abundant basophilic cytoplasm containing pale Golgi zones in an aspirate smear of bone marrow from a dog with multiple myeloma and a biclonal hyperglobulinemia migrating in the gamma region on serum protein electrophoresis. A binucleated plasma cell is present near the center. Wright-Giemsa stain.   **B.**   Infiltrate of plasma cells with eccentric nuclei and abundant cytoplasm in an aspirate smear of bone marrow from the same dog with multiple myeloma as presented in Figure 67A. These cells have been called flame cells because of their red-staining cytoplasm. A binucleated plasma cell is present near the bottom left corner. Diff-Quik stain.   **C.** Infiltrate of plasma cells with eccentric nuclei and abundant cytoplasm in a section of bone marrow collected as a core biopsy from the same dog with multiple myeloma as presented in Figures 67A and 67B. H&E stain.   **D.**   Infiltrate of basophilic lymphoid cells in an aspirate smear of bone marrow from a dog with macroglobulinemia (IgM hyperglobulinemia). Neoplastic cells were also present in the spleen but not in lymph nodes. Wright-Giemsa stain.   **E.**   Basophilic plasmacytoid blast cell infiltrate in an aspirate smear of bone marrow from a cat. Similar blast cells were present in blood, skin, lungs, and liver. A monoclonal IgA hyperglobulinemia was present. Wright-Giemsa stain.   **F.**   Marked infiltrate of plasmacytoid blast cells in a postmortem bone marrow section from the same cat as presented in Figure 67E. H&E stain.

mals.[101,303,309,425,514,603–606] The unitary concept of myeloproliferative disorders was developed because all nonlymphoid blood cells are derived from a common myeloid stem cell and neoplastic transformations in these disorders usually occur in pluripotent progenitor cells.[607] Although the proliferation of one cell type may predominate, a marrow cell line is seldom singly affected. Morphologic or functional disorders of other cell lines can usually be detected. In addition, some of these disorders appear to evolve into one another. For example, MDS with excessive proliferation of nucleated erythrocytes (MDS-Er) in cats may evolve into erythroleukemia and eventually myeloblastic leukemia.[17,603]

Cats with myeloproliferative disorders are generally infected with FeLV and/or FIV viruses.[17,559,560,606,608] Irradiation has been experimentally shown to cause myeloproliferative disorders in dogs.[339,514] Myeloproliferative disorders are rare in domestic animal species other than cats and dogs and their causes are unknown.

Myelodysplastic Syndromes

The bone marrow in MDS is usually normocellular or hypercellular (Figs. 46D–46F), but cytopenias (especially anemia and thrombocytopenia) are present in the blood. This apparent ineffective hematopoiesis appears to result from extensive apoptosis.[309] Apoptosis or physiologic cell death is a mechanism of gene-directed cellular self-destruction in which intracellular endonucleases initially cut DNA into fragments.[369] Recognizable apoptotic cells with fragmented nuclei exist for only 10 to 15 minutes before removal by phagocytic cells.[309] MDS may result from FeLV and/or FIV infections in cats,[426,431,450,451] but one study indicates that many cats with MDS have negative tests for these viruses.[609]

Evidence of dyserythropoiesis, dysgranulopoiesis, and/or dysmegakaryocytopoiesis is present in the marrow.[58,183] These proliferative abnormalities are presented in more detail elsewhere in this text. Erythroid abnormalities that may be present include megaloblastic cells, abnormal nuclear shapes, premature nuclear pyknosis, nuclear fragmentation, multinucleated cells, nuclear and cytoplasmic asynchrony, maturation arrest, and siderotic inclusions (Figs. 51E, 52A–52M).[11,58,101–103,303,404,424–426,430,432] Neutrophilic abnormalities that may be present include increased numbers (5% to 29%) of myeloblasts; maturation arrest in the neutrophilic series at the myelocyte-metamyelocyte stage; giant metamyelocytes, bands, and mature neutrophils; abnormal granulation such as large primary granules or granules surrounded by vacuoles; hyposegmented neutrophils (pseudo-Pelger-Huet); hypersegmented neutrophils; and neutrophils with bizarre nuclear shapes (Figs. 52N–52P, 55A–55F).[101,103,131,178,303,404,430,431,451] Increased numbers of eosinophilic cells are also commonly observed in MDS in cats and dogs.[236] Megakaryocytic abnormalities that may be present include dwarf granular megakaryocytes with single or multiple nuclei and large megakaryocytes with nuclear abnormalities including hypolobulation, hyperlobulation, or multiple round nuclei (Figs. 57A–57C).[131,178,303,425,431,514] Some cats with MDS have stainable iron in their marrow (Fig. 46D).[605]

Additional abnormalities that may be present in blood include nonregenerative anemia with erythrocyte macrocytosis, anisocytosis, and/or poikilocytosis; nucleated erythrocytes (normoblastemia) out of proportion to the number of reticulocytes present; nucleated erythrocytes with lobulated or fragmented nuclei; large bizarre platelets; immature granulocytes; and abnormal granulocyte morphology (large size, hyposegmentation, hypersegmentation).[70,101,102,424,431,605] The total leukocyte counts and absolute neutrophil counts vary from low to high.[238]

Classification of MDS into three subtypes has been suggested in animals based on blood and bone marrow findings.[183] MDS with erythroid predominance in the bone marrow (M:E ratio below 1) may be classified as MDS-Er.[101,236,238,303] Cases previously diagnosed as erythremic myelosis would now be placed in this category, as long as the number of blast cells in the marrow was less than 30% of all nucleated cells. Cases with refractory anemia and M:E ratio above 1, with or without other refractory cytopenias, may be described as myelodysplastic syndrome-refractory cytopenia (MDS-RC).[425,431,605] Myeloblasts account for less than 5% of all nucleated cells in this subtype. When myeloblasts are increased (5% to 29% of bone marrow nucleated cells), the term "myelodysplastic syndrome-excess blasts" (MDS-EB) may be used.[430] Animals with bone marrow blast counts slightly below 30% may represent animals in transition between MDS and AML, or they may represent animals that have AML which is not diagnosed as such, because the blast count does not exceed the arbitrary number previously established.[238]

Dogs and cats with MDS may subsequently develop AML,[101,303,425,514,603–606] and FeLV-positive cats with MDS may also develop lymphoid neoplasms.[604] It is unknown what percentage of MDS cases represent a preleukemic state. Extended and costly supportive care is generally required for the survival of animals with MDS, and many animals with MDS die or are euthanized before sufficient time has elapsed for an acute leukemia to develop. Although rare, animals with MDS may recover spontaneously, as occurred in a FeLV-positive cat that became FeLV negative.[610]

Acute Myeloid Leukemias

A classification system for acute myeloid leukemia (AML) has been proposed by the American Society for Veterinary Clinical Pathology Animal Leukemia Study Group for use in dogs and cats.[236] It was adapted from the French-American-British (FAB) system established by a National Cancer Institute workshop for use in humans.[611] AML is diagnosed when the percentage of nonlymphoid hematopoietic blast cells in the bone marrow equals or exceeds 30% of all nucleated cells (ANC), excluding lymphocytes, macrophages, plasma cells, and mast cells. Dyserythropoiesis, dysgranulopoiesis, and/or dysmegakaryocytopoiesis are also usually present, with megaloblastic nucleated erythroid cells being most commonly observed.[236] If blast cells account for less than 30% of all nucleated cells and dysplastic changes are present, a diagnosis of MDS is made. Some

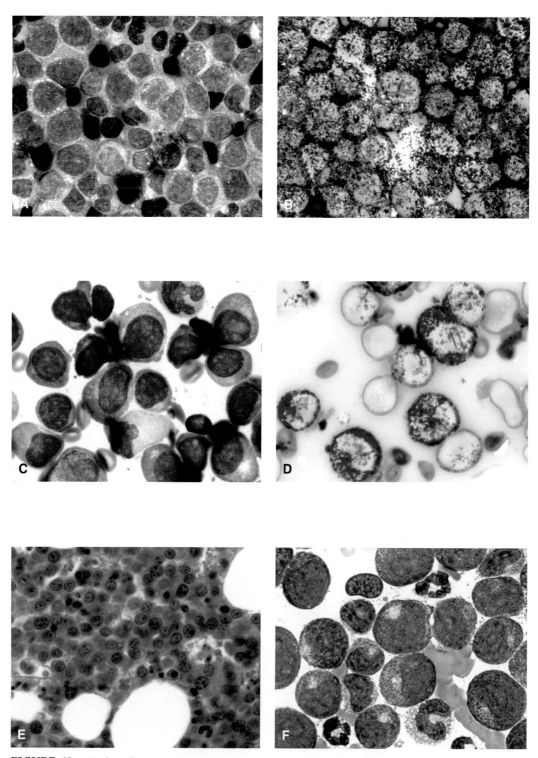

FIGURE 68.   *See legend on opposite page.*

cases of erythroleukemia (AML-M6) are exceptions to these guidelines, as will be discussed subsequently. Cytochemistry, immunocytochemistry, and electron microscopy may be used to help identify the type(s) of blast cells present. Several subtypes of AML have been recognized in animals.[183,236,238,602,612] In addition to quantifying cells as a percentage of ANC, they may also be quantified based on the total nonerythroid cells (NEC), which is determined by subtracting the nucleated erythroid cells from the ANC count.[183]

AML-M1. Myeloblastic leukemia without maturation is designated as AML-M1. Myeloblasts (primarily type I myeloblasts) account for 90% or more of NEC. Type I myeloblasts appear as large round cells with round to oval nuclei that are generally centrally located in the cell. The N:C ratio is high (>1.5) and the nuclear outline is usually regular and smooth. Nuclear chromatin is finely stippled, containing one or more nucleoli or nucleolar rings. The cytoplasm is generally moderately basophilic.[236] Differentiated granulocytes (promyelocytes through mature neutrophils and eosinophils) and monocytes account for the remaining NEC.

AML-M2. Myeloblastic leukemia with differentiation is designated AML-M2. Myeloblasts account for 30% to 89% of NEC (Figs. 68A–68F, 69A, 69B). In addition to type I myeloblasts, variable numbers of type II myeloblasts, containing a few (<15) small, magenta-staining granules in the cytoplasm, may be present. Differentiated granulocytes account for 10% or more of NEC and monocytic cells account for less than 20% of NEC. Increased marrow basophil and/or eosinophil precursors may be seen in some cats with myeloproliferative disorders (Fig. 54B), and variants of AML-M2 with basophilic differentiation and eosinophilic differentiation have been reported in cats and classified as M2-B and M2-Eos, respectively.[238,613]

AML-M3. Promyelocytic leukemia has not been reported in animals. In humans, the predominant cells involved are abnormal-appearing promyelocytes with folded, reniform, or bilobed nuclei. Type III myeloblasts may also be present in this disorder. These cells have distinct nucleoli and abundant cyto-

FIGURE 68. Acute myeloid leukemia (AML) in bone marrow aspirate smears and a core biopsy section. A. Proliferation of myeloblasts, promyelocytes, and myelocytes in an aspirate smear of bone marrow from a cat with AML-M2. Approximately 35% of all nucleated cells were myeloblasts. Few band or mature neutrophils were present and rare erythroid precursors were recognized. Wright-Giemsa stain. **B.** Proliferation of myeloblasts, promyelocytes, and myelocytes in an aspirate smear of bone marrow from the same cat with AML-M2 as presented in Figure 68A. The strongly peroxidase-positive nature of the cells present rules out a lymphoproliferative disorder and indicates that these cells are granulocytic precursors. Peroxidase stain. **C.** Proliferation of myeloblasts in an aspirate smear of bone marrow from a dog with AML-M2. Nucleoli were easily recognized in many cells. Wright-Giemsa stain. **D.** Proliferation of myeloblasts in an aspirate smear of bone marrow from the same dog with AML-M2 as presented in Figure 68C. Most of these cells were peroxidase positive, ruling out a lymphoproliferative disorder. Peroxidase stain. **E.** Proliferation of myeloblasts in a section of bone marrow collected as a core biopsy from the same dog with AML-M2 as presented in Figures 68C and 68D. H&E stain. **F.** Proliferation of myeloblasts and promyelocytes in an aspirate smear of bone marrow from a dog with AML-M2. Many of the cells contain primary magenta-staining granules. Wright-Giemsa stain.

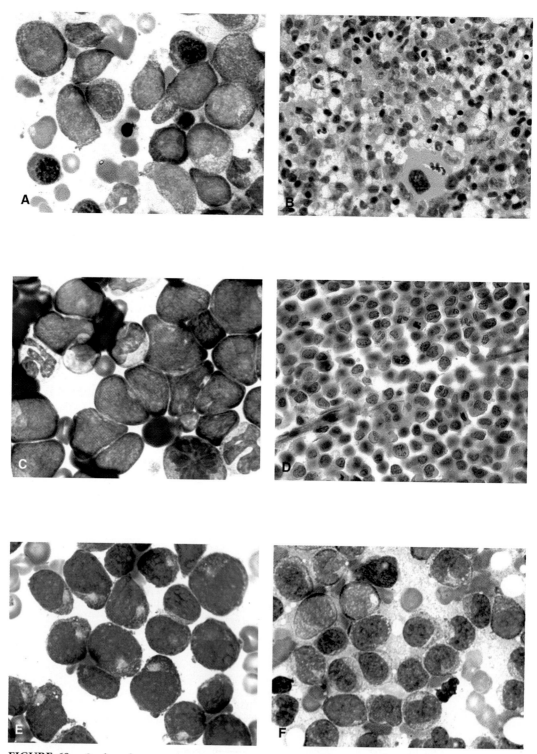

FIGURE 69.   *See legend on opposite page.*

plasm containing many magenta-staining cytoplasmic granules. Type III myelo-blasts appear to represent blast cells with asynchronous cytoplasmic maturation. Low numbers of these cells may be present in cats with AML.[238]

AML-M4.   Acute myelomonocytic leukemia is diagnosed when combined num-bers of myeloblasts and monoblasts equal or exceed 30% of ANC, and differen-tiated granulocytes and monocytes each account for 20% or more of NEC. Monoblasts resemble myeloblasts except that their nuclear shape is irregularly round to convoluted in appearance (Figs. 69C, 69D). A clear area in the cytoplasm, representing the Golgi zone, is often observed, especially near the site of nuclear indentation. The N:C ratio is high but may be somewhat lower than that in myeloblasts.[236]

AML-M5.   Acute monocytic leukemia is diagnosed when monoblasts are in-creased, but myeloblasts are not (Figs. 69E, 69F). It may be separated into subtypes depending on the maturity of the monocytic cells present. Little matu-ration to monocytes is present in M5a, with monoblasts and promonocytes accounting for 80% or more of all NEC. When 30% to 79% of NEC are monoblasts and promonocytes and maturation to monocytes is prominent, the leukemia is classified as M5b. Granulocytes account for less than 20% of NEC.

AML-M6.   "Erythroleukemia" is a term used to describe myeloproliferative disorders in which erythroid abnormalities are prominent.[183,236,238] In contrast to the subtypes of AML discussed previously, the M:E ratio is less than 1 in AML-M6, and blasts cells (myeloblasts, monoblasts, and megakaryoblasts com-bined) may not equal or exceed 30% of ANC, but they will equal or exceed 30% of the NEC (Fig. 70A). The designation "AML-M6Er" is used when the M:E ratio is less than 1 and rubriblasts are included with myeloblast, mono-blasts, and megakaryoblasts in the blast count to equal or exceed 30% of ANC. In some cases, most of the blasts present appear to be rubriblasts (Figs. 70B, 70C). Rubriblasts have deeply basophilic cytoplasm that is devoid of granules.

FIGURE 69.   Myeloblastic leukemia (AML-M2), acute myelomonocytic leukemia (AML-M4), and acute monocytic leukemia (AML-M5) in bone marrow aspirate smears and core biopsy sections.   **A.**   Increased numbers of myeloblasts (large round cells with medium-blue cytoplasm) in an aspirate smear of bone marrow from a horse with AML-M2. The smaller and more darkly staining cells present are erythroid precursors. Wright-Giemsa stain.   **B.**   Proliferation of myeloblasts in a section of bone marrow collected as a core biopsy from the same horse with AML-M2 as presented in Figure 69A. Darker cells are erythroid precursors. Several red-staining eosinophils are also present. A megakaryocyte is present at bottom center. H&E stain.   **C.**   Proliferation of myeloblasts (generally round nuclei) and monoblasts (frequently indented nuclei) in an aspirate smear of bone marrow from a dog with AML-M4. Wright-Giemsa stain.   **D.**   Proliferation of myeloblasts and monoblasts in a section of bone marrow collected as a core biopsy from the same dog with AML-M4 as presented in Figure 69C. H&E stain.   **E.**   Proliferation of monoblasts (frequently indented nuclei) in an aspirate smear of bone marrow from a dog with acute monocytic leukemia (AML-M5). Wright-Giemsa stain.   **F.**   Proliferation of monoblasts (fre-quently indented nuclei) in an aspirate smear of bone marrow from a dog with acute monocytic leukemia (AML-M5) different from the one presented in Figure 69E. Wright-Giemsa stain.

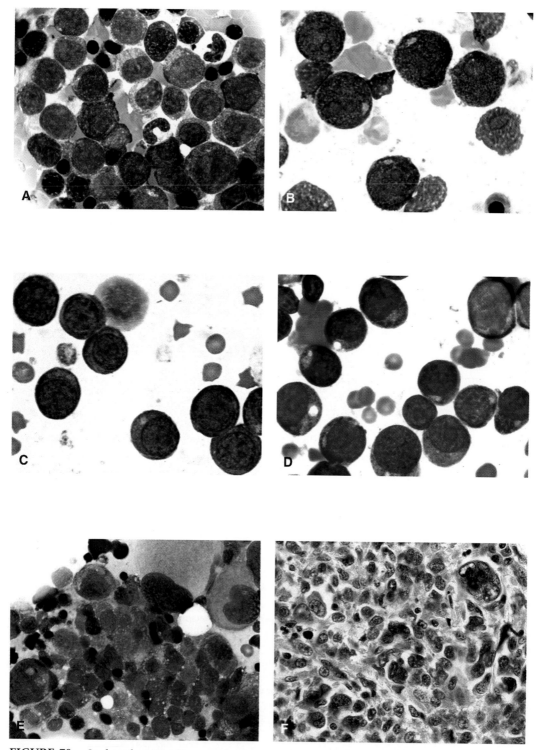

FIGURE 70. *See legend on opposite page.*

The nucleus of a rubriblast is usually nearly perfectly round and has finely stippled chromatin, with one or more distinct nucleoli.

AML-M7. Megakaryoblastic leukemia is diagnosed when megakaryoblasts account for 30% or more of ANC or NEC in bone marrow (Figs. 70E, 70F).[183,241–244,614–616] Nuclei of megakaryoblasts are nearly as round as rubriblast nuclei, but their cytoplasm is typically less basophilic. Unique features that are present in some of these cells include multiple discrete vacuoles[241,242] and cytoplasmic projections.[183,243,244] Some differentiation with morphologically abnormal multinucleated megakaryocytes is also generally present. Immunocytochemical stains for factor VIII or for platelet specific glycoprotein GP IIIa may be used to identify the blast cells as megakaryoblasts.[244,614–616]

Acute Undifferentiated Leukemia (AUL). AUL is diagnosed when the blast cells cannot be identified with certainty using routine blood stains or cytochemical markers (Fig. 70D). This term may be used as a temporary category in some cases pending the use of specialized cell markers. As more cellular markers are developed, the percentage of cases classified as AUL will decrease. The hallmark of AUL is the presence of blast cells with broad cytoplasmic pseudopods and/or some magenta-staining cytoplasmic granules.[238] Cats with a myeloproliferative disorder previously referred to as reticuloendotheliosis may be included in this category. However, some cases previously diagnosed as reticuloendotheliosis would now be included in AML-M6Er, because the blast cells present had deeply basophilic cytoplasm without granules and nuclei that were characteristic of those present in rubriblasts.[131]

Peripheral Blood Findings. Peripheral blood findings for AML are similar to those described previously for MDS, except that blast cells and marked leukocytosis are more likely to be present in the circulation in AML. However, leukopenia occurs in nearly one third of AML-M2 cats.[238] Monocytosis is generally marked in M4 and M5 types of AML. Additionally, some cases of AML-M7 have a thrombocytosis,[243,381,616] while others have a thrombocytopenia, as is commonly seen in all other types of AML.[238]

FIGURE 70. Erythroleukemia (AML-M6), megakaryoblastic leukemia (AML-M7), and acute unclassified leukemia (AUL) in bone marrow aspirate smears and a core biopsy section. **A.** Increased myeloblasts and rubriblasts in an aspirate smear of bone marrow from a cat with AML-M6. Wright-Giemsa stain. **B.** Rubriblasts in an aspirate smear of bone marrow from a dog with erythroleukemia with erythroid predominance (AML-M6Er). Several free nuclei (basket cells) are also present. Wright-Giemsa stain. **C.** Rubriblasts in an aspirate smear of bone marrow from a cat with AML-M6Er. Wright-Giemsa stain. **D.** Predominance of blast cells in an aspirate smear of bone marrow from a cat with an AUL in which the neoplastic cells could not be classified with certainty. Wright-Giemsa stain. **E.** Predominance of megakaryoblasts and abnormal megakaryocytes in an aspirate smear of bone marrow from a dog with AML-M7. Wright-Giemsa stain. **F.** Predominance of megakaryoblasts and abnormal megakaryocytes in a section of bone marrow collected as a core biopsy from a dog with AML-M7. H&E stain.

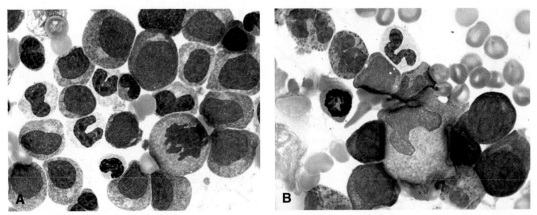

FIGURE 71. Chronic myeloid leukemia (CML), basophilic leukemia, and mast cell infiltrates in bone marrow aspirate smears. Wright-Giemsa stain.   **A.** Granulocytic hyperplasia with left shift in an aspirate smear of bone marrow from a dog with CML. Myeloblasts accounted for less than 30% of all nucleated cells in the marrow preparation.   **B.** Increased numbers of basophils and blast cells in an aspirate smear of bone marrow from a dog with basophilic leukemia. Basophils accounted for nearly half and blast cells accounted for less than 30% of all nucleated cells in the hypercellular marrow preparation (Photograph taken from a stained smear provided by Dr. R.E. Raskin).[469]

Frequency in Animal Species. AML is seen most commonly in cats, with myeloblastic leukemia (M1 and M2 combined) being most common.[238] Myeloblastic leukemia (M1 and M2 combined) and myelomonocytic leukemia (M4) are the most commonly reported types in dogs. Although rare, most horses reported with AML have had either AML-M4 or AML-M5.[567] Erythroleukemia (M6 and M6Er combined) has been reported primarily in cats.[238] Megakaryoblastic leukemia (M7) is rare, being reported in dogs and cats. AML is rarely reported in cattle.[617,618]

Chronic Myeloproliferative Disorders

Chronic myeloproliferative disorders are neoplastic proliferations of hematopoietic cells resulting in high numbers of differentiated cells in blood. Like MDS, animals with chronic myeloproliferative disorders have less than 30% blast cells in the bone marrow with few or no blast cells in the blood. Dysplastic changes may be present in both disorders, but they tend to be more noticeable in MDS. The major difference between these disorders is that high numbers of one or more blood cell type(s) occur in chronic myeloproliferative disorders, and cytopenias frequently occur in MDS.

Chronic Myeloid Leukemia (CML). CML is a rare disorder in animals, occurring primarily in dogs.[130-132,447-449,461] It presents with a high total leukocyte count (greater than 50,000/μL) with a marked neutrophilic left shift in blood. Increased numbers of monocytes, eosinophils, and/or basophils may also be present. If monocytes predominate, a diagnosis of chronic monocytic leukemia may be considered. Myeloblasts are either absent or present in low numbers in blood. Nucleated erythrocytes are often present in blood in the presence of nonregenerative anemia. Platelet counts may be low, normal, or increased.

Granulocytic hyperplasia is present in bone marrow, with or without erythroid and megakaryocytic hypoplasia. The percentage of immature granulocytic cells is increased, but the percentage of myeloblasts does not exceed 30% of all nucleated cells (Fig. 71A). Dysplastic changes are typically also present in one or more marrow cell lines.

CML must be differentiated from severe inflammatory leukemoid reactions. The presence of cytoplasmic toxicity, increased inflammatory plasma proteins, and physical evidence of inflammation suggest a leukemoid reaction is present. The presence of myelodysplasia suggests that CML is present. In some canine cases, CML has been recognized to terminate in a "blast" crisis, in which maturation of granulocytic cells is greatly diminished and blast cells predominate in blood and bone marrow.[130,449]

Chronic Myelomonocytic Leukemia.   Chronic myelomonocytic leukemia has been considered a variant of CML in humans but is now generally classified as a form of MDS.[619] A case has been reported in a cat that exhibited marked monocytosis along with dyshematopoiesis and increased blast cells in bone marrow.[178] Based on the MDS scheme listed above, this case could also be classified as MDS-EB.

Eosinophilic Leukemia.   Eosinophilic leukemia is a variant of CML in which eosinophilic cells predominate in blood and marrow. Differentiation of eosinophilic leukemia and the hypereosinophilic syndrome in cats can be difficult. The hypereosinophilic syndrome is characterized by a mature eosinophilia with frequent involvement of the intestines. Eosinophilic leukemia is characterized by marked eosinophilic left shifts in bone marrow, blood, and organ infiltrates.[184–186,459]

Basophilic Leukemia.   Basophilic leukemia is a variant of CML in which basophilic cells predominate in blood and marrow. It has rarely been reported in dogs.[189,190,469] Early reports of basophilic leukemia in animals represented misdiagnosed cases of systemic mastocytosis with mastocytemia. Basophilic leukemia is characterized by marked basophilia with many immature basophilic cells in blood and bone marrow (Fig. 71B).

Primary Erythrocytosis.   Primary erythrocytosis (polycythemia vera) in adult dogs and cats is considered to be a chronic myeloproliferative disorder that results from an autonomous (erythropoietin-independent) proliferation of erythroid precursor cells, resulting in high numbers of mature erythrocytes in blood. In contrast to polycythemia vera in humans, granulocyte and platelet numbers are generally not increased.[602,612] The bone marrow is hyperplastic with orderly maturation of cells. Erythroid hyperplasia may be accompanied by megakaryocytic and/or granulocytic hyperplasia in some cases.[298,620] The M : E ratio is often normal but may be decreased secondary to erythroid hyperplasia.[602] Marrow iron stores may be low, presumably as a result of increased demands for erythrocyte production.[298]

Thrombocythemia. Thrombocythemia is a myeloproliferative disorder that is characterized by persistent, markedly increased (usually above $1 \times 10^6/\mu L$) platelet counts and megakaryocytic hyperplasia in the bone marrow (Figs. 56C, 56D) in the absence of iron deficiency, recovery from severe hemorrhage, rebound from a thrombocytopenia, splenectomy, an underlying chronic inflammatory condition, or another myeloproliferative disorder.[468,501–505,621] Megakaryocyte morphology may appear normal or dysplastic when examined by light microscopy. Thrombocythemia is viewed as the platelet counterpart of primary erythrocytosis and, as in primary erythrocytosis, a diagnosis of thrombocythemia is ultimately made by ruling out other causes of the high cell counts.

CHAPTER 10

NONHEMATOPOIETIC NEOPLASMS

Nonhematopoietic neoplasms of bone marrow develop in other tissues and metastasize to the marrow. A metastasis to bone marrow is relatively common, but it is rarely diagnosed because the multi-focal distributions of neoplastic infiltrates are easily missed using a small biopsy needle. Recognition of metastatic neoplasms within the marrow is increased if biopsies are collected from lesions identified using diagnostic imaging techniques.[622]

■ MAST CELL TUMORS

Mast cells are round cells with round nuclei. They typically have large numbers of purple granules in the cytoplasm, although the granules may not stain with the Diff-Quik or other aqueous-based Wright stains. Mast cell precursors are produced in the bone marrow but rarely develop into mast cells there.[196] Rather, these precursors leave the marrow, circulate in blood, and migrate into tissue sites, where they develop into mast cells.[280] Mast cell tumors, originating in the skin, the spleen, and other peripheral sites, may metastasize to bone marrow; consequently, bone marrow examination may be a part of staging this neoplasm (Figs. 72A, 72B). Bone marrow involvement is especially likely in noncutaneous systemic mastocytosis.[316–319]

■ METASTATIC CARCINOMAS

Metastatic carcinomas are rarely recognized in routine bone marrow biopsies (Figs. 73A–73D)[70,99] but are identified more commonly in necropsy material or in instances in which biopsy needles are directed at bone lesions identified using diagnostic imaging.[622–625] The morphology of cells observed varies with the tumor type present. A disseminated adenocarcinoma, diagnosed in a dog using a routine bone marrow biopsy, appeared as cohesive clusters of epithelial cells, exhibiting morphologic abnormalities that may include anisocytosis, anisokaryosis, high N:C ratios, coarse nuclear chromatin, multiple nucleoli, deeply

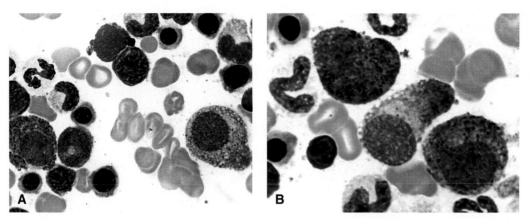

FIGURE 72.   A. Mast cell infiltrate (slightly below center at right and left edges) in an aspirate smear of bone marrow from a dog with a metastatic mast cell tumor.   **B.**   Mast cell infiltrate in an aspirate smear of bone marrow from a dog with a metastatic mast cell tumor. Three mast cells with round nuclei and purple granules are located diagonally from top left to bottom right.

basophilic cytoplasm, discrete cytoplasmic vacuoles, mitotic figures, and acinar formation.[99] Histologic sections are preferred to aspirate smears in the diagnosis of metastatic carcinomas in human bone marrow.[626]

■ SARCOMAS OF BONE

Bone tumors often spread into the marrow space. Osteogenic sarcoma is a common bone tumor of dogs that is easily diagnosed using exfoliative cytology of biopsy material collected from bone lesions (Figs. 73E, 73F). Malignant osteoblasts are polygonal to fusiform, with abundant foamy basophilic cytoplasm. Nuclei are often eccentrically located and variable in size, exhibiting coarse chromatin patterns and multiple nucleoli. These cells produce osteoid, and consequently, they may contain reddish granules in the cytoplasm and may

FIGURE 73.   Metastatic adenocarcinoma and osteogenic sarcoma in bone marrow.   A. Cohesive clusters of basophilic epithelial cells in an aspirate smear of bone marrow from a dog with a metastatic pancreatic adenocarcinoma. Wright-Giemsa stain.   **B.**   Cohesive clusters of basophilic epithelial cells in an aspirate smear of bone marrow from a second dog with a metastatic adenocarcinoma of unknown origin. Wright-Giemsa stain.   **C.**   Cohesive clusters of basophilic epithelial cells in an aspirate smear of bone marrow from a third dog with a disseminated metastatic adenocarcinoma. The origin could not be determined even after necropsy examination. Wright-Giemsa stain.   **D.**   Metastatic foci of neoplastic epithelial cells (right) in a section of bone marrow collected as a core biopsy from the dog with an adenocarcinoma as presented in Figure 73C. The remaining marrow is hypocellular with myelofibrosis. H&E stain.   **E.**   A multinucleated osteoclast (left) and osteoblasts with eccentric nuclei in an aspirate smear of bone marrow from a dog with osteogenic sarcoma. Wright-Giemsa stain.   **F.**   A multinucleated osteoclast (bottom) and many osteoblasts in an aspirate smear of bone marrow from a second dog with osteogenic sarcoma. Wright-Giemsa stain.

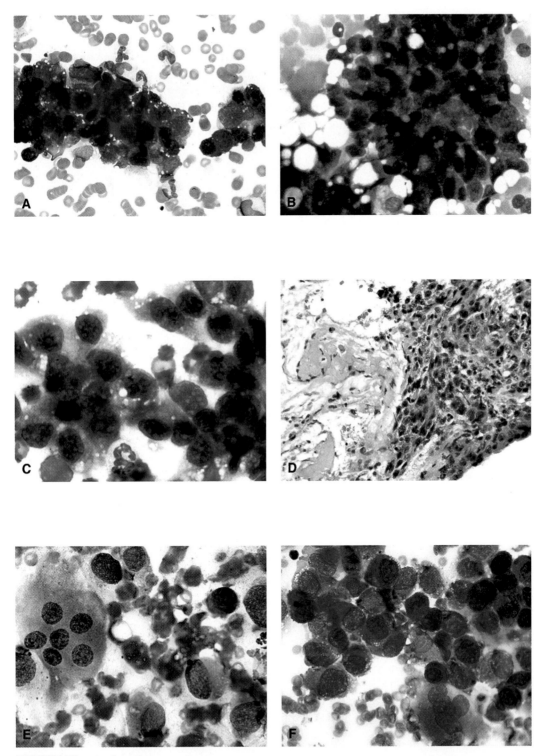

FIGURE 73. *See legend on opposite page.*

be found embedded in an eosinophilic osteoid matrix. Variable numbers of nonneoplastic osteoclasts are also usually present.[627]

Chondrosarcomas of bone appear similar to osteogenic sarcomas on exfoliative cytology, except they are usually associated with more eosinophilic matrix material than are osteogenic sarcomas. Other potential bone tumors that might be diagnosed by aspirate or core biopsy include fibrosarcomas, hemangiosarcomas, and giant cell tumors of bone.[627]

Example of Bone Marrow Evaluation and Interpretation

Patient: A nine-year-old castrated male mixed-breed cat.

History: Decreased appetite, lethargy, and weight loss were recognized two weeks ago. The referring veterinarian diagnosed severe periodontal disease. In-house tests for FeLV and FIV were negative. Four teeth were pulled and antibiotic therapy was initiated. The animal had intermittent fever, exhibited variable anorexia, became dehydrated, and was referred to the Veterinary Medical Teaching Hospital for evaluation.

Clinical Findings: The cat was lethargic, slightly dehydrated, and thin, with a dry hair coat. The gums were hyperemic in association with continuing periodontal disease.

Laboratory Findings: Abnormal hematology findings included a hematocrit of 27% and total leukocyte count of 1,300/μL, most of which were lymphocytes. Platelets were not counted, but numbers appeared normal during stained blood film examination. Erythrocyte morphology was normal. Urinalysis and clinical chemistry values were within normal limits. The FeLV test was negative, but the FIV test was positive.

Bone Marrow Aspirate Smear Evaluation

13% Immature myeloid cells[a]	4% Immature erythroid cells[b]
63% Mature myeloid cells	13% Mature erythroid cells
1% Eosinophilic cells	4% Lymphocytes
<1% Monocytoid cells	<1% Plasma cells

M : E Ratio = 4.5

Multiple particles were present and their cellularity appeared to be increased. Megakaryocyte numbers appeared normal, a majority of which were mature. The myeloid series was left-shifted, with a depletion of mature neutrophils. The erythroid series was complete, with orderly maturation, but a decreased amount of polychromasia was present. Lymphocytes, plasma cells, and macrophages were present in normal numbers. Hemosiderin was not observed, but this is a normal finding in cats. Erythrophagocytosis and leukophagocytosis were rarely observed.

Interpretation: Granulocytic hyperplasia with abnormal maturation.

[a] Immature myeloid cells include myeloblasts and promyelocytes. Mature myeloid cells include neutrophilic myelocytes, neutrophilic metamyelocytes, neutrophilic bands, and mature neutrophils.
[b] Immature erythroid cells include rubriblasts and prorubricytes. Mature erythroid cells include basophilic rubricytes, polychromatophilic rubricytes, and metarubricytes.

Comment: An increased M : E ratio in a severely leukopenic and mildly anemic animal with hypercellular marrow and disordered myeloid maturation is most likely secondary to FIV infection in this cat. This pattern could also be detected transiently during a recovery phase after severe granulocytic depletion, although this is less likely based on the history. If the animal is in a recovery phase from neutropenia, the leukocyte count should increase in the peripheral blood within a few days.

Bibliography

1. Meyer DJ, Harvey JW: Veterinary Laboratory Medicine. Interpretation and Diagnosis, 2nd ed. W.B. Saunders Co., Philadelphia, PA, 1998.

2. Harenberg J, Malsch R, Piazolo L, Huhle G, Heene DL: Preferential binding of heparin to granulocytes of various species. Am J Vet Res 57:1016–1020, 1996.

3. Hinchcliff KW, Kociba GJ, Mitten LA: Diagnosis of EDTA-dependent pseudothrombocytopenia in a horse. J Am Vet Med Assoc 203:1715–1716, 1993.

4. Savage RA: Pseudoleukocytosis due to EDTA-induced platelet clumping. Am J Clin Pathol 81:317–322, 1984.

5. Deol I, Hernandez AM, Pierre RV: Ethylenediamine tetraacetic acid-associated leukoagglutination. Am J Clin Pathol 103:338–340, 1995.

6. Bizzaro N: EDTA-dependent pseudothrombocytopenia: a clinical and epidemiological study of 112 cases, with 10-year follow-up. Am J Hematol 50:103–109, 1995.

7. Ragan HA: Platelet agglutination induced by ethylenediaminetetraacetic acid in blood samples from a miniature pig. Am J Vet Res 33:2601–2603, 1972.

8. Moraglio D, Banfi G, Arnelli A: Association of pseudothrombocytopenia and pseudoleukopenia: evidence for different pathogenic mechanisms. Scand J Clin Lab Invest 54:257–265, 1994.

9. Harvey JW: The erythrocyte: physiology, metabolism and biochemical disorders. In: Clinical Biochemistry of Domestic Animals, 5th ed. Kaneko JJ, Harvey JW, Bruss ML, eds. pp 157–203, Academic Press, San Diego, CA, 1997.

10. Harvey JW, King RR, Berry CR, Blue JT: Methaemoglobin reductase deficiency in dogs. Comp Haematol Int 1:55–59, 1991.

11. Jain NC: Essentials of Veterinary Hematology. Lea & Febiger, Philadelphia, PA, 1993.

12. Engelking LR: Evaluation of equine bilirubin and bile acid metabolism. Comp Cont Ed Pract Vet 11:328–336, 1989.

13. Whitney MS: Evaluation of hyperlipidemia in dogs and cats. Sem Vet Med Surg Small Anim 7:292–300, 1992.

14. Watson TDG, Gaffney D, Mooney CT, Thompson H, Packard CJ, Shepherd J: Inherited hyperchylomicronaemia in the cat: lipoprotein lipase function and gene structure. J Small Anim Pract 33:207–212, 1992.

15. Jeffcott LB, Field JR: Current concepts of hyperlipaemia in horses and ponies. Vet Rec 116:461–466, 1985.

16. Mogg TD, Palmer JE: Hyperlipidemia, hyperlipemia, and hepatic lipidosis in American miniature horses: 23 cases (1990–1994). J Am Vet Med Assoc 207:604–607, 1995.

17. Jain NC: Schalm's Veterinary Hematology, 4th ed. Lea & Febiger, Philadelphia, PA, 1986.

18. Dintenfass L, Kammer S: Re-evaluation of heat precipitation method for plasma fibrinogen estimation: effect of abnormal proteins and plasma viscosity. J Clin Pathol 29:130–134, 1976.

19. Blaisdell FS, Dodds WJ: Evaluation of two microhematocrit methods for quantitating plasma fibrinogen. J Am Vet Med Assoc 171:340–342, 1977.

20. Burkhard MJ, Baxter G, Thrall MA: Blood precipitate associated with intra-abdominal carboxymethylcellulose administration. Vet Clin Pathol 25:114–117, 1996.

21. Harvey JW: Hematology tip—stains for distemper inclusions. Vet Clin Pathol 11(1):12, 1982.

22. Alsaker RD, Laber J, Stevens JB, Perman V: A comparison of polychromasia and

reticulocyte counts in assessing erythrocyte regenerative response in the cat. J Am Vet Med Assoc 170:39–41, 1977.

23. Perkins PC, Grindem CB, Cullins LD: Flow cytometric analysis of punctate and aggregate reticulocyte responses in phlebotomized cats. Am J Vet Res 56:1564–1569, 1995.

24. Cramer DV, Lewis RM: Reticulocyte response in the cat. J Am Vet Med Assoc 160:61–67, 1972.

25. Fan LC, Dorner JL, Hoffman WE: Reticulocyte response and maturation in experimental acute blood loss anemia in the cat. J Am Anim Hosp Assoc 14:219–224, 1978.

26. Grindem CB: Blood cell markers. Vet Clin N Am Small Anim Pract 26:1043–1064, 1996.

27. Raskin RE, Valenciano A: Cytochemical tests for diagnosis of leukemia. In: Schalm's Veterinary Hematology, 5th ed. Feldman BF, Zinkl JG, Jain NC, eds. pp 755–763, Lippincott Williams & Wilkins, Philadelphia, PA, 2000.

28. Raskin RE, Valenciano A: Cytochemistry of normal leukocytes. In: Schalm's Veterinary Hematology, 5th ed. Feldman BF, Zinkl JG, Jain NC, eds. pp 337–346, Lippincott Williams & Wilkins, Baltimore, MD, 2000.

29. Weiss DJ: Uniform evaluation and semiquantitative reporting of hematologic data in veterinary laboratories. Vet Clin Pathol 13:27–31, 1984.

30. Tasker S, Cripps PJ, Macklin AJ: Estimation of platelet counts on feline blood smears. Vet Clin Pathol 28:42–45, 1999.

31. Moore JN, Mahaffey EA, Zboran M: Heparin-induced agglutination of erythrocytes in horses. Am J Vet Res 48:68–71, 1987.

32. Monreal L, Villatoro AJ, Monreal M, Espada Y, Angles AM, Ruiz-Gopegui R: Comparison of the effects of low-molecular-weight and unfractioned heparin in horses. Am J Vet Res 56:1281–1285, 1995.

33. Laber J, Perman V, Stevens JB: Polychromasia or reticulocytes—an assessment of the dog. J Am Anim Hosp Assoc 10:399–406, 1974.

34. Harvey JW: Canine bone marrow: normal hematopoiesis, biopsy techniques, and cell identification and evaluation. Comp Cont Ed Pract Vet 6:909–926, 1984.

35. Harvey JW: Microcytic anemias. In: Schalm's Veterinary Hematology, 5th ed. Feldman BF, Zinkl JG, Jain NC, eds. pp 200–204, Lippincott Williams & Wilkins, Philadelphia, PA, 2000.

36. Morin DE, Garry FB, Weiser MG: Hematologic responses in llamas with experimentally-induced iron deficiency anemia. Vet Clin Pathol 22:81–85, 1993.

37. Holman HH, Drew SM: The blood picture of the goat. II. Changes in erythrocyte shape, size and number associated with age. Res Vet Sci 5:274–285, 1964.

38. Sato T, Mizuno M: Poikilocytosis of newborn calves. Nippon Juigaku Zasshi 44:801–805, 1982.

39. Okabe J, Tajima S, Yamato O, Inaba M, Hagiwara S, Maede Y: Hemoglobin types, erythrocyte membrane skeleton and plasma iron concentration in calves with poikilocytosis. J Vet Med Sci 58:629–634, 1996.

40. Rebar AH, Lewis HB, DeNicola DB, Halliwell WH, Boon GD: Red cell fragmentation in the dog: an editorial review. Vet Pathol 18:415–426, 1981.

41. Badylak SF, Van Vleet JF, Herman EH, Ferrans VJ, Myers CE: Poikilocytosis in dogs with chronic doxorubicin toxicosis. Am J Vet Res 46:505–508, 1985.

42. O'Keefe DA, Schaeffer DJ: Hematologic toxicosis associated with doxorubicin administration in cats. J Vet Intern Med 6:276–283, 1992.

43. Holland CT, Canfield PJ, Watson ADJ, Allan GS: Dyserythropoiesis, polymyopathy, and cardiac disease in three related English springer spaniels. J Vet Intern Med 5:151–159, 1991.

44. Weiss DJ, Kristensen A, Papenfuss N, McClay CB: Quantitative evaluation of echinocytes in the dog. Vet Clin Pathol 19:114–118, 1990.

45. Brown DE, Meyer DJ, Wingfield WE, Walton RM: Echinocytosis associated with rattlesnake envenomation in dogs. Vet Pathol 31:654–657, 1994.

46. Walton RM, Brown DE, Hamar DW, Meador VP, Horn JW, Thrall MA: Mechanisms of echinocytosis induced by *Crotalus atrox* venom. Vet Pathol 34:442–449, 1997.

47. Marks SL, Mannella C, Schaer M: Coral snake envenomation in the dog: report of four cases and review of the literature. J Am Anim Hosp Assoc 26:629–634, 1990.

48. Chandler FW, Prasse KW, Callaway CS: Surface ultrastructure of pyruvate kinase-deficient erythrocytes in the basenji dog. Am J Vet Res 36:1477–1480, 1975.

49. Rebar AH: Hemogram Interpretation for Dogs and Cats. Ralston Purina Co. St. Louis, 1998.

50. Geor RJ, Lund EM, Weiss DJ: Echinocytosis in horses: 54 cases (1990). J Am Vet Med Assoc 202:976–980, 1993.

51. Weiss DJ, Geor RJ: Clinical and rheological implications of echinocytosis in the horse: a review. Comp Haematol Int 3:185–189, 1993.

52. Bessis M: Living Blood Cells and Their Ultrastructure. Springer-Verlag, New York, NY, 1973.

53. Cooper RA, Leslie MH, Knight D, Detweiler DK: Red cell cholesterol enrichment and spur cell anemia in dogs fed a cholesterol-enriched atherogenic diet. J Lipid Res 21:1082–1089, 1980.

54. Weiss DJ, Kristensen A, Papenfuss N: Quantitative evaluation of irregularly spiculated red blood cells in the dog. Vet Clin Pathol 22:117–121, 1993.

55. Christopher MM, Lee SE: Red cell morphologic alterations in cats with hepatic disease. Vet Clin Pathol 23:7–12, 1994.

56. McGillivray SR, Searcy GP, Hirsch VM: Serum iron, total iron binding capacity, plasma copper and hemoglobin types in anemic and poikilocytic calves. Can J Comp Med 49:286–290, 1985.

57. Jain NC, Kono CS, Myers A, Bottomly K: Fusiform erythrocytes resembling sickle cells in angora goats: observations on osmotic and mechanical fragilities and reversal of shape during anaemia. Res Vet Sci 28:25–35, 1980.

58. Weiss DJ, Lulich J: Myelodysplastic syndrome with sideroblastic differentiation in a dog. Vet Clin Pathol 28:59–63, 1999.

59. Fletch SM, Pinkerton PH, Brueckner PJ: The Alaskan Malamute chondrodysplasia (dwarfism—anemia) syndrome—in review. J Am Anim Hosp Assoc 11:353–361, 1975.

60. Slappendel RJ, Renooij W, De Bruijne JJ: Normal cations and abnormal membrane lipids in the red blood cells of dogs with familial stomatocytosis-hypertrophic gastritis. Blood 84:904–909, 1994.

61. Brown DE, Weiser MG, Thrall MA, Giger U, Just CA: Erythrocyte indices and volume distribution in a dog with stomatocytosis. Vet Pathol 31:247–250, 1994.

62. Smith JE, Mohandas N, Shohet SB: Interaction of amphipathic drugs with erythrocytes from various species. Am J Vet Res 43:1041–1048, 1982.

63. Klag AR, Giger U, Shofer FS: Idiopathic immune-mediated hemolytic anemia in dogs: 42 cases (1986–1990). J Am Vet Med Assoc 202:783–788, 1993.

64. Noble S, Armstrong PJ: Bee sting envenomation resulting in secondary immune-mediated hemolytic anemia in two dogs. J Am Vet Med Assoc 214:1026–1027, 1999.

65. Breitschwerdt EB, Armstrong PJ, Robinette CL, Dillman RC, Karl ML: Three cases of acute zinc toxicosis in dogs. Vet Hum Toxicol 28:109–117, 1986.

66. Swenson C, Jacobs R: Spherocytosis associated with anaplasmosis in two cows. J Am Vet Med Assoc 188:1061–1063, 1986.

67. Ban A, Ogata Y, Kato T, et al: Erythrocyte morphology and the frequency of spherocytes in hereditary erythrocyte membrane protein disorder in Japanese Black cattle. Bulletin of Nippon Veterinary and Animal Science University 44:21–27, 1995.

68. English RV, Breitschwerdt EB, Grindem CB, Thrall DE, Gainsburg L: Zollinger-Ellison syndrome and myelofibrosis in a dog. J Am Vet Med Assoc 192:1430–1434, 1988.

69. Shelly SM: Causes of canine pancytopenia. Comp Cont Ed Pract Vet 10:9–16, 1988.

70. Lewis HB, Rebar AH: Bone Marrow Evaluation in Veterinary Practice. Ralston Purina Co., St. Louis, 1979.

71. Hammer AS, Couto CG, Swardson C, Getzy D: Hemostatic abnormalities in dogs with hemangiosarcoma. J Vet Intern Med 5:11–14, 1991.

72. Prasse KW, Crouser D, Beutler E, Walker M, Schall WD: Pyruvate kinase deficiency anemia with terminal myelofibrosis and osteosclerosis in a beagle. J Am Vet Med Assoc 166:1170–1175, 1975.

73. Schaer M, Harvey JW, Calderwood Mays MB, Giger U: Pyruvate kinase deficiency causing hemolytic anemia with secondary hemochromatosis in a Cairn terrier dog. J Am Anim Hosp Assoc 28:233–239, 1992.

74. Cooper RA, Diloy-Puray M, Lando P, Greenberg MS: An analysis of lipoproteins, bile acids, and red cell membranes associated with target cells and spur cells in patients with liver disease. J Clin Invest 51:3182–3192, 1972.

75. Harvey JW: Methemoglobinemia and Heinz-body hemolytic anemia. In: Kirk's Current Veterinary Therapy XII, Small Animal Practice. Bonagura JD, ed. pp 443–446, W.B. Saunders Co., Philadelphia, PA, 1995.

76. Reagan WJ, Carter C, Turek J: Eccentrocytosis in equine red maple leaf toxicosis. Vet Clin Pathol 23:123–127, 1994.

77. MacWilliams P, Meadows R: Unpublished case submitted to the 1993 ASVCP microscopic slide review, 1993.

78. Stockham SL, Harvey JW, Kinden DA: Equine glucose-6–phosphate dehydrogenase deficiency. Vet Pathol 31:518–527, 1994.

79. Harvey JW, Stockham SL, Johnson PJ, Scott MA: Methemoglobinemia and eccentrocytosis in a horse with erythrocyte flavin adenine dinucleotide (FAD) deficiency (abstract) Revue Med Vet 151:710, 2000.

80. Scavelli TD, Hornbuckle WE, Roth L, et al: Portosystemic shunts in cats: seven cases (1976–1984). J Am Vet Med Assoc 189:317–325, 1986.

81. Hoff B, Lumsden JH, Valli VE: An appraisal of bone marrow biopsy in assessment of sick dogs. Can J Comp Med 49:34–42, 1985.

82. Smith JE, Moore K, Arens M, Rinderknecht GA, Ledet A: Hereditary elliptocytosis with protein band 4.1 deficiency in the dog. Blood 61:373–377, 1983.

83. Reagan WJ: A review of myelofibrosis in dogs. Toxicol Pathol 21:164–169, 1993.

84. Kuehn NF, Gaunt SD: Hypocellular marrow and extramedullary hematopoiesis in a dog: hematologic recovery after splenectomy. J Am Vet Med Assoc 188:1313–1315, 1986.

85. Taylor WJ: Sickled red cells in the Cervidae. Adv Vet Sci Comp Med 27:77–98, 1983.

86. Jain NC, Kono CS: Fusiform erythrocytes in angora goats resembling sickle cells: influence of temperature, pH, and oxygenation on cell shape. Am J Vet Res 38:983–990, 1977.

87. Rees Evans ET: Sickling phenomenon in sheep. Nature 217:74–75, 1968.

88. Altman NH, Melby EC, Squire RA: Intraerythrocytic crystalloid bodies in cats. Blood 39:801–803, 1972.

89. Altman NH: Intraerythrocytic crystalloid bodies in cats and their comparison with hemoglobinopathies of man. Ann N Y Acad Sci 241:589–593, 1974.

90. Simpson CF, Gaskin JM, Harvey JW: Ultrastructure of erythrocytes parasitized by *Haemobartonella felis*. J Parasitol 64:504–511, 1978.

91. Tvedten HW: What is your diagnosis? Vet Clin Pathol 19(3):77–78, 1990.

92. Van Houten D, Weiser MG, Johnson L, Garry F: Reference hematologic values and morphologic features of blood cells in healthy adult llamas. Am J Vet Res 53:1773–1775, 1992.

93. Lund JE: Hemoglobin crystals in canine blood. Am J Vet Res 35:575–577, 1974.

94. Tyler RD, Cowell RL: Normoblastemia. In: Consultations in Feline Internal Medicine 3. August JR, ed. pp 483–487, W.B. Saunders Co., Philadelphia, PA, 1997.

95. Mandell CP, Jain NC, Farver TB: The significance of normoblastemia and leukoerythroblastic reaction in the dog. J Am Anim Hosp Assoc 25:665–672, 1989.

96. George JW, Duncan JR: The hematology of lead poisoning in man and animals. Vet Clin Pathol 8:23–30, 1979.

97. Morgan RV, Moore FM, Pearce LK, Rossi T: Clinical and laboratory findings in small companion animals with lead poisoning: 347 cases (1977–1986). J Am Vet Med Assoc 199:93–97, 1991.

98. Deldar A, Lewis H, Bloom J, Weiss L: Cephalosporin-induced changes in the ultrastructure of canine bone marrow. Vet Pathol 25:211–218, 1988.

99. Henson KL, Alleman AR, Fox LE, Richey LJ, Castleman WL: Diagnosis of disseminated adenocarcinoma by bone marrow aspiration in a dog with leukoerythroblastosis and fever of unknown origin. Vet Clin Pathol 27:80–84, 1998.

100. Steffen DJ, Elliott GS, Leipold HW, Smith JE: Congenital dyserythropoiesis and progressive alopecia in Polled Hereford calves: hematologic, biochemical, bone marrow cytologic, electrophoretic, and flow cytometric findings. J Vet Diagn Invest 4:31–37, 1992.

101. Couto CG, Kallet AJ: Preleukemic syndrome in a dog. J Am Vet Med Assoc 184:1389–1392, 1984.

102. Durando MM, Alleman AR, Harvey JW: Myelodysplastic syndrome in a quarter horse gelding. Equine Vet J 26:83–85, 1994.

103. Searcy GP, Orr JP: Chronic granulocytic leukemia in a horse. Can Vet J 22:148–151, 1981.

104. Christopher MM, Broussard JD, Peterson ME: Heinz body formation associated with ketoacidosis in diabetic cats. J Vet Intern Med 9:24–31, 1995.

105. Blue J, Weiss L: Vascular pathways in nonsinusal red pulp—an electron microscope study of the cat spleen. Am J Anat 161:135–168, 1981.

106. Christopher MM: Relation of endogenous Heinz bodies to disease and anemia in cats: 120 cases (1978–1987). J Am Vet Med Assoc 194:1089–1095, 1989.

107. Robertson JE, Christopher MM, Rogers QR: Heinz body formation in cats fed baby food containing onion powder. J Am Vet Med Assoc 212:1260–1266, 1998.

108. Desnoyers M, Hebert P: Heinz body anemia in a dog following possible naphthalene ingestion. Vet Clin Pathol 24:124–125, 1995.

109. Harvey JW: Unpublished findings, 2000.

110. Plier M: Unpublished findings, 2000.

111. De Waal DT: Equine piroplasmosis: a review. Br Vet J 148:6–14, 1992.

112. Kuttler KL: World-wide impact of babesiosis. In: Babesiosis of Domestic Animals and Man. Ristic M, ed. pp 2–22, CRC Press, Inc., Boca Raton, FL, 1988.

113. Taboada J: Babesiosis. In: Infectious Diseases of the Dog and Cat, 2nd ed. Greene CE, ed. pp 473–481, W.B. Saunders Co., Philadelphia, PA, 1998.

BIBLIOGRAPHY

114. Urquhart GM, Armour J, Duncan JL, Dunn AM, Jennings FW: Veterinary Parasitology, 2nd ed. Blackwell Science, Cambridge, MA, 1996.

115. Stockham SL, Kjemtrup AM, Conrad PA, et al: Theilerosis in a Missouri beef herd caused by *Theileria buffeli:* case report, herd investigation, ultrastructure, phylogenetic analysis, and experimental transmission. Vet Pathol 37:11–21, 2000.

116. Kier AB, Greene CE: Cytauxzoonosis. In: Infectious Diseases of the Dog and Cat, 2nd ed. Greene CE, ed. pp 470–473, W.B. Saunders Co., Philadelphia, PA, 1998.

117. Wanduragala L, Ristic M: Anaplasmosis. In: Rickettsial and Chlamydial Diseases of Domestic Animals. Woldehiwet Z, Ristic M, eds. pp 65–87, Pergamon Press, New York, NY, 1993.

118. Watson ADJ, Wright RG: The ultrastructure of inclusions in blood cells of dogs with distemper. J Comp Pathol 84:417–427, 1974.

119. Gossett KA, MacWilliams PS, Fulton RW: Viral inclusions in hematopoietic precursors in a dog with distemper. J Am Vet Med Assoc 181:387–388, 1982.

120. Harvey JW: Haemobartonellosis. In: Infectious Diseases of the Dog and Cat, 2nd ed. Greene CE, ed. pp 166–171, W.B. Saunders Co., Philadelphia, PA, 1998.

121. Rikihisa Y, Kawahara M, Wen BH, Kociba G, Fuerst P, Kawamori F, Suto C, Shibata S, Futohashi M: Western immunoblot analysis of *Haemobartonella muris* and comparison of 16S rRNA gene sequences of *H-muris, H-felis,* and *Eperythrozoon suis.* J Clin Microbiol 35:823–829, 1997.

122. Messick JB, Berent LM, Cooper SK: Development and evaluation of a PCR-based assay for detection of *Haemobartonella felis* in cats and differentiation of *H. felis* from related bacteria by restriction fragment length polymorphism analysis. J Clin Microbiol 36:462–466, 1998.

123. Reagan WJ, Garry F, Thrall MA, Colgan S, Hutchison J, Weiser MG: The clinicopathologic, light, and scanning electron microscopic features of eperythrozoonosis in four naturally infected llamas. Vet Pathol 27:426–431, 1990.

124. Scott GR, Woldehiwet Z: Eperythrozoonoses. In: Rickettsial and Chlamydial Diseases of Domestic Animals. Woldehiwet Z, Ristic M, eds. pp 111–129, Pergamon Press, New York, NY, 1993.

125. Welles EG, Tyler JW, Wolfe DF: Hematologic and semen quality changes in bulls with experimental eperythrozoon infection. Theriogenology 43:427–437, 1995.

126. Smith JA, Thrall MA, Smith JL, Salman MD, Ching SV, Collins JK: *Eperythrozoon wenyonii* infection in dairy cattle. J Am Vet Med Assoc 196:1244–1250, 1990.

127. Neimark H, Kocan KM: The cell wall-less rickettsia *Eperythrozoon wenyonii* is a Mycoplasma. FEMS Microbiol Let 156:287–291, 1997.

128. Breitschwerdt EB, Greene CE: Bartonellosis. In: Infectious Diseases of the Dog and Cat, 2nd ed. Greene CE, ed. pp 337–343, W.B. Saunders Co., Philadelphia, PA, 1998.

129. Kordick DL, Breitschwerdt EB: Intraerythrocytic presence of *Bartonella henselae.* J Clin Microbiol 33:1655–1656, 1995.

130. Leifer CE, Matus RE, Patnaik AK, MacEwen EG: Chronic myelogenous leukemia in the dog. J Am Vet Med Assoc 183:686–689, 1983.

131. Harvey JW: Myeloproliferative disorders in dogs and cats. Vet Clin N Am Small Anim Pract 11:349–381, 1981.

132. Grindem CB, Stevens JB, Brost DR, Johnson DD: Chronic myelogenous leukaemia with meningeal infiltration in a dog. Comp Haematol Int 2:170–174, 1992.

133. Latimer KS, Duncan JR, Kircher IM: Nuclear segmentation, ultrastructure and cytochemistry of blood cells from dogs with Pelger-Huet anomaly. J Comp Pathol 97:61–72, 1987.

134. Latimer KS, Robertson SL: Inherited leukocyte disorders. In: Consultations in Feline Internal Medicine 2. August JR, ed. pp 503–507, W.B. Saunders Co., Philadelphia, PA, 1994.

135. Gossett KA, MacWilliams PS: Ultrastructure of canine toxic neutrophils. Am J Vet Res 43:1634–1637, 1982.

136. Gossett KA, MacWilliams PS, Cleghorn B: Sequential morphological and quantitative changes in blood and bone marrow neutrophils in dogs with acute inflammation. Can J Comp Med 49:291–297, 1985.

137. Duncan JR, Mahaffey EA: Unpublished case submitted to the 1983 ASVCP microscopic slide review, 1983.

138. Jolly RD, Walkley SU: Lysosomal storage diseases of animals: an essay in comparative pathology. Vet Pathol 34:527–548, 1998.

139. Neer TM, Dial SM, Pechman R, Wang P, Oliver JL, Giger U: Mucopolysaccharidosis VI in a miniature Pinscher. J Vet Intern Med 9:429–433, 1995.

140. Alroy J, Freden GO, Goyal V, Raghavan SS, Schunk KL: Morphology of leukocytes from cats affected with α-mannosidosis and mucopolysaccharidosis VI (MPS VI). Vet Pathol 26:294–302, 1989.

141. Cowell KR, Jezyk PF, Haskins ME, Patterson DF: Mucopolysaccharidosis in a cat. J Am Vet Med Assoc 169:334–339, 1976.

142. Haskins ME, Aguirre GD, Jezyk PF, Schuchman EH, Desnick RJ, Patterson DF: Mucopolysaccharidosis type VII (Sly syndrome): beta-glucuronidase-deficient. Am J Physiol 138:1553–1555, 1991.

143. Gitzelmann R, Bosshard NU, Superti-Furga A, et al: Feline mucopolysaccharidosis VII due to β-glucuronidase deficiency. Vet Pathol 31:435–443, 1994.

144. Haskins ME, Desnick RJ, DiFerrante N, Jezyk PF, Patterson DF: β-glucuronidase deficiency in a dog: a model of human mucopolysaccharidosis VII. Pediatr Res 18:980–984, 1984.

145. Johnsrude JD, Alleman AR, Schumacher J, et al: Cytologic findings in cerebrospinal fluid from two animals with GM_2-gangliosidosis. Vet Clin Pathol 25:80–83, 1996.

146. Kosanke SD, Pierce KR, Bay WW: Clinical and biochemical abnormalities in porcine GM_2-gangliosidosis. Vet Pathol 15:685–699, 1978.

147. Hirsch VM, Cunningham TA: Hereditary anomaly of neutrophil granulation in Birman cats. Am J Vet Res 45:2170–2174, 1984.

148. Padgett GA, Gorham JR, O'Mary CC: The familial occurrence of Chediak-Higashi syndrome in mink and cattle. Genetics 49:505–512, 1964.

149. Ayers JR, Leipold HW, Padgett GA: Lesions in Brangus cattle with Chediak-Higashi syndrome. Vet Pathol 25:432–436, 1988.

150. Ogawa H, Tu CH, Kagamizono H, et al: Clinical, morphologic, and biochemical characteristics of Chediak-Higashi syndrome in fifty-six Japanese black cattle. Am J Vet Res 58:1221–1226, 1997.

151. Rothenbacher HJ, Ishida K, Barner RD: Equine infectious anemia—part II. The sideroleukocyte test as an aid in the clinical diagnosis. Vet Med 57:886–890, 1962.

152. Henson JB, McGuire TC, Kobayashi K, Gorman JR: The diagnosis of equine infectious anemia using the complement-fixation test, siderocyte counts, hepatic biopsies, and serum protein alterations. J Am Vet Med Assoc 151:1830–1839, 1967.

153. Cello RM, Moulton JE, McFarland S: The occurrence of inclusion bodies in the circulating neutrophils of dogs with canine distemper. Cornell Vet 49:127–146, 1959.

154. Anderson BE, Greene CE, Jones DC, Dawson JE: Ehrlichia ewingii spp. nov., the etiologic agent of canine granulocytic ehrlichiosis. Int J Syst Bacteriol 42:299–302, 1992.

155. Engvall EO, Pettersson B, Persson M, Artursson K, Johansson KE: A 16S rRNA-based PCR assay for detection and identification of granulocytic *Ehrlichia* species in dogs, horses, and cattle. J Clin Microbiol 34:2170–2174, 1996.

156. Stockham SL, Schmidt DA, Curtis KS, Schauf BG, Tyler JW, Simpson ST: Evaluation of granulocytic ehrlichiosis in dogs of Missouri, including serologic status to *Ehrlichia canis, Ehrlichia equi,* and *Borrelia burgdorferi.* Am J Vet Res 53:63–68, 1992.

157. Madigan JE, Gribble D: Equine ehrlichiosis in northern California: 49 cases (1968–1981). J Am Vet Med Assoc 190:445–448, 1987.

158. Madigan JE, Richter PJ Jr, Kimsey RB, Barlough JE, Bakken JS: Transmission and passage in horses of the agent of human granulocytic ehrlichiosis. J Infect Dis 172: 1141–1144, 1995.

159. Madigan JE, Barlough JE, Dumler JS, Schankman NS, DeRock E: Equine granulocytic ehrlichiosis in Connecticut caused by an agent resembling the human granulocytotropic Ehrlichia. J Clin Microbiol 34:434–435, 1996.

160. Pusterla N, Wolfensberger C, Gerber-Bretscher R, Lutz H: Comparison of indirect immunofluorescence for *Ehrlichia phagocytophila* and *Ehrlichia equi* in horses. Equine Vet J 29:490–492, 1997.

161. Lewis GE Jr, Huxsoll DL, Ristic M, Johnson AJ: Experimentally induced infection of dogs, cats, and nonhuman primates with *Ehrlichia equi,* etiologic agent of equine ehrlichiosis. Am J Vet Res 36:85–88. 1975.

162. Johansson K-E, Pettersson B, Uhlén M, Gunnarsson A, Malmqvist M, Olsson E: Identification of the causative agent of granulocytic ehrlichiosis in Swedish dogs and horses by direct solid phase sequencing of PCR products from the 16S rRNA gene. Res Vet Sci 58:109–112, 1995.

163. Greig B, Asanovich KM, Armstrong PJ, Dumler JS: Geographic, clinical, serologic, and molecular evidence of granulocytic ehrlichiosis, a likely zoonotic disease, in Minnesota and Wisconsin dogs. J Clin Microbiol 34:44–48, 1996.

164. Lilliehook I, Egenvall A, Tvedten HW: Hematopathology in dogs experimentally infected with a Swedish granulocytic *Ehrlichia* species. Vet Clin Pathol 27:116–122, 1998.

165. Woldehiwet Z, Scott GR: Tick-borne (pasture) fever. In: Rickettsial and Chlamydial Diseases of Domestic Animals. Woldehiwet Z, Ristic M, eds. pp 233–254, Pergamon Press, New York, NY, 1993.

166. Barlough JE, Madigan JE, Turoff DR, Clover JR, Shelly SM, Dumler S: An *Ehrlichia* strain from a llama (*Lama glama*) and llama-associated ticks (*Ixodes pacificus*). J Clin Microbiol 35:1005–1007, 1997.

167. Craig TM: Hepatozoonosis. In: Infectious Diseases of the Dog and Cat, 2nd ed. Greene CE, ed. pp 458–465, W.B. Saunders Co., Philadelphia, PA, 1998.

168. Vincent Johnson NA, Macintire DK, Lindsay DS, et al: A new Hepatozoon species from dogs: description of the causative agent of canine hepatozoonosis in North America. J Parasitol 83:1165–1172, 1997.

169. Mercer SH, Craig TM: Comparisons of various staining procedures in the identification of *Hepatozoon canis.* Vet Clin Pathol 17:63–65, 1988.

170. Pedersen NC: Feline infectious diseases. American Veterinary Publication, Goeleta, CA, 1988.

171. Jordan HL, Cohn LA, Armstrong PJ: Disseminated *Mycobacterium avium* complex infection in three Siamese cats. J Am Vet Med Assoc 204:90–93, 1994.

172. Latimer KS, Jameson PH, Crowell WA, Duncan JR, Currin KP: Disseminated *Mycobacterium avium* complex infection in a cat: presumptive diagnosis by blood smear examination. Vet Clin Pathol 26:85–89, 1997.

173. Blischok D, Bender H: What is your diagnosis? 15-year-old male domestic shorthair cat [disseminated histoplasmosis]. Vet Clin Pathol 25:113,152, 1996.

174. Clinkenbeard KD, Wolf AM, Cowell RL, Tyler RD: Feline disseminated histoplasmosis. J Am Anim Hosp Assoc 11:1223–1233, 1989.

175. Schalm OW: Uncommon hematologic disorders: spirochetosis, trypanosomiasis, leishmaniasis, and Pelger-Huet anomaly. Can Pract 6:46–49, 1979.

176. Ruiz-Gopegui R, Espada Y: What is your diagnosis? Peripheral blood and abdominal fluid from a dog with abdominal distention [leishmaniasis]. Vet Clin Pathol 27:64, 67, 1998.

177. Eichacker P, Lawrence C: Steroid-induced hypersegmentation in neutrophils. Am J Hematol 18:41–45, 1985.

178. Raskin RE, Krehbiel JD: Myelodysplastic changes in a cat with myelomonocytic leukemia. J Am Vet Med Assoc 187:171–174, 1985.

179. Prasse KW, George LW, Whitlock RH: Idiopathic hypersegmentation of neutrophils in a horse. J Am Vet Med Assoc 303–305, 1981.

180. Fyfe JC, Giger U, Hall CA, et al: Inherited selective intestinal cobalamin malabsorption and cobalamin deficiency in dogs. Pediatr Res 29:24–31, 1991.

181. Meyers S, Wiks K, Giger U: Macrocytic anemia caused by naturally occurring folate-deficiency in the cat (abstract). Vet Clin Pathol 25:30, 1996.

182. Gossett KA, Carakostas MC: Effect of EDTA on morphology of neutrophils of healthy dogs and dogs with inflammation. Vet Clin Pathol 13:22–25, 1984.

183. Raskin RE: Myelopoiesis and myeloproliferative disorders. Vet Clin N Am Small Anim Pract 26:1023–1042, 1996.

184. Toth SR, Nash AS, McEwan AM, Jarrett O: Chronic eosinophilic leukaemia in blast crises in a cat negative for feline leukaemia virus. Vet Rec 117:471–472, 1985.

185. Swenson CL, Carothers MA, Wellman ML, Kociba GJ: Eosinophilic leukemia in a cat with naturally acquired feline leukemia virus infection. J Am Anim Hosp Assoc 29:467–501, 1993.

186. Huibregtse BA, Turner JL: Hypereosinophilic syndrome and eosinophilic leukemia: a comparison of 22 hypereosinophilic cats. J Am Anim Hosp Assoc 30:591–599, 1994.

187. Aroch I, Ofri R, Aizenberg I: Haematological, ocular and skeletal abnormalities in a Samoyed family. J Small Anim Pract 37:333–339, 1996.

188. Clinkenbeard KD, Cowell RL, Tyler RD: Identification of *Histoplasma* organisms in circulating eosinophils of a dog. J Am Vet Med Assoc 192:217–218, 1988.

189. MacEwen EG, Drazner FH, McClelland AJ, Wilkins RJ: Treatment of basophilic leukemia in a dog. J Am Vet Med Assoc 166:376–380, 1975.

190. Mahaffey EA, Brown TP, Duncan JR, Latimer KS, Brown SA: Basophilic leukaemia in a dog. J Comp Pathol 97:393–399, 1987.

191. Moulton JE, Harvey JW: Tumors of lymphoid and hematopoietic system. In: Tumors of Domestic Animals, 3rd ed. Moulton JE, ed. pp 231–307, University of California Press, Berkley, CA, 1990.

192. Takahashi T, Kadosawa T, Nagase M, et al: Visceral mast cell tumors in dogs: 10 cases (1982–1997). J Am Vet Med Assoc 216:222–226, 2000.

193. Madewell BR, Munn RJ, Phillips LP: Endocytosis of erythrocytes *in vivo* and particulate substances *in vitro* by feline neoplastic mast cells. Can J Vet Res 51:517–520, 1987.

194. Madewell BR, Gunn C, Gribble DH: Mast cell phagocytosis of red blood cells in a cat. Vet Pathol 20:638–640, 1983.

195. Stockham SL, Basel DL, Schmidt DA: Mastocytemia in dogs with acute inflammatory diseases. Vet Clin Pathol 15(1):16–21, 1986.

196. Bookbinder PF, Butt MT, Harvey HJ: Determination of the number of mast cells in lymph node, bone marrow, and buffy coat cytologic specimens from dogs. J Am Vet Med Assoc 200:1648–1650, 1992.

197. Cayatte SM, McManus PM, Miller WH Jr, Scott DW: Identification of mast cells in buffy coat preparations from dogs with inflammatory skin diseases. J Am Vet Med Assoc 206:325–326, 1995.

198. McManus PM: Frequency and severity of mastocytemia in dogs with and without mast cell tumors: 120 cases (1995–1997). J Am Vet Med Assoc 215:355–357, 1999.

199. Ziemer EL, Whitlock RH, Palmer JE, Spencer PA: Clinical and hematologic variables in ponies with experimentally induced equine ehrlichial colitis (Potomac horse fever). Am J Vet Res 48:63–67, 1987.

200. Dutta SK, Penney BE, Myrup AC, Robl MG, Rice RM: Disease features in horses with induced equine monocytic ehrlichiosis (Potomac horse fever). Am J Vet Res 49:1747–1751, 1988.

201. Ristic M, Dawson J, Holland CJ, Jenny A: Susceptibility of dogs to infection with *Ehrlichia risticii,* causative agent of equine monocytic ehrlichiosis (Potomac horse fever). Am J Vet Res 49:1497–1500, 1988.

202. Dawson JE, Abeygunawardena I, Holland CJ, Buese MM, Ristic M: Susceptibility of cats to infection with *Ehrlichia risticii,* causative agent of equine monocytic ehrlichiosis. Am J Vet Res 49:2096–2100, 1988.

203. Kakoma I, Hansen RD, Anderson BE, et al: Cultural, molecular, and immunological characterization of the etiologic agent for atypical canine ehrlichiosis. J Clin Microbiol 32:170–175, 1994.

204. Wolf AM: Histoplasmosis. In: Infectious Diseases of the Dog and Cat, 2nd ed. Greene CE, ed. pp 378–383, W.B. Saunders Co., Philadelphia, PA, 1998.

205. Greene CE, Gunn-Moore DA: Tuberculous mycobacterial infections. In: Infectious Diseases of the Dog and Cat, 2nd ed. Greene CE, ed. pp 313–321, W.B. Saunders Co., Philadelphia, PA, 1998.

206. Hammer RF, Weber AF: Ultrastructure of agranular leukocytes in peripheral blood of normal cows. Am J Vet Res 35:527–536, 1974.

207. Dascanio JJ, Zhang CH, Antczak DF, Blue JT, Simmons TR: Differentiation of chronic lymphocytic leukemia in the horse. J Vet Intern Med 6:225–229, 1992.

208. Peterson JL, Couto CG: Lymphoid leukemias. In: Consultations in Feline Internal Medicine 2. August JR, ed. pp 509–513, W.B. Saunders Co., Philadelphia, PA, 1994.

209. Leifer CE, Matus RE: Lymphoid leukemia in the dog. Acute lymphoblastic leukemia and chronic lymphocytic leukemia. Vet Clin N Am Small Anim Pract 15:723–739, 1985.

210. Hodgkins EM, Zinkl JG, Madewell BR: Chronic lymphocytic leukemia in the dog. J Am Vet Med Assoc 177:704–707, 1980.

211. Vernau W, Moore PF: An immunophenotypic study of canine leukemias and preliminary assessment of clonality by polymerase chain reaction. Vet Immunol Immunopathol 69:145–164, 1999.

212. Ferrer JF, Marshak RR, Abt DA, Kenyon SJ: Relationship between lymphosarcoma and persistent lymphocytosis in cattle: a review. J Am Vet Med Assoc 175:705–708, 1979.

213. Weiser MG, Thrall MA, Fulton R, Beck ER, Wise LA, Van Steenhouse JL: Granular lymphocytosis and hyperproteinemia in dogs with chronic ehrlichiosis. J Am Anim Hosp Assoc 27:84–88, 1991.

214. Wellman ML: Lymphoproliferative disorders of large granular lymphocytes. In: Proc 15th ACVIM Forum, pp 20–21, Lake Buena Vista, FL, 1997.

215. Wellman ML, Couto CG, Starkey RJ, Rojko JL: Lymphocytosis of large granular lymphocytes in three dogs. Vet Pathol 26:158–163, 1989.

216. Kramer J, Tornquist S, Erfle J, Sloeojan G: Large granular lymphocyte leukemia in a horse. Vet Clin Pathol 22:126–128, 1993.

217. Franks PT, Harvey JW, Mays MC, Senior DF, Bowen DJ, Hall BJ: Feline large granular lymphoma. Vet Pathol 23:200–202, 1986.

218. Kariya K, Konno A, Ishida T: Perforin-like immunoreactivity in four cases of lymphoma of large granular lymphocytes in the cat. Vet Pathol 34:156–159, 1997.

219. Darbès J, Majzoub M, Breuer W, Hermanns W: Large granular lymphocytic leukemia/lymphoma in six cats. Vet Pathol 35:370–379, 1998.

220. Neuwelt EA, Johnson WG, Blank NK, et al: Characterization of a new model of G_{M2}-gangliosidosis (Sandloff's disease) in Korat cats. J Clin Invest 76:482–490, 1985.

221. Dial SM, Mitchell TW, LeCouteur RA, Wenger DA, Roberts SM, Gasper PW, Thrall MA: GM_1-gangliosidosis (Type II) in three cats. J Am Anim Hosp Assoc 30:355–359, 1994.

222. Alroy J, Orgad U, Ucci AA, et al: Neurovisceral and skeletal GM_1–gangliosidosis in dogs with beta-galactosidase deficiency. Science 229:470–472, 1985.

223. Pearce RD, Callahan JW, Little PB, Klunder LR, Clarke JTR: Caprine β-D-mannosidosis: Characterization of a model lysosomal storage disorder. Can J Vet Res 54:22–29, 1990.

224. Brown DE, Thrall MA, Walkley SU, et al: Feline Niemann-Pick disease type C. Am J Pathol 144:1412–1415, 1994.

225. Keller CB, Lamarre J: Inherited lysosomal storage disease in an English Springer Spaniel. J Am Vet Med Assoc 200:194–195, 1992.

226. Matus RE, Leifer CE, MacEwen EG: Acute lymphoblastic leukemia in the dog: a review of 30 cases. J Am Vet Med Assoc 183:859–862, 1983.

227. Grindem CB, Stevens JB, Perman V: Morphological classification and clinical and pathological characteristics of spontaneous leukemia in 17 dogs. J Am Anim Hosp Assoc 21:219–226, 1985.

228. Lester GD, Alleman AR, Raskin RE, Meyer JC: Pancytopenia secondary to lymphoid leukemia in three horses. J Vet Intern Med 7:360–363, 1993.

229. Carlson GP: Lymphosarcoma in horses. Leukemia 9:S101, 1995.

230. Raskin RE, Krehbiel JD: Prevalence of leukemic blood and bone marrow in dogs with multicentric lymphoma. J Am Vet Med Assoc 194:1427–1429, 1989.

231. Weber WT: Cattle leukemia—hematologic and biochemical studies. Ann N Y Acad Sci 108:1270–1283, 1963.

232. Madewell BR, Munn RJ: Canine lymphoproliferative disorders. An ultrastructural study of 18 cases. J Vet Intern Med 4:63–70, 1990.

233. Thrall MA, Macy DW, Snyder SP, Hall RL: Cutaneous lymphosarcoma and leukemia in a dog resembling Sezary syndrome in man. Vet Pathol 21:182–186, 1984.

234. Foster AP, Evans E, Kerlin RL, Vail DM: Cutaneous T-cell lymphoma with Sezary syndrome in a dog. Vet Clin Pathol 26:188–192, 1997.

235. Schick RO, Murphy GF, Goldschmidt MH: Cutaneous lymphosarcoma and leukemia in a cat. J Am Vet Med Assoc 203:1155–1158, 1993.

236. Jain NC, Blue JT, Grindem CB, et al: Proposed criteria for classification of acute myeloid leukemia in dogs and cats. Vet Clin Pathol 20:63–82, 1991.

237. Grindem CB, Perman V, Stevens JB: Morphological classification and clinical and

pathological characteristics of spontaneous leukemia in 10 cats. J Am Anim Hosp Assoc 21:227–236, 1985.

238. Jain NC: Classification of myeloproliferative disorders in cats using criteria proposed by the animal leukaemia study group: a retrospective study of 181 cases (1969–1992). Comp Haematol Int 3:125–134, 1993.

239. Bienzle D, Hughson SL, Vernau W: Acute myelomonocytic leukemia in a horse. Can Vet J 34:36–37, 1993.

240. Latimer KS, White SL: Acute monocytic leukemia (M5a) in a horse. Comp Haematol Int 6:111–114, 1996.

241. Shull RM, DeNovo RC, McCraken MD: Megakaryoblastic leukemia in a dog. Vet Pathol 23:533–536, 1986.

242. Bolon B, Buergelt CD, Harvey JW, Meyer DJ, Kaplan-Stein D: Megakaryoblastic leukemia in a dog. Vet Clin Pathol 18:69–72, 1989.

243. Michel RL, O'Handley P, Dade AW: Megakaryocytic myelosis in a cat. J Am Vet Med Assoc 168:1021–1025, 1976.

244. Messick J, Carothers M, Wellman M: Identification and characterization of megakaryoblasts in acute megakaryoblastic leukemia in a dog. Vet Pathol 27:212–214, 1990.

245. Russell KE, Perkins PC, Grindem CB, Walker KM, Sellon DC: Flow cytometric method for detecting thiazole orange-positive (reticulated) platelets in thrombocytopenic horses. Am J Vet Res 58:1092–1096, 1997.

246. Wolf RF, Peng J, Friese P, Gilmore LS, Burstein SA, Dale GL: Erythropoietin administration increases production and reactivity of platelets in dogs. Thromb Haemost 78:1505–1509, 1997.

247. Dunn JK, Heath MF, Jefferies AR, Blackwood L, McKay JS, Nicholls PK: Diagnosis and hematologic features of probable essential thrombocythemia in two dogs. Vet Clin Pathol 28:131–138, 1999.

248. Brown SJ, Simpson KW, Baker S, Spagnoletti MA, Elwood CM: Macrothrombocytosis in cavalier King Charles spaniels. Vet Rec 135:281–283, 1994.

249. Dodds WJ: Familial canine thrombocytopathy. Thromb Diath Haemorrh 26:241–247, 1967.

250. Cain GR, Feldman BF, Kawakami TG, Jain NC: Platelet dysplasia associated with megakaryoblastic leukemia in a dog. J Am Vet Med Assoc 188:529–530, 1986.

251. Weiser MG, Cockerell GL, Smith JA, Jensen WA: Cytoplasmic fragmentation associated with lymphoid leukemia in ruminants: interference with electronic determination of platelet concentration. Vet Pathol 26:177–178, 1989.

252. Harvey JW: Canine thrombocytic ehrlichiosis. In: Infectious Diseases of the Dog and Cat, 2nd ed. Greene CE, ed. pp 147–149, W.B. Saunders Co., Philadelphia, PA, 1998.

253. Santarém VA, Laposy CB, Farias MR: Ehrlichia platys–like inclusions bodies and morulae in platelets of a cat. Brazilian J Vet Science (abstract) 7:130, 2000.

254. Roszel J, Prier JE, Koprowska I: The occurrence of megakaryocytes in the peripheral blood of dogs. J Am Vet Med Assoc 147:133–137, 1965.

255. Matthews DM, Kingston N, Maki L, Nelms G: Trypanosoma theileri Laveran, 1902, in Wyoming cattle. Am J Vet Res 40:623–629, 1979.

256. Schlafer DH: Trypanosoma theileri: a literature review and report of incidence in New York cattle. Cornell Vet 69:411–425, 1979.

257. Barr SC: American trypanosomiasis. In: Infectious Diseases of the Dog and Cat, 2nd ed. Greene CE, ed. pp 445–448, W.B. Saunders Co., Philadelphia, PA, 1998.

258. Breitschwerdt EB, Nicholson WL, Kiehl AR, Steers C, Meuten DJ, Levine JF: Natural infections with Borrelia spirochetes in two dogs in Florida. J Clin Microbiol 32:352–357, 1994.

259. Quesenberry PJ: Hemopoietic stem cells, progenitor cells, and cytokines. In: Williams Hematology, 5th ed. Beutler E, Lichtman MA, Coller BS, Kipps TJ, eds. pp 211–228, McGraw-Hill, New York, NY, 1995.

260. Waller EK, Olweus J, Lund-Johansen F, et al: The "common stem cell" hypothesis reevaluated: human fetal bone marrow contains separate populations of hematopoietic and stromal progenitors. Blood 85:2422–2435, 1995.

261. Hayase Y, Muguruma Y, Lee MY: Osteoclast development from hematopoietic stem cells: apparent divergence of the osteoclast lineage prior to macrophage commitment. Exp Hematol 25:19–25, 1997.

262. Mbalaviele G, Jaiswal N, Meng A, Cheng L, Van den Bos C, Thiede M: Human mesenchymal stem cells promote osteoclast differentiation from CD34+ bone marrow hematopoietic progenitors. Endocrinology 140:3736–3743, 1999.

263. Kirshenbaum AS, Goff JP, Semere T, Foster B, Scott LM, Metcalfe DD: Demonstration that human mast cells arise from a progenitor cell population that is CD34(+), c-kit(+), and expresses aminopeptidase N (CD13). Blood 94:2333–2342, 1999.

264. Rosenzwajg M, Canque B, Gluckman JC: Human dendritic cell differentiation pathway from CD34(+) hematopoietic precursor cells. Blood 87:535–544, 1996.

265. Herbst B, Köhler G, Mackensen A, Veelken H, Lindemann A: GM-CSF promotes differentiation of a precursor cell of monocytes and Langerhans-type dendritic cells from CD34+ haemopoietic progenitor cells. Br J Haematol 101:231–241, 1998.

266. Herbst B, Köhler G, Mackensen A, et al: In vitro differentiation of CD34(+) hemato-poietic progenitor cells toward distinct dendritic cell subsets of the Birbeck granule and MIIC-positive Langerhans cell and the interdigitating dendritic cell type. Blood 88: 2541–2548, 1996.

267. Yoder MC, Williams DA: Matrix molecule interactions with hematopoietic stem cells. Exp Hematol 23:961–967, 1995.

268. Pantel K, Nakeff A: The role of lymphoid cells in hematopoietic regulation. Exp Hematol 21:738–742, 1993.

269. Campbell AD: The role of hemonectin in the cell adhesion mechanisms of bone marrow. Hematol Pathol 6:51–60, 1992.

270. Gordon MY: Physiology and function of the haemopoietic microenvironment. Br J Haematol 86:241–243, 1994.

271. Asahara T, Masuda H, Takahashi T, et al: Bone marrow origin of endothelial progeni-tor cells responsible for postnatal vasculogenesis in physiological and pathological neo-vascularization. Circ Res 85:221–228, 1999.

272. Park SR, Oreffo RO, Triffitt JT: Interconversion potential of cloned marrow adipocytes in vitro. Bone 24:549–554, 1999.

273. Pittenger MF, Mackay AM, Beck SC, et al: Multilineage potential of adult human mesenchymal stem cells. Science 284:143–147, 1999.

274. Majumdar MK, Thiede MA, Mosca JD, Moorman MA, Gerson SL: Phenotypic and functional comparison of cultures of marrow-derived mesenchymal stem cells (MSCs) and stromal cells. J Cell Physiol 176:57–66, 1998.

275. Metcalf D: Hematopoietic regulators: redundancy or subtlety. Blood 82:3515–3523, 1993.

276. Erslev AJ, Beutler E: Production and destruction of erythrocytes. In: Williams Hematol-ogy, 5th ed. Beutler E, Lichtman MA, Coller BS, Kipps TJ, eds. pp 425–441, McGraw-Hill, New York, NY, 1995.

277. Babior BM, Golde DW: Production, distribution, and fate of neutrophils. In: Williams Hematology, 5th ed. Beutler E, Lichtman MA, Coller BS, Kipps TJ, eds. pp 773–779, McGraw-Hill, New York, NY, 1995.

278. Wardlaw AJ, Kay AB: Eosinophils: production, biochemistry and function. In: Williams Hematology, 5th ed. Beutler E, Lichtman MA, Coller BS, Kipps TJ, eds. pp 798–805, McGraw-Hill, New York, NY, 1995.

279. Galli SJ, Dvorak AM: Production, biochemistry, and function of basophils and mast cells. In: Williams Hematology, 5th ed. Beutler E, Lichtman MA, Coller BS, Kipps TJ, eds. pp 805–810, McGraw-Hill, New York, NY, 1995.

280. Födinger M, Fritsch G, Winkler K, et al: Origin of human mast cells: development from transplanted hematopoietic stem cells after allogeneic bone marrow transplantation. Blood 84:2954–2959, 1994.

281. Lebien TW: Lymphocyte otogeny and homing receptors. In: Williams Hematology, 5th ed. Beutler E, Lichtman MA, Coller BS, Kipps TJ, eds. pp 921–929, McGraw-Hill, New York, NY, 1995.

282. Spits H, Lanier LL, Phillips JH: Development of human T and natural killer cells. Blood 85:2654–2670, 1995.

283. Burstein SA, Breton-Gorius J: Megakaryopoiesis and platelet formation. In: Williams Hematology, 5th ed. Beutler E, Lichtman MA, Coller BS, Kipps TJ, eds. pp 1149–1161, McGraw-Hill, New York, NY, 1995.

284. Perman V, Osborne CA, Stevens JB: Bone marrow biopsy. Vet Clin North Am 4:293–310, 1974.

285. Grindem CB: Bone marrow biopsy and evaluation. Vet Clin North Am Small Anim Pract 19:669–696, 1989.

286. Schalm OW, Lasmanis J: Cytologic features of bone marrow in normal and mastitic cows. Am J Vet Res 37:359–363, 1976.

287. Russell KE, Sellon DC, Grindem CB: Bone marrow in horses: indications, sample handling, and complications. Comp Cont Ed Pract Vet 16:1359–1365, 1994.

288. Berggren PC: Aplastic anemia in a horse. J Am Vet Med Assoc 179:1400–1402, 1981.

289. Brunning RD, Bloomfield CD, McKenna RW, Peterson L: Bilateral trephine bone marrow biopsies in lymphoma and other neoplastic diseases. Ann Intern Med 82:365–366, 1975.

290. El-Okda M, Ko YH, Xie SS, Hsu SM: Russell bodies consist of heterogenous glycoproteins in B-cell lymphoma cells. Am J Clin Pathol 97:866–871, 1992.

291. Zinkl JG, LeCouteur RA, Davis DC, Saunders GK: "Flaming" plasma cells in a dog with IgA multiple myeloma. Vet Clin Pathol 12(3):15–19, 1983.

292. Altman DH, Meyer DJ, Thompson JP, Bailey EA: Canine IgG_{2c} myeloma with Mott and flame cells. J Am Anim Hosp Assoc 27:419–423, 1991.

293. Norrdin RW, Powers BE: Bone changes in hypercalcemia of malignancy in dogs. J Am Vet Med Assoc 183:441–444, 1983.

294. Rozman C, Reverter JC, Feliu E, Rozman M, Climent C: Variations of fat tissue fractions in abnormal human bone marrow depend both on size and number of adipocytes: a stereologic study. Blood 76:892–895, 1990.

295. Tyler RD, Cowell RL, Meador V: Bone marrow evaluation. In: Consultations in Feline Internal Medicine 2. August JR, ed. pp 515–523, W.B. Saunders, Co., Philadelphia, PA, 1994.

296. Penny RH, Carlisle CH: The bone marrow of the dog: a comparative study of biopsy material obtained from the iliac crest, rib and sternum. J Small Anim Pract 11:727–734, 1970.

297. Stokol T, Blue JT: Pure red cell aplasia in cats: 9 cases (1989–1997). J Am Vet Med Assoc 214:75–79, 1999.

298. Weiss DJ: Histopathology of canine nonneoplastic bone marrow. Vet Clin Pathol 15(2):7–11, 1986.

299. Blue JT: Myelofibrosis in cats with myelodysplastic syndrome and acute myelogenous leukemia. Vet Pathol 25:154–160, 1988.

300. Fauci AS: Mechanisms of corticosteroid action on lymphocyte subpopulations. I. Redistribution of circulating T and B lymphocytes to the bone marrow. Immunology 28: 669–680, 1975.

301. Bloemena E, Weinreich S, Schellekens PTA: The influence of prednisolone on the recirculation of peripheral blood lymphocytes *in vivo.* Clin Exp Immunol 80:460–466, 1990.

302. Jasper DE, Jain NC: The influence of adrenocorticotropic hormone and prednisolone upon marrow and circulating leukocytes in the dog. Am J Vet Res 26:844–850, 1965.

303. Weiss DJ, Raskin RE, Zerbe C: Myelodysplastic syndrome in two dogs. J Am Vet Med Assoc 187:1038–1040, 1985.

304. Holloway SA, Meyer DJ, Mannella C: Prednisolone and danazol for treatment of immune-mediated anemia, thrombocytopenia, and ineffective erythroid regeneration in a dog. J Am Vet Med Assoc 197:1045–1048, 1990.

305. Walton RM, Modiano JF, Thrall MA, Wheeler SL: Bone marrow cytological findings in 4 dogs and a cat with hemophagocytic syndrome. J Vet Intern Med 10:7–14, 1996.

306. Canfield PJ, Watson ADJ, Ratcliffe RCC: Dyserythropoiesis, sideroblasts/siderocytes and hemoglobin crystallization in a dog. Vet Clin Pathol 16(1):21–28, 1987.

307. Weiss DJ, Reidarson TH: Idiopathic dyserythropoiesis in a dog. Vet Clin Pathol 18:43–46, 1989.

308. Bloom JC, Thiem PA, Sellers TS, Deldar A, Lewis HB: Cephalosporin-induced immune cytopenia in the dog: demonstration of erythrocyte-, neutrophil-, and platelet-associated IgG following treatment with cefazedone. Am J Hematol 28:71–78, 1988.

309. Raza A, Mundle S, Iftikhar A, et al: Simultaneous assessment of cell kinetics and programmed cell death in bone marrow biopsies of myelodysplastics reveals extensive apoptosis as the probable basis for ineffective hematopoiesis. Am J Hematol 48:143–154, 1995.

310. Weiss DJ, Armstrong PJ, Reimann K: Bone marrow necrosis in the dog. J Am Vet Med Assoc 187:54–59, 1985.

311. Felchle LM, McPhee LA, Kerr ME, Houston DM: Systemic lupus erythematosus and bone marrow necrosis in a dog. Can Vet J 37:742–744, 1996.

312. Terpstra V, van Berkel TJC: Scavenger receptors on liver Kupffer cells mediate the in vivo uptake of oxidatively damaged red cells in mice. Blood 95:2157–2163, 2000.

313. Alleman AR, Harvey JW: The morphologic effects of vincristine sulfate on canine bone marrow cells. Vet Clin Pathol 22:36–41, 1993.

314. Walker D, Cowell RL, Clinkenbeard KD, Feder B, Meinkoth JH: Bone marrow mast cell hyperplasia in dogs with aplastic anemia. Vet Clin Pathol 26:106–111, 1997.

315. Sheridan WP, Hunt P, Simonet S, Ulich TR: Hematologic effects of cytokines. In: Cytokines in Health and Disease, 2nd ed. Remick DG, Friedland JS, eds. pp 487–505, Marcel Dekker, Inc. New York, NY, 1997.

316. Garner FM, Lingeman CH: Mast-cell neoplasms in the domestic cat. Pathol Vet 7:517–530, 1970.

317. Liska WD, MacEwen EG, Zaki FA, Garvey M: Feline systemic mastocytosis: a review and results of splenectomy in seven cases. J Am Anim Hosp Assoc 15:589–597, 1979.

318. Davies AP, Hayden DW, Klausner JS, Perman V: Noncutaneous systemic mastocytosis and mast cell leukemia in a dog: case report and literature review. J Am Anim Hosp Assoc 17:361–368, 1981.

319. O'Keefe DA, Couto CG, Burke Schwartz C, Jacobs RM: Systemic mastocytosis in 16 dogs. J Vet Intern Med 1:75–80, 1987.

320. Schalm OW: Autoimmune hemolytic anemia in the dog. Can Pract 2:37–45, 1975.

321. Weiss DJ, Evanson O, Sykes J: A retrospective study of canine pancytopenia. Vet Clin Pathol 28:83–88, 1999.

322. Khanna C, Bienzle D: Polycythemia vera in a cat: bone marrow culture in erythropoietin-deficient medium. J Am Anim Hosp Assoc 30:45–49, 1994.

323. Shadduck RK: Aplastic anemia. In: Williams Hematology, 5th ed. Beutler E, Lichtman MA, Coller BS, Kipps TJ, eds. pp 238–251, McGraw-Hill, New York, NY, 1995.

324. Bowen RA, Olson PN, Behrendt MD, Wheeler SL, Husted PW, Nett TM: Efficacy and toxicity of estrogens commonly used to terminate canine pregnancy. J Am Vet Med Assoc 186:783–788, 1985.

325. Miura N, Sasaki N, Ogawa H, Takeuchi A: Bone marrow hypoplasia induced by administration of estradiol benzoate in male beagle dogs. Jpn J Vet Sci 47:731–739, 1985.

326. Weiss DJ, Klausner JS: Drug-associated aplastic anemia in dogs: eight cases (1984–1988). J Am Vet Med Assoc 196:472–475, 1990.

327. Watson AD, Wilson JT, Turner DM, Culvenor JA: Phenylbutazone-induced blood dyscrasias suspected in three dogs. Vet Rec 107:239–241, 1980.

328. Dunavant ML, Murry ES: Clinical evidence of phenylbutazone induced hypoplastic anemia. In: Proceedings First International Symposium on Equine Hematology. Kitchen H, Krehbiel JD, eds. pp 383–385, American Association of Equine Practitioners, Golden, CO, 1975.

329. Fox LE, Ford S, Alleman AR, Homer BL, Harvey JW: Aplastic anemia associated with prolonged high-dose trimethoprim-sulfadiazine administration in two dogs. Vet Clin Pathol 22:89–92, 1993.

330. Sippel WL: Bracken fern poisoning. J Am Vet Med Assoc 121:9–13, 1952.

331. Parker WH, McCrea CT: Bracken (Pteris aquilina) poisoning of sheep in the North York moors. Vet Rec 77:861–865, 1965.

332. Strafuss AC, Sautter JH: Clinical and general pathologic findings of aplastic anemia associated with S-(dichlorovinyl)-L-cysteine in calves. Am J Vet Res 28:25–37, 1967.

333. Stokol T, Randolph JF, Nachbar S, Rodi C, Barr SC: Development of bone marrow toxicosis after albendazole administration in a dog and cat. J Am Vet Med Assoc 1753–1756, 1997.

334. Helton KA, Nesbitt GH, Caciolo PL: Griseofulvin toxicity in cats: literature and report of seven cases. J Am Anim Hosp Assoc 22:453–458, 1986.

335. Rottman JB, English RV, Breitschwerdt EB, Duncan DE: Bone marrow hypoplasia in a cat treated with griseofulvin. J Am Vet Med Assoc 198:429–431, 1991.

336. Weiss DJ: Leukocyte response to toxic injury. Toxicol Pathol 21:135–140, 1993.

337. Rosenthal RC: Chemotherapy induced myelosuppression. In: Current Veterinary Therapy X, Small Animal Practice. Kirk RW, ed. pp 494–496, W.B. Saunders Co., Philadelphia, PA, 1989.

338. Phillips B: Severe, prolonged bone marrow hypoplasia secondary to the use of carboplatin in an azotemic dog. J Am Vet Med Assoc 215:1250–1252, 1999.

339. Seed TM, Carnes BA, Tolle DV, Fritz TE: Blood responses under chronic low daily dose gamma irradiation: I. Differential preclinical responses of irradiated male dogs in progression to either aplastic anemia or myeloproliferative disease. Leuk Res 13:1069–1084, 1989.

340. Seed TM, Kaspar LV: Changing patterns of radiosensitivity of hematopoietic progenitors from chronically irradiated dogs prone either to aplastic anemia or to myeloproliferative disease. Leuk Res 14:299–307, 1990.

341. Nash RA, Schuening FG, Seidel K, et al: Effect of recombinant canine granulocyte-macrophage colony-stimulating factor on hematopoietic recovery after otherwise lethal total body irradiation. Blood 83:1963–1970, 1994.

342. Watson ADJ: Bone marrow failure in a dog. J Small Anim Pract 20:681–690, 1979.

343. Morgan RV: Blood dyscrasias associated with testicular tumors in the dog. J Am Anim Hosp Assoc 18:970–975, 1982.

344. Sherding RG, Wilson GP, Kociba GJ: Bone marrow hypoplasia in eight dogs with Sertoli cell tumor. J Am Vet Med Assoc 178:497–501, 1981.

345. Suess RP, Jr, Barr SC, Sacre BJ, French TW: Bone marrow hypoplasia in a feminized dog with an interstitial cell tumor. J Am Vet Med Assoc 200:1346–1348, 1992.

346. McCandlish IAP, Munro CD, Breeze RG, Nash AS: Hormone producing ovarian tumour in the dog. Vet Rec 105:9–11, 1979.

347. Brockus CW: Endogenous estrogen myelotoxicity associated with functional cystic ovaries in a dog. Vet Clin Pathol 27:55–56, 1998.

348. Kociba GJ, Caputo CA: Aplastic anemia associated with estrus in pet ferrets. J Am Vet Med Assoc 178:1293–1294, 1981.

349. Bernard SL, Leathers CW, Brobst DF, Gorham JR: Estrogen-induced bone marrow depression in ferrets. Am J Vet Res 44:657–661, 1983.

350. Robinson WF, Wilcox GE, Fowler RLP: Canine parvoviral disease: experimental reproduction of the enteric form with a parvovirus isolated from a case of myocarditis. Vet Pathol 17:589–599, 1980.

351. Potgieter LN, Jones JB, Patton CS, Webb Martin TA: Experimental parvovirus infection in dogs. Can J Comp Med 45:212–216, 1981.

352. Brock KV, Jones JB, Shull RM, Potgieter LND: Effect of canine parvovirus on erythroid progenitors in phenylhydrazine-induced regenerative hemolytic anemia in dogs. Am J Vet Res 50:965–969, 1989.

353. Larsen S, Flagstad A, Aalbaek B: Experimental panleukopenia in the conventional cat. Vet Pathol 13:216–240, 1976.

354. Langheinrich KA, Nielsen SW: Histopathology of feline panleukopenia: a report of 65 cases. J Am Vet Med Assoc 158:863–872, 1971.

355. Cotter SM: Anemia associated with feline leukemia virus infection. J Am Vet Med Assoc 175:1191–1194, 1979.

356. Rojko JL, Olsen RG: The immunobiology of the feline leukemia virus. Vet Immunol Immunopathol 6:107–165, 1984.

357. Lutz H, Castelli I, Ehrensperger F, et al: Panleukopenia-like syndrome of FeLV caused by co-infection with FeLV and feline panleukopenia virus. Vet Immunol Immunopathol 46:21–33, 1995.

358. Buhles WC, Jr, Huxsoll DL, Hildebrandt PK: Tropical canine pancytopenia: role of aplastic anaemia in the pathogenesis of severe disease. J Comp Pathol 85:511–521, 1975.

359. Neer TM: Canine monocytic and granulocytic ehrlichiosis. In: Infectious Diseases of the Dog and Cat, 2nd ed. Greene CE, ed. pp 139–147, W.B. Saunders Co., Philadelphia, PA, 1998.

360. Toribio RE, Bain FT, Mrad DR, Messer NT IV, Sellers RS, Hinchcliff KW: Congenital defects in newborn foals of mares treated for equine protozoal myeloencephalitis during pregnancy. J Am Vet Med Assoc 212:697–701, 1998.

361. Ammann VJ, Fecteau G, Helie P, Desnoyers M, Hebert P, Babkine M: Pancytopenia associated with bone marrow aplasia in a Holstein heifer. Can Vet J 37:493–495, 1996.

362. Milne EM, Pyrah ITG, Smith KC, Whitewell KE: Aplastic anemia in a Clydesdale foal: a case report. J Equine Vet Sci 15:129–131, 1995.

363. Kohn CW, Swardson C, Provost P, Gilbert RO, Couto CG: Myeloid and megakaryocytic hypoplasia in related standardbreds. J Vet Intern Med 9:315–323, 1995.

364. Eldor A, Hershko C, Bruchim A: Androgen-responsive aplastic anemia in a dog. J Am Vet Med Assoc 173:304–305, 1978.

365. Weiss DJ, Christopher MM: Idiopathic aplastic anemia in a dog. Vet Clin Pathol 14(2): 23–25, 1985.

366. Lavoie JP, Morris DD, Zinkl JG, Lloyd K, Divers TJ: Pancytopenia caused by marrow aplasia in a horse. J Am Vet Med Assoc 191:1462–1464, 1987.

367. Ward MV, Mountan PC, Dodds WJ: Severe idiopathic refractory anemia and leukopenia in a horse. Calif Vet 12:19–22, 1980.

368. Nakao S: Immune mechanism of aplastic anemia. Int J Hematol 66:127–134, 1997.

369. Cohen JJ: Apoptosis: physiologic cell death. J Lab Clin Med 124:761–765, 1994.

370. Hoshi H, Weiss L: Rabbit bone marrow after administration of saponin. Lab Invest 38: 67–80, 1978.

371. Hoenig M: Six dogs with features compatible with myelonecrosis and myelofibrosis. J Am Anim Hosp Assoc 25:335–339, 1989.

372. Rebar AH: General responses of the bone marrow to injury. Toxicol Pathol 21:118–129, 1993.

373. Doige CE: Bone and bone marrow necrosis associated with the calf form of sporadic bovine leukosis. Vet Pathol 24:186–188, 1987.

374. Weiss DJ, Armstrong PJ: Secondary myelofibrosis in three dogs. J Am Vet Med Assoc 187:423–425, 1985.

375. Bloom JC, Lewis HB, Sellers TS, Deldar A, Morgan DG: The hematopathology of cefonicid- and cefazedone-induced blood dyscrasias in the dog. Toxicol Appl Pharmacol 90:143–155, 1987.

376. Scruggs DW, Fleming SA, Maslin WR, Groce AW: Osteopetrosis, anemia, thrombocytopenia, and marrow necrosis in beef calves naturally infected with bovine virus diarrhea virus. J Vet Diagn Invest 7:555–559, 1995.

377. Boosinger TR, Rebar AH, DeNicola DB, Boon GD: Bone marrow alterations associated with canine parvoviral enteritis. Vet Pathol 19:558–561, 1982.

378. Weiss DJ, Miller DC: Bone marrow necrosis associated with pancytopenia in a cow. Vet Pathol 22:90–92, 1985.

379. Fenger CK, Bertone JJ, Biller D, Merryman J: Generalized medullary infarction of the long bones in a horse. J Am Vet Med Assoc 202:621–623, 1993.

380. Villiers EJ, Dunn JK: Clinicopathological features of seven cases of canine myelofibrosis and the possible relationship between the histological findings and prognosis. Vet Rec 145:222–228, 1999.

381. Canfield PJ, Church DB, Russ IG: Myeloproliferative disorder involving the megakaryocytic line. J Small Anim Pract 34:296–301, 1993.

382. Breuer W, Darbès J, Hermanns W, Thiele J: Idiopathic myelofibrosis in a cat and in three dogs. Comp Haematol Int 9:17–24, 1999.

383. Angel KL, Spano JS, Schumacher J, Kwapien RP: Myelophthisic pancytopenia in a pony mare. J Am Vet Med Assoc 198:1039–1042, 1991.

384. Cain GR, East N, Moore PF: Myelofibrosis in young pygmy goats. Comp Haematol Int 4:167–172, 1994.

385. Hoff B, Lumsden JH, Valli VEO, Kruth SA: Myelofibrosis: review of clinical and pathological features in fourteen dogs. Can Vet J 32:357–361, 1991.

386. Searcy GP, Tasker JB, Miller DR: Animal model: pyruvate kinase deficiency in dogs. Am J Physiol 94:689–692, 1979.

387. Randolph JF, Center SA, Kallfelz FA, et al: Familial nonspherocytic hemolytic anemia in poodles. Am J Vet Res 47:687–695, 1986.

388. Bader R, Bode G, Rebel W, Lexa P: Stimulation of bone marrow by administration of excessive doses of recombinant human erythropoietin. Pathol Res Pract 188:676–679, 1992.

389. Whyte MP: Skeletal disorders characterized by osteosclerosis or hyperostosis. In: Metabolic Bone Disease and Clinically Related Disorders, 3rd ed. Avioli LV, Krane SM, eds. pp 697–738, Academic Press, San Diego, CA, 1998.

390. Lees GE, Sautter JH: Anemia and osteopetrosis in a dog. J Am Vet Med Assoc 175:820–824, 1979.

391. O'Brien SE, Riedesel EA, Miller LD: Osteopetrosis in an adult dog. J Am Anim Hosp Assoc 23:213–216, 1987.

392. Kramers P, Fluckiger MA, Rahn BA, Cordey J: Osteopetrosis in cats. J Small Anim Pract 29:153–164, 1988.

393. Berry CR, House JK, Poulos PP, et al: Radiographic and pathologic features of osteopetrosis in two Peruvian Paso foals. Vet Radiol Ultrasound 35:355–361, 1994.

394. Leipold HW, Cook JE: Animal model: osteopetrosis in Angus and Hereford calves. Am J Pathol 86:745–748, 1977.

395. Dunn JK, Doige CE, Searcy GP, Tamke P: Myelofibrosis-osteosclerosis syndrome associated with erythroid hypoplasia in a dog. J Small Anim Pract 27:799–806, 1986.

396. Hoover EA, Kociba GJ: Bone lesions in cats with anemia induced by feline leukemia virus. J Natl Cancer Inst 53:1277–1284, 1974.

397. Smith JE, Agar NS: The effect of phlebotomy on canine erythrocyte metabolism. Res Vet Sci 18:231–236, 1975.

398. Bremner KC: The reticulocyte response in calves made anaemic by phlebotomy. Aust J Exp Biol Med Sci 44:251–258, 1966.

399. Ulich TR, Del Castillo J, Yin S, Egrie JC: The erythropoietic effects of interleukin 6 and erythropoietin in vivo. Exp Hematol 19:29–34, 1991.

400. McGrath C: Polycythemia vera in dogs. J Am Vet Med Assoc 164:1117–1122, 1974.

401. Hasler AH, Giger U: Serum erythropoietin values in polycythemic cats. J Am Anim Hosp Assoc 32:294–301, 1996.

402. Couto CG, Boudrieau RJ, Zanjani ED: Tumor-associated erythrocytosis in a dog with nasal fibrosarcoma. J Vet Intern Med 3:183–185, 1989.

403. Waters DJ, Prueter JC: Secondary polycythemia associated with renal disease in the dog: two case reports and review of literature. J Am Anim Hosp Assoc 24:109–114, 1988.

404. Miyamoto T, Horie T, Shimada T, Kuwamura M, Baba E: Long-term case study of myelodysplastic syndrome in a dog. J Am Anim Hosp Assoc 35:475–481, 1999.

405. Jonas LD, Thrall MA, Weiser MG: Nonregenerative form of immune-mediated hemolytic anemia in dogs. J Am Anim Hosp Assoc 23:201–204, 1987.

406. Stockham SL, Ford RB, Weiss DJ: Canine autoimmune hemolytic disease with delayed erythroid regeneration. J Am Anim Hosp Assoc 16:927–931, 1980.

407. Dessypris EN: The biology of pure red cell aplasia. Semin Hematol 28:275–284, 1991.

408. Erslev AJ, Soltan A: Pure red-cell aplasia: a review. Blood Rev 10:20–28, 1996.

409. Weiss DJ: Antibody-mediated suppression of erythropoiesis in dogs with red blood cell aplasia. Am J Vet Res 47:2646–2648, 1986.

410. Weiss DJ, Stockham SL, Willard MD, Schirmer RG: Transient erythroid hypoplasia in the dog: report of five cases. J Am Anim Hosp Assoc 18:353–359, 1982.

411. Dodds WJ: Immune-mediated diseases of the blood. Adv Vet Sci Comp Med 27:163–196, 1983.

412. Watson AD: Chloramphenicol toxicity in dogs. Res Vet Sci 23:66–69, 1977.

413. Watson AD, Middleton DJ: Chloramphenicol toxicosis in cats. Am J Vet Res 39:1199–1203, 1978.

414. Hotston Moore A, Day MJ, Graham MWA: Congenital pure red blood cell aplasia (Diamond-Blackfan anaemia) in a dog. Vet Rec 132:414–415, 1993.

415. Lange RD, Jones JB, Chambers C, Quirin Y, Sparks JC: Erythropoiesis and erythrocytic survival in dogs with cyclic hematopoiesis. Am J Vet Res 37:331–334, 1976.

416. Abkowitz JL, Holly RD: Cyclic hematopoiesis in dogs: studies of erythroid burst-forming cells confirm an early stem cell defect. Exp Hematol 16:941–945, 1988.

417. Scott RE, Dale DC, Rosenthal AS, Wolff SM: Cyclic neutropenia in grey collie dogs. Ultrastructural evidence for abnormal neutrophil granulopoiesis. Lab Invest 28:514–525, 1973.

418. Rojko JL, Hartke JR, Cheney CM, Phipps AJ, Neil JC: Cytopathic feline leukemia viruses cause apoptosis in hemolymphatic cells. Prog Mol Subcell Biol 16:13–43, 1996.

419. Cowgill LD, James KM, Levy JK, et al: Use of recombinant human erythropoietin for management of anemia in dogs and cats with renal failure. J Am Vet Med Assoc 212:521–528, 1998.

420. Piercy RJ, Swardson CJ, Hinchcliff KW: Erythroid hypoplasia and anemia following administration of recombinant human erythropoietin to two horses. J Am Vet Med Assoc 212:244–247, 1998.

421. Woods PR, Campbell G, Cowell RL: Nonregenerative anaemia associated with administration of recombinant human erythropoietin to a thoroughbred racehorse. Equine Vet J 29:326–328, 1997.

422. Means RT, Jr, Krantz SB: Progress in understanding the pathogenesis of the anemia of chronic disease. Blood 80:1639–1647, 1992.

423. Anderson TD: Cytokine-induced changes in the leukon. Toxicol Pathol 21:147–157, 1993.

424. Hirsch V, Dunn J: Megaloblastic anemia in the cat. J Am Anim Hosp Assoc 19:873–880, 1983.

425. McManus PM, Hess RS: Myelodysplastic changes in a dog with subsequent acute myeloid leukemia. Vet Clin Pathol 27:112–115, 1998.

426. Shelton GH, Linenberger ML, Grant CK, Abkowitz JL: Hematologic manifestations of feline immunodeficiency virus infection. Blood 76:1104–1109, 1990.

427. Thenen SW, Rasmussen SD: Megaloblastic erythropoiesis and tissue depletion of folic acid in the cat. Am J Vet Res 39:1205–1207, 1978.

428. Canfield PJ, Watson ADJ: Investigations of bone marrow dyscrasia in a poodle with macrocytosis. J Comp Pathol 101:269–278, 1989.

429. Schalm OW: Erythrocyte macrocytosis in miniature and toy poodles. Can Pract 3(6):55–57, 1976.

430. Baker RJ, Valli VEO: Dysmyelopoiesis in the cat: a hematological disorder resembling anemia with excess blasts in man. Can J Vet Res 50:3–6, 1985.

431. Blue JT, French TW, Kranz JS: Non-lymphoid hematopoietic neoplasia in cats: a retrospective study of 60 cases. Cornell Vet 78:21–42, 1988.

432. Schalm OW: Bone marrow cytology as an aid to diagnosis. Vet Clin North Am Small Anim Pract 11:383–404, 1981.

433. Harvey JW, Wolfsheimer KJ, Simpson CF, French TW: Pathologic sideroblasts and siderocytes associated with chloramphenicol therapy in a dog. Vet Clin Pathol 14(1):36–42, 1985.

434. Thompson JP, Christopher MM, Ellison GW, Homer BL, Buchanan BA: Paraneoplastic

leukocytosis associated with a rectal adenomatous polyp in a dog. J Am Vet Med Assoc 201:737–738, 1992.

435. Finco DR, Duncan JR, Schall WD, Prasse KW: Acetaminophen toxicosis in the cat. J Am Vet Med Assoc 166:469–472, 1975.

436. Obradovich JE, Ogilvie GK, Powers BE, Boone T: Evaluation of recombinant canine granulocyte colony-stimulating factor as an inducer of granulopoiesis. J Vet Intern Med 5:75–79, 1991.

437. Nash RA, Schuening F, Appelbaum F, Hammond WP, Boone T, Morris CF, Slichter SJ, Storb R: Molecular cloning and in vivo evaluation of canine granulocyte-macrophage colony-stimulating factor. Blood 78:930–937, 1991.

438. Cullor JS, Smith W, Zinkl JG, Dellinger JD, Boone T: Hematologic and bone marrow changes after short- and long-term administration of two recombinant bovine granulocyte colony-stimulating factors. Vet Pathol 29:521–527, 1992.

439. Lappin MR, Latimer KS: Hematuria and extreme neutrophilic leukocytosis in a dog with renal tubular carcinoma. J Am Vet Med Assoc 192:1289–1292, 1988.

440. Sharkey LC, Rosol IJ, Gröne A, Ward H, Steinmeyer C: Production of granulocyte colony-stimulating factor and granulocyte-macrophage colony-stimulating factor by carcinomas in a dog and a cat with paraneoplastic leukocytosis. J Vet Intern Med 10:405–408, 1996.

441. Trowald-Wigh G, Håkansson L, Johannisson A, Norrgren L, Hård af Segerstad C: Leucocyte adhesion protein deficiency in Irish setter dogs. Vet Immunol Immunopathol 32:261–280, 1992.

442. Nagahata H, Nochi H, Tamoto K, Yamashita K, Noda H, Kociba GJ: Characterization of functions of neutrophils from bone marrow of cattle with leukocyte adhesion deficiency. Am J Vet Res 56:167–171, 1995.

443. Giger U, Boxer LA, Simpson PJ, Lucchesi BR, Dodd RF: Deficiency of leukocyte surface glycoproteins Mo1, LFA-1, and Leu M5 in a dog with recurrent bacterial infections: an animal model. Blood 69:1622–1630, 1987.

444. Nagahata H, Kehrli ME, Jr, Murata H, Okada H, Noda H, Kociba GJ: Neutrophil function and pathologic findings in Holstein calves with leukocyte adhesion deficiency. Am J Vet Res 55:40–48, 1994.

445. Cheville NF: The gray collie syndrome. J Am Vet Med Assoc 152:620–630, 1968.

446. Dale DC, Alling DW, Wolff SM: Cyclic hematopoiesis: the mechanism of cyclic neutropenia in grey collie dogs. J Clin Invest 51:2197–2204, 1972.

447. Cooper BJ, Watson ADJ: Myeloid neoplasia in a dog. Aust Vet J 51:150–154, 1975.

448. Joiner GN, Fraser CJ, Jardine JH, Trujillo JM: A case of chronic granulocytic leukemia in a dog. Can J Comp Med 40:153–160, 1976.

449. Pollet L, Van Hove W, Mattheeuws D: Blastic crisis in chronic myelogenous leukaemia in a dog. J Small Anim Pract 19:469–475, 1978.

450. Mandell CP, Sparger EE, Pedersen NC, Jain NC: Long-term haematological changes in cats experimentally infected with feline immunodeficiency virus (FIV). Comp Haematol Int 2:8–17, 1992.

451. Beebe AM, Gluckstern TG, George J, Pedersen NC, Dandekar S: Detection of feline immunodeficiency virus infection in bone marrow of cats. Vet Immunol Immunopathol 35:37–49, 1992.

452. Jacobs G, Calvert C, Kaufman A: Neutropenia and thrombocytopenia in three dogs treated with anticonvulsants. J Am Vet Med Assoc 212:681–684, 1998.

453. Maddison JE, Hoff B, Johnson RP: Steroid responsive neutropenia in a dog. J Am Anim Hosp Assoc 19:881–886, 1982.

454. Duckett WM, Matthews HK: Hypereosinophilia in a horse with intestinal lymphosarcoma. Can Vet J 38:719–720, 1997.

455. Pollack MJ, Flanders JA, Johnson RC: Disseminated malignant mastocytoma in a dog. J Am Anim Hosp Assoc 27:435–440, 1991.

456. Sellon RK, Rottman JB, Jordan HL, et al: Hypereosinophilia associated with transitional cell carcinoma in a cat. J Am Vet Med Assoc 201:591–593, 1992.

457. Latimer KS, Bounous DI, Collatos C, Charmichael KP, Howerth EW: Extreme eosinophilia with disseminated eosinophilic granulomatous disease in a horse. Vet Clin Pathol 25:23–26, 1996.

458. Jensen AL, Nielsen OL: Eosinophilic leukaemoid reaction in a dog. J Small Anim Pract 33:337–340, 1992.

459. Ndikuwera J, Smith DA, Obwolo MJ, Masvingwe C: Chronic granulocytic leukaemia/eosinophilic leukaemia in a dog? J Small Anim Pract 33:553–557, 1992.

460. Morris DD, Bloom JC, Roby KA, Woods K, Tablin F: Eosinophilic myeloproliferative disorder in a horse. J Am Vet Med Assoc 185:993–996, 1984.

461. Fine DM, Tvedten H: Chronic granulocytic leukemia in a dog. J Am Vet Med Assoc 214:1809–1812, 1999.

462. Deldar A, Lewis H, Bloom J, Weiss L: Cephalosporin-induced alterations in erythroid (CFU-E) and granulocyte-macrophage (CFU-GM) colony-forming capacity in canine bone marrow. Fundam Appl Toxicol 11:450–463, 1988.

463. Rawlings CA: Clinical laboratory evaluations of seven heartworm infected beagles: during disease development and following treatment. Cornell Vet 72:49–56, 1982.

464. Atkins CE, DeFrancesco TC, Miller MW, Meurs KM, Keene B: Prevalence of heartworm infection in cats with signs of cardiorespiratory abnormalities. J Am Vet Med Assoc 212:517–520, 1998.

465. Allan GS, Watson AD, Duff BC, Howlett CR: Disseminated mastocytoma and mastocytemia in a dog. J Am Vet Med Assoc 165:346–349, 1974.

466. Bortnowski HB, Rosenthal RC: Gastrointestinal mast cell tumors and eosinophilia in two cats. J Am Anim Hosp Assoc 28:271–275, 1992.

467. Postorino NC, Wheeler SL, Park RD, Powers BE, Withrow SJ: A syndrome resembling lymphomatoid granulomatosis in the dog. J Vet Intern Med 3:15–19, 1989.

468. Hopper PE, Mandell CP, Turrel JM, Jain NC, Tablin F, Zinkl JG: Probable essential thrombocythemia in a dog. J Vet Intern Med 3:79–85, 1989.

469. Mears EA, Raskin RE, Legendre AM: Basophilic leukemia in a dog. J Vet Intern Med 11:92–94, 1997.

470. Juliá A, Olona M, Bueno J, et al: Drug-induced agranulocytosis: prognostic factors in a series of 168 episodes. Br J Haematol 79:366–371, 1991.

471. Dale DC: Neutropenia. In: Williams Hematology, 5th ed. Beutler E, Lichtman MA, Coller BS, Kipps TJ, eds. pp 815–824, McGraw-Hill, New York, NY, 1995.

472. Chickering WR, Prasse KW: Immune-mediated neutropenia in man and animals: a review. Vet Clin Pathol 10(1):6–16, 1981.

473. Beale KM, Altman D, Clemmons RR, Bolon B: Systemic toxicosis associated with azathioprine administration in domestic cats. Am J Vet Res 53:1236–1240, 1992.

474. Kunkle GA, Meyer DJ: Toxicity of high doses of griseofulvin in cats. J Am Vet Med Assoc 191:322–323, 1987.

475. Shelton GH, Grant CK, Linenberger ML, Abkowitz JL: Severe neutropenia associated with griseofulvin therapy in cats with feline immunodeficiency virus infection. J Vet Intern Med 4:317–319, 1990.

476. Peterson ME, Kintzer PP, Hurvitz AI: Methimazole treatment of 262 cats with hyperthyroidism. J Vet Intern Med 2:150–157, 1988.

477. Moreb J, Shemesh O, Manor C, Hershko C: Transient methimazole-induced bone marrow aplasia: in vitro evidence of a humoral mechanism of bone marrow suppression. Acta Haematol 69:127–131, 1983.

478. Reagan WJ, Murphy D, Battaglino M, Bonney P, Boone TC: Antibodies to canine granulocyte colony-stimulating factor induce persistent neutropenia. Vet Pathol 32:374–378, 1995.

479. Hammond WP, Csiba E, Canin A, et al: Chronic neutropenia. A new canine model induced by human granulocyte colony-stimulating factor. J Clin Invest 87:704–710, 1991.

480. Machado EA, Jones JB, Aggio MC, Chernoff AI, Maxwell PA, Lange RD: Ultrastructural changes of bone marrow in canine cyclic hematopoiesis (CH dog). A sequential study. Virchows Arch Pathol Anat 390:93–108, 1981.

481. Swenson CL, Kociba GJ, O'Keefe DA, Crisp MS, Jacobs RM, Rojko JL: Cyclic hematopoiesis associated with feline leukemia virus infection in two cats. J Am Vet Med Assoc 191:93–96, 1987.

482. Morley A, Stohlman F: Cyclophosphamide-induced cyclical neutropenia: an animal model of human periodic disease. N Engl J Med 12:643–646, 1970.

483. Dieringer TM, Brown SA, Rogers KS, Lees GE, Whitney MS, Weeks BR: Effects of lithium carbonate administration to healthy cats. Am J Vet Res 53:721–726, 1992.

484. Nasisse MP, Dorman DC, Jamison KC, Weigler BJ, Hawkins EC, Stevens JB: Effects of valacyclovir in cats infected with feline herpesvirus. Am J Vet Res 58:1141–1144, 1997.

485. Fyfe JC, Jezyk PF, Giger U, Patterson DF: Inherited selective malabsorption of vitamin B12 in giant schnauzers. J Am Anim Hosp Assoc 25:533–539, 1989.

486. Hill RJ, Levin J: Regulators of thrombopoiesis: their biochemistry and physiology. Blood Cells 15:141–166, 1989.

487. Kaushansky K: Thrombopoietin: in vitro predictions, in vivo realities. Am J Hematol 53:188–191, 1996.

488. Joshi BC, Raplee RG, Powell AL, Hancock F: Autoimmune thrombocytopenia in a cat. J Am Anim Hosp Assoc 15:585–588, 1979.

489. Peterson ME, Hurvitz AI, Leib MS, Cavanaugh PG, Dutton RE: Propylthiouracil-associated hemolytic anemia, thrombocytopenia, and antinuclear antibodies in cats with hyperthyroidism. J Am Vet Med Assoc 184:806–808, 1984.

490. Williams DA, Maggio Price L: Canine idiopathic thrombocytopenia: clinical observations and long-term follow-up in 54 cases. J Am Vet Med Assoc 185:660–663, 1984.

491. Grindem CB, Breitschwerdt EB, Corbett WT, Page RL, Jans HE: Thrombocytopenia associated with neoplasia in dogs. J Vet Intern Med 8:400–405, 1994.

492. Lewis DC: Canine idiopathic thrombocytopenia purpura. J Vet Intern Med 10:207–218, 1996.

493. Breitschwerdt EB: Infectious thrombocytopenia in dogs. Comp Cont Ed Pract Vet 10:1177–1190, 1988.

494. Reardon MJ, Pierce KR: Acute experimental canine ehrlichiosis. I. Sequential reaction of the hemic and lymphoreticular systems. Vet Pathol 18:48–61, 1981.

495. Edwards JF, Dodds WJ, Slauson DO: Megakaryocytic infection and thrombocytopenia in African swine fever. Vet Pathol 22:171–176, 1985.

496. McAnulty JF, Rudd RG: Thrombocytopenia associated with vaccination of a dog with a modified-live paramyxovirus vaccine. J Am Vet Med Assoc 186:1217–1219, 1985.

497. Handagama PJ, Feldman BF: Drug-induced thrombocytopenia. Vet Res Commun 10:1–20, 1986.

498. Bloom JC, Blackmer SA, Bugelski PJ, Sowinski JM, Saunders LZ: Gold-induced immune thrombocytopenia in the dog. Vet Pathol 22:492–499, 1985.

499. Davis WM: Hapten-induced immune-mediated thrombocytopenia in a dog. J Am Vet Med Assoc 184:976–977, 1984.

500. Harrus S, Waner T, Weiss DJ, Keysary A, Bark H: Kinetics of serum antiplatelet antibodies in experimental acute canine ehrlichiosis. Vet Immunol Immunopathol 51: 13–20, 1996.

501. Nimer SD: Essential thrombocythemia: another "heterogeneous disease" better understood? Blood 93:415–416, 1999.

502. Evans RJ, Jones DRE, Gruffydd-Jones TJ: Essential thrombocythaemia in the dog and cat: a report of four cases. J Small Anim Pract 23:457–467, 1982.

503. Mandell CP, Goding B, Degen MA, Hopper PE, Zinkl JG: Spurious elevation of serum potassium in two cases of thrombocythemia. Vet Clin Pathol 17:32–33, 1988.

504. Hammer AS, Couto CG, Getzy D, Bailey MQ: Essential thrombocythemia in a cat. J Vet Intern Med 4:87–91, 1990.

505. Bass MC, Schultze AE: Essential thrombocythemia in a dog: case report and literature review. J Am Anim Hosp Assoc 34:197–203, 1998.

506. Hoffman R: Acquired pure amegakaryocytic thrombocytopenic purpura. Semin Hematol 28:303–312, 1991.

507. Joshi BC, Jain NC: Detection of antiplatelet antibody in serum and on megakaryocytes in dogs with autoimmune thrombocytopenia. J Am Vet Med Assoc 681–685, 1976.

508. Murtaugh RJ, Jacobs RM: Suspected immune-mediated megakaryocytic hypoplasia or aplasia in a dog. J Am Vet Med Assoc 186:1313–1315, 1985.

509. Gaschen FP, Smith Meyer B, Harvey JW: Amegakaryocytic thrombocytopenia and immune-mediated haemolytic anaemia in a cat. Comp Haematol Int 2:175–178, 1992.

510. Sockett DC, Traub Dargatz J, Weiser MG: Immune-mediated hemolytic anemia and thrombocytopenia in a foal. J Am Vet Med Assoc 190:308–310, 1987.

511. Lees GE, McKeever PJ, Ruth GR: Fatal thrombocytopenic hemorrhagic diathesis associated with dapsone administration to a dog. J Am Vet Med Assoc 175:49–52, 1979.

512. Weiss RC, Cox NR, Boudreaux MK: Toxicologic effects of ribavirin in cats. J Vet Pharmacol Ther 16:301–316, 1993.

513. Joshi BC, Jain NC: Experimental immunologic thrombocytopenia in dogs: a study of thrombocytopenia and megakaryocytopoiesis. Res Vet Sci 22:11–17, 1977.

514. Tolle DV, Cullen SM, Seed TM, Fritz TE: Circulating micromegakaryocytes preceding leukemia in three dogs exposed to 2.5 R/day gamma radiation. Vet Pathol 20:111–114, 1983.

515. Sahebekhtiari HA, Tavassoli M: Marrow cell uptake by megakaryocytes in routine bone marrow smears during blood loss. Scand J Haematol 16:13–17, 1976.

516. Cashell AW, Buss DH: The frequency and significance of megakaryocytic emperipolesis in myeloproliferative and reactive states. Ann Hematol 64:273–276, 1992.

517. Lee KP: Emperipolesis of hematopoietic cells within megakaryocytes in bone marrow of the rat. Vet Pathol 26:473–478, 1989.

518. Tavassoli M: Modulation of megakaryocyte emperipolesis by phlebotomy: megakaryocytes as a component of marrow-blood barrier. Blood Cells 12:205–216, 1986.

519. Stahl CP, Zucker Franklin D, Evatt BL, Winton EF: Effects of human interleukin-6 on megakaryocyte development and thrombocytopoiesis in primates. Blood 78:1467–1475, 1991.

520. Stenberg PE, McDonald TP, Jackson CW: Disruption of microtubules in vivo by vincristine induces large membrane complexes and other cytoplasmic abnormalities in megakaryocytes and platelets of normal rats like those in human and Wistar Furth rat hereditary macrothrombocytopenias. J Cell Physiol 162:86–102, 1995.

521. Tanaka M, Aze Y, Fujita T: Adhesion molecule LFA-1/ICAM-1 influences on LPS-induced megakaryocytic emperipolesis in the rat bone marrow. Vet Pathol 34:463–466, 1997.

522. Prater MR, De Gopegui RR, Burdette K, Veit H, Feldman B: Bone marrow aspirate from a cat with cutaneous lesions. Vet Clin Pathol 28:52, 57–58, 1999.

523. Woda BA, Sullivan JL: Reactive histiocytic disorders. Am J Clin Pathol 99:459–463, 1993.

524. Walsh KM, Losco PE: Canine mycobacteriosis: a case report. J Am Anim Hosp Assoc 20:295–299, 1984.

525. Meinkoth J, Crystal M, Cowell R, Thiessen A: What is your diagnosis? Cytology of post-treatment histoplasmosis. Vet Clin Pathol 26:118,133–134, 1997.

526. Clinkenbeard KD, Cowell RL, Tyler RD: Disseminated histoplasmosis in cats: 12 cases (1981–1986). J Am Vet Med Assoc 190:1445–1448, 1987.

527. Clinkenbeard KD, Cowell RL, Tyler RD: Disseminated histoplasmosis in dogs: 12 cases (1981–1986). J Am Vet Med Assoc 193:1443–1447, 1988.

528. Slappendel RJ, Ferrer L: Leishmaniasis. In: Infectious Diseases of the Dog and Cat, 2nd ed. Greene CE, ed. pp 450–458, W.B. Saunders Co., Philadelphia, PA, 1998.

529. Ciaramella P, Oliva G, Luna RD, et al: A retrospective clinical study of canine leishmaniasis in 150 dogs naturally infected by Leishmania infantum. Vet Rec 141:539–543, 1997.

530. Ozon C, Marty P, Pratlong F, et al: Disseminated feline leishmaniosis due to Leishmania infantum in Southern France. Vet Parasitol 75:273–277, 1998.

531. Franks PT, Harvey JW, Shields RP, Lawman MJP: Hematological findings in experimental feline cytauxzoonosis. J Am Anim Hosp Assoc 24:395–401, 1988.

532. Smith AN, Spencer JA, Stringfellow JS, Vygantas KR, Welch JA: Disseminated infection with Phialemonium obovatum in a German Shepherd dog. J Am Vet Med Assoc 216:708–712, 2000.

533. Cork LC, Munnell JF, Lorenz MD: The pathology of feline G_{M2} gangliosidosis. Am J Pathol 90:723–734, 1978.

534. Hanichen T, Breuer W, Hermanns W: Lipid storage disease. Lab Anim Sci 47:275–279, 1997.

535. Chang CS, Wang CH, Su IJ, Chen YC, Shen MC: Hematophagic histiocytosis: a clinicopathologic analysis of 23 cases with special reference to the association with peripheral T-cell lymphoma. J Formos Med Assoc 93:421–428, 1994.

536. Majluf Cruz A, Sosa Camas R, Perez Ramirez O, Rosas Cabral A, Vargas Vorackova F, Labardini Mendez J: Hemophagocytic syndrome associated with hematological neoplasias. Leuk Res 22:893–898, 1998.

537. Risti B, Flury RF, Schaffner A: Fatal hematophagic histiocytosis after granulocyte-macrophage colony-stimulating factor and chemotherapy for high-grade malignant lymphoma. Clin Investig 72:457–461, 1994.

538. Stockhaus C, Slappendel RJ: Haemophagocytic syndrome with disseminated intravascular coagulation in a dog. J Small Anim Pract 39:203–206, 1998.

539. Reiner AP, Spivak JL: Hematophagic histiocytosis. A report of 23 new patients and a review of the literature. Medicine (Baltimore) 67:369–388, 1988.

540. Cline MJ: Histiocytes and histiocytosis. Blood 84:2840–2853, 1994.

541. Peastron AE, Munn RJ, Madewell BR: Malignant histiocytosis. J Vet Intern Med 7:101–103, 1993.

542. Court EA, Earnest-Koons KA, Barr SC, Gould WJ II: Malignant histiocytosis in a cat. J Am Vet Med Assoc 203:1300–1302, 1993.

543. Newlands CE, Houston DM, Vasconcelos DY: Hyperferritinemia associated with malignant histiocytosis in a dog. J Am Vet Med Assoc 205:849–851, 1994.

544. Freeman L, Stevens J, Loughman C, Tompkins M: Malignant histiocytosis in a cat. J Vet Intern Med 9:171–173, 1995.

545. Brown DE, Thrall MA, Getzy DM, Weiser MG, Ogilvie GK: Cytology of canine malignant histiocytosis. Vet Clin Pathol 23:118–122, 1994.

546. Moore PF, Rosin A: Malignant histiocytosis of Bernese mountain dogs. Vet Pathol 23: 1–10, 1986.

547. Lester GD, Alleman AR, Raskin RE, Calderwood Mays MB: Malignant histiocytosis in an Arabian filly. Equine Vet J 25:471–473, 1993.

548. Wellman ML, Davenport DJ, Morton D, Jacobs RM: Malignant histiocytosis in four dogs. J Am Vet Med Assoc 187:919–921, 1985.

549. Moore P: Systemic histiocytosis of Bernese mountain dogs. Vet Pathol 21:554–563, 1984.

550. Weiss DJ, Greig B, Aird B, Geor RJ: Inflammatory disorders of bone marrow. Vet Clin Pathol 21:79–84, 1992.

551. Johnson KA: Osteomyelitis in dogs and cats. J Am Vet Med Assoc 204:1882–1887, 1994.

552. Fossum TW, Hulse DA: Osteomyelitis. Semin Vet Med Surg Small Anim 7:85–97, 1992.

553. Perdue BD, Collier MA, Dzata GK, Mosier DA: Multisystemic granulomatous inflammation in a horse. J Am Vet Med Assoc 198:663–664, 1991.

554. Brearley MJ, Jeffery N: Cryptococcal osteomyelitis in a dog. J Small Anim Pract 33:601–604, 1992.

555. Canfield PJ, Malik R, Davis PE, Martin P: Multifocal idiopathic pyogranulomatous bone disease in a dog. J Small Anim Pract 35:370–373, 1994.

556. Lehrer RI, Ganz T: Biochemistry and function of monocytes and macrophages. In: Williams Hematology, 5th ed. Beutler E, Lichtman MA, Coller BS, Kipps TJ, eds. pp 869–875, McGraw-Hill, New York, NY, 1995.

557. MacEwen EG: Feline lymphoma and leukemias. In: Small Animal Clinical Oncology. Withrow SJ, MacEwen EG, eds. pp 479–495, W.B. Saunders Co., Philadelphia, PA, 1996.

558. MacEwen EG, Young KM: Canine lymphoma and lymphoid leukemias. In: Small Animal Clinical Oncology. Withrow SJ, MacEwen EG, eds. pp 451–479, W.B. Saunders Co., Philadelphia, PA, 1996.

559. Hopper CD, Sparkes AH, Gruffydd-Jones TJ, et al: Clinical and laboratory findings in cats infected with feline immunodeficiency virus. Vet Rec 125:341–346, 1989.

560. Sparkes AH, Hopper CD, Millard WG, Gruffydd-Jones TJ, Harbour DA: Feline immunodeficiency virus infection. Clinicopathologic findings in 90 naturally occurring cases. J Vet Intern Med 7:85–90, 1993.

561. Ruslander DA, Gebhard DH, Tompkins MB, Grindem CB, Page RL: Immunophenotypic characterization of canine lymphoproliferative disorders. In Vivo 11:169–172, 1997.

562. Leifer CE, Matus RE: Chronic lymphocytic leukemia in the dog: 22 cases (1974–1984). J Am Vet Med Assoc 214–217, 1986.

563. MacEwen EG, Hurvitz AI, Hayes A: Hyperviscosity syndrome associated with lymphocytic leukemia in three dogs. J Am Vet Med Assoc 170:1309–1312, 1977.

564. Vernau W, Jacobs RM, Valli VEO, Heeney JL: The immunophenotypic characterization of bovine lymphomas. Vet Pathol 34:222–225, 1997.

565. Vernau W, Valli VEO, Dukes TW, Jacobs RM, Shoukri M, Heeney JL: Classification of

1,198 cases of bovine lymphoma using the National Cancer Institute Working Formulation for human non-Hodgkin's lymphomas. Vet Pathol 29:183–195, 1992.

566. Callanan JJ, Jones BA, Irvine J, Willett BJ, McCandlish IAP, Jarrett O: Histologic classification and immunophenotype of lymphosarcomas in cats with naturally and experimentally acquired feline immunodeficiency virus infections. Vet Pathol 33:264–272, 1996.

567. Savage CJ: Lymphoproliferative and myeloproliferative disorders. Vet Clin North Am Equine Pract 14:563–578, 1998.

568. van den Hoven R, Franken P: Clinical aspects of lymphosarcoma in the horse: a clinical report of 16 cases. Equine Vet J 15:49–53, 1983.

569. Madewell BR: Hematologic and bone marrow cytological abnormalities in 75 dogs with malignant lymphoma. J Am Anim Hosp Assoc 22:235–240, 1986.

570. Raskin RE, Krehbiel JD: Histopathology of canine bone marrow in malignant lymphoproliferative disorders. Vet Pathol 25:83–88, 1988.

571. Wellman ML, Hammer AS, DiBartola SP, Carothers MA, Kociba GJ, Rojko JL: Lymphoma involving large granular lymphocytes in cats: 11 cases (1982–1991). J Am Vet Med Assoc 201:1265–1269, 1992.

572. McEntee MF, Horton S, Blue J, Meuten DJ: Granulated round cell tumor of cats. Vet Pathol 30:195–203, 1993.

573. Drobatz KJ, Fred R, Waddle J: Globule leukocyte tumor in six cats. J Am Anim Hosp Assoc 29:391–396, 1993.

574. Grindem CB, Roberts MC, McEntee MF, Dillman RC: Large granular lymphocyte tumor in a horse. Vet Pathol 26:86–88, 1989.

575. Drazner FH: Multiple myeloma in the cat. Comp Cont Ed Pract Vet 4:206–216, 1982.

576. Matus RE, Leifer CE: Immunoglobulin-producing tumors. Vet Clin North Am Small Anim Pract 15:741–753, 1985.

577. Matus RE, Leifer CE, MacEwen EG, Hurvitz AI: Prognostic factors for multiple myeloma in the dog. J Am Vet Med Assoc 188:1288–1292, 1986.

578. Forrester SD, Greco DS, Relford RL: Serum hyperviscosity syndrome associated with multiple myeloma in two cats. J Am Vet Med Assoc 200:79–82, 1992.

579. Edwards DF, Parker JW, Wilkinson JE, Helman RG: Plasma cell myeloma in the horse. J Vet Intern Med 7:169–176, 1993.

580. Kato H, Momoi Y, Omori K, et al: Gammopathy with two M-components in a dog with IgA-type multiple myeloma. Vet Immunol Immunopathol 49:161–168, 1995.

581. Vail DM: Plasma cell neoplasms. In: Small Animal Clinical Oncology. Withrow SJ, MacEwen EG, eds. pp 509–520, W.B. Saunders Co., Philadelphia, PA, 1996.

582. Sheafor SE, Gamblin RM, Couto CG: Hypercalcemia in two cats with multiple myeloma. J Am Anim Hosp Assoc 32:503–508, 1996.

583. MacEwen EG, Patnaik AK, Hurvitz AI, et al: Nonsecretory multiple myeloma in two dogs. J Am Vet Med Assoc 184:1283–1286, 1984.

584. Marks SL, Moore PF, Taylor DW, Munn RJ: Nonsecretory multiple myeloma in a dog: immunohistologic and ultrastructural observations. J Vet Intern Med 9:50–54, 1995.

585. Jacobs RM, Couto CG, Wellman ML: Biclonal gammopathy in a dog with myeloma and cutaneous lymphoma. Vet Pathol 23:211–213, 1986.

586. Peterson EN, Meininger AC: Immunoglobulin A and immunoglobulin G biclonal gammopathy in a dog with multiple myeloma. J Am Anim Hosp Assoc 33:45–47, 1997.

587. Hurvitz AI, Kehoe JM, Capra JD, Prata R: Bence Jones proteinemia and proteinuria in a dog. J Am Vet Med Assoc 159:1112–1116, 1971.

588. Hoenig M: Multiple myeloma associated with the heavy chains of immunoglobulin A in a dog. J Am Vet Med Assoc 190:1191–1192, 1987.

589. MacEwen EG, Patnaik AK, Johnson GF, Hurvitz AI, Erlandson RA, Lieberman PH: Extramedullary plasmacytoma of the gastrointestinal tract in two dogs. J Am Vet Med Assoc 184:1396–1398, 1984.

590. Carothers MA, Johnson GC, DiBartola SP, Liepnicks J, Benson MD: Extramedullary plasmacytoma and immunoglobulin-associated amyloidosis in a cat. J Am Vet Med Assoc 195:1593–1597, 1989.

591. Kyriazidou A, Brown PJ, Lucke VM: An immunohistochemical study of canine extramedullary plasma cell tumours. J Comp Pathol 100:259–266, 1989.

592. Rakich PM, Latimer KS, Weiss R, Steffens WL: Mucocutaneous plasmacytomas in dogs: 75 cases (1980–1987). J Am Vet Med Assoc 194:803–810, 1989.

593. Trevor PB, Saunders GK, Waldron DR, Leib MS: Metastatic extramedullary plasmacytoma of the colon and rectum in a dog. J Am Vet Med Assoc 203:406–409, 1993.

594. Brunnert SR, Dee LA, Herron AJ, Altman NH: Gastric extramedullary plasmacytoma in a dog. J Am Vet Med Assoc 200:1501–1502, 1992.

595. Jackson MW, Helfand SC, Smedes SL, Bradley GA, Schultz RD: Primary IgG secreting plasma cell tumor in the gastrointestinal tract of a dog. J Am Vet Med Assoc 204:404–406, 1994.

596. Mandel NS, Esplin DG: A retroperitoneal extramedullary plasmacytoma in a cat with a monoclonal gammopathy. J Am Anim Hosp Assoc 30:603–608, 1994.

597. Larsen AE, Carpenter JL: Hepatic plasmacytoma and biclonal gammopathy in a cat. J Am Vet Med Assoc 205:708–710, 1994.

598. Lester SJ, Mesfin GM: A solitary plasmacytoma in a dog with progression to a disseminated myeloma. Can Vet J 21:284–286, 1980.

599. Kipps TJ: Macroglobulinemia. In: Williams Hematology, 5th ed. Beutler E, Lichtman MA, Coller BS, Kipps TJ, eds. pp 1127–1131, McGraw-Hill, New York, NY, 1995.

600. Hurvitz AI, Haskins SC, Fischer CA: Macroglobulinemia with hyperviscosity syndrome in a dog. J Am Vet Med Assoc 157:455–460, 1970.

601. Hurvitz AI, MacEwen EG, Middaugh CR, Litman GW: Monoclonal cryoglobulinemia with macroglobulinemia in a dog. J Am Vet Med Assoc 170:511–513, 1977.

602. Young KM, MacEwen EG: Canine myeloproliferative disorders and malignant histiocytosis. In: Small Animal Clinical Oncology. Withrow SJ, MacEwen EG, eds. pp 495–509, W.B. Saunders Co., Philadelphia, PA, 1996.

603. Harvey JW, Shields RP, Gaskin JM: Feline myeloproliferative disease. Changing manifestations in the peripheral blood. Vet Pathol 15:437–448, 1978.

604. Maggio L, Hoffman R, Cotter SM, Dainiak N, Mooney S, Maffei LA: Feline preleukemia: an animal model of human disease. Yale J Biol Med 51:469–476, 1978.

605. Madewell BR, Jain NC, Weller RE: Hematologic abnormalities preceding myeloid leukemia in three cats. Vet Pathol 16:510–519, 1979.

606. Toth SR, Onions DE, Jarrett O: Histopathological and hematological findings in myeloid leukemia induced by a new feline leukemia virus isolate. Vet Pathol 23:462–470, 1986.

607. Raskind WH, Steinmann L, Najfeld V: Clonal development of myeloproliferative disorders: clues to hematopoietic differentiation and multistep pathogenesis of cancer. Leukemia 12:108–116, 1998.

608. Shelton GH, Linenberger ML, Abkowitz JL: Hematologic abnormalities in cats seropositive for feline immunodeficiency virus. J Am Vet Med Assoc 199:1353–1357, 1991.

609. Ford SL, Raskin RE, Snyder PS: Clinical implications of feline bone marrow dysplasia—a retrospective study of 16 cats (abstract). J Vet Intern Med 12:226, 1998.

610. Lester SJ, Searcy GP: Hematologic abnormalities preceding apparent recovery from feline leukemia virus infection. J Am Vet Med Assoc 178:471–474, 1981.

611. Cheson BD, Cassileth PA, Head DR, et al: Report of the National Cancer Institute-sponsored workshop on definitions of diagnosis and response in acute myeloid leukemia. J Clin Oncol 8:813–819, 1990.

612. Grindem CB: Classification of myeloproliferative diseases. In: Consultations in Feline Medicine 3. August JR, ed. pp 499–508, W.B. Saunders Co., Philadelphia, PA, 1997.

613. Bounous DI, Latimer KS, Campagnoli RP, Hynes PF: Acute myeloid leukemia with basophilic differentiation (AML, M-2B) in a cat. Vet Clin Pathol 23:15–18, 1994.

614. Colbatzky F, Hermanns W: Acute megakaryoblastic leukemia in one cat and two dogs. Vet Pathol 30:186–194, 1993.

615. Pucheu-Haston CM, Camus A, Taboada J, Gaunt SD, Snider TG III, Lopez MK: Megakaryoblastic leukemia in a dog. J Am Vet Med Assoc 207:194–196, 1995.

616. Burton S, Miller L, Horney B, Marks C, Shaw D: Acute megakaryoblastic leukemia in a cat. Vet Clin Pathol 25:6–9, 1996.

617. Woods PR, Gossett RE, Jain NC, Smith R III, Rappaport ES, Kasari TR: Acute myelo-monocytic leukemia in a calf. J Am Vet Med Assoc 203:1579–1582, 1993.

618. Takayama H, Gejima S, Honma A, Ishikawa Y, Kadota K: Acute myeloblastic leukaemia in a cow. J Comp Pathol 115:95–101, 1996.

619. Lichtman MA, Brennan JK: Myelodysplastic disorders. In: Williams Hematology, 5th ed. Beutler E, Lichtman MA, Coller BS, Kipps TJ, eds. pp 257–272, McGraw-Hill, New York, NY, 1995.

620. Peterson ME, Randolph JF: Diagnosis of canine primary polycythemia and management with hydroxyurea. J Am Vet Med Assoc 180:415–418, 1982.

621. Degen MA, Feldman BF, Turrel JM, Goding B, Kitchell B, Mandell CP: Thrombocytosis associated with a myeloproliferative disorder in a dog. J Am Vet Med Assoc 194:1457–1459, 1989.

622. Powers BE, LaRue SM, Withrow SJ, Straw RC, Richter SL: Jamshidi needle biopsy for diagnosis of bone lesions in small animals. J Am Vet Med Assoc 193:205–210, 1988.

623. Wykes PM, Withrow SJ, Powers BE, Park RD: Closed biopsy for diagnosis of long bone tumors: accuracy and results. J Am Anim Hosp Assoc 21:489–494, 1985.

624. Durham SK, Dietze AE: Prostatic adenocarcinoma with and without metastasis to bone in dogs. J Am Vet Med Assoc 188:1432–1436, 1986.

625. Hahn KA, Matlock CL: Nasal adenocarcinoma metastatic to bone in two dogs. J Am Vet Med Assoc 197:491–494, 1990.

626. Roeckel IE: Diagnosis of metastatic carcinoma by bone marrow biopsy versus bone marrow aspiration. Ann Clin Lab Sci 4:193–197, 1974.

627. Mahaffey EA: Cytology of the musculoskeletal system. In: Diagnostic Cytology and Hematology of the Dog and Cat, 2nd ed. Cowell RL, Tyler RD, Meinkoth JH, eds. pp 120–124, Mosby, St. Louis, MO, 1999.

Index

Note: Page numbers in *italics* refer to illustrations; page numbers followed by t refer to tables.